SPORTS EMERGENCY

CARE A TEAM APPROACH
Second Edition

SPORTS EMERGENCY CARE

A TEAM APPROACH
Second Edition

ROBB S. REHBERG, PhD, ATC, CSCS, NREMT
ASSOCIATE PROFESSOR
COORDINATOR OF CLINICAL EDUCATION
ATHLETIC TRAINING EDUCATION PROGRAM
WILLIAM PATERSON UNIVERSITY
CO-FOUNDER AND EXECUTIVE DIRECTOR
SPORT SAFETY INTERNATIONAL
WAYNE, NEW JERSEY

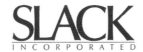

SLACK
INCORPORATED

www.Healio.com/books

ISBN: 978-1-61711-005-4

Copyright © 2013 by SLACK Incorporated

Sports Emergency Care: A Team Approach, Second Edition, Instructor's Manual is also available from SLACK Incorporated. Don't miss this important companion to *Sports Emergency Care: A Team Approach, Second Edition.* To obtain the *Instructor's Manual*, please visit http://www.efacultylounge.com.

The procedures and practices described in this publication should be implemented in a manner consistent with the professional standards set for the circumstances that apply in each specific situation. Every effort has been made to confirm the accuracy of the information presented and to correctly relate generally accepted practices. The authors, editors, and publisher cannot accept responsibility for errors or exclusions or for the outcome of the material presented herein. There is no expressed or implied warranty of this book or information imparted by it. Care has been taken to ensure that drug selection and dosages are in accordance with currently accepted/recommended practice. Off-label uses of drugs may be discussed. Due to continuing research, changes in government policy and regulations, and various effects of drug reactions and interactions, it is recommended that the reader carefully review all materials and literature provided for each drug, especially those that are new or not frequently used. Some drugs or devices in this publication have clearance for use in a restricted research setting by the Food and Drug and Administration or FDA. Each professional should determine the FDA status of any drug or device prior to use in their practice.

Any review or mention of specific companies or products is not intended as an endorsement by the author or publisher.

SLACK Incorporated uses a review process to evaluate submitted material. Prior to publication, educators or clinicians provide important feedback on the content that we publish. We welcome feedback on this work.

Published by: SLACK Incorporated
                   6900 Grove Road
                   Thorofare, NJ 08086 USA
                   Telephone: 856-848-1000
                   Fax: 856-848-6091
                   www.Healio.com/books

Contact SLACK Incorporated for more information about other books in this field or about the availability of our books from distributors outside the United States.

Library of Congress Cataloging-in-Publication Data

Sports emergency care : a team approach / [edited by] Robb S. Rehberg. -- 2nd ed.
      p. ; cm.
   Includes bibliographical references and index.
   ISBN 978-1-61711-005-4 (alk. paper)
   I. Rehberg, Robb S.
   [DNLM: 1. Athletic Injuries--therapy. 2. Emergency Treatment. QT 261]

   617.1'027--dc23
                           2012047755

For permission to reprint material in another publication, contact SLACK Incorporated. Authorization to photocopy items for internal, personal, or academic use is granted by SLACK Incorporated provided that the appropriate fee is paid directly to Copyright Clearance Center. Prior to photocopying items, please contact the Copyright Clearance Center at 222 Rosewood Drive, Danvers, MA 01923 USA; phone: 978-750-8400; website: www.copyright.com; email: info@copyright.com

Printed in the United States of America.

Last digit is print number: 10   9   8   7   6   5   4   3   2

DEDICATION

For my beautiful wife, Joelle,
for her love, encouragement, and patience.
This project would not have been possible without you;

For my wonderful children, Anna and Joseph,
for never letting me forget what is most important in life.
Watching you grow (too fast!) is the greatest joy in my life;

For my parents,
who always told me that I could do anything if I put my mind to it;

For my teachers, professors, and clinical instructors,
who inspired me to learn;

And for my colleagues, the athletic trainers and EMTs,
who, day in and day out, selflessly help others in need.
You are the inspiration for this book.

CONTENTS

Dedication .... *v*

Acknowledgments .... *ix*

About the Author .... *xi*

Contributing Authors .... *xiii*

Preface .... *xv*

Foreword to the First Edition by Ron Courson, ATC, PT, NREMT-I, CSCS .... *xvii*

Chapter 1   Introduction to Sports Emergency Care 1
               Robb S. Rehberg, PhD, ATC, CSCS, NREMT

Chapter 2   Preparing for Sports Emergencies 7
               Robb S. Rehberg, PhD, ATC, CSCS, NREMT

Chapter 3   Assessment of Sports Emergencies 19
               Robb S. Rehberg, PhD, ATC, CSCS, NREMT

Chapter 4   Airway Management and Breathing 37
               Robb S. Rehberg, PhD, ATC, CSCS, NREMT

Chapter 5   Cardiovascular Emergencies 51
               Robb S. Rehberg, PhD, ATC, CSCS, NREMT

Chapter 6   Management of Spinal Injuries 59
               Robb S. Rehberg, PhD, ATC, CSCS, NREMT

Chapter 7   Unconsciousness and Seizures 95
               David A. Middlemas, EdD, ATC

Chapter 8   Management of Traumatic Brain Injury 109
               Casey Christy, MA, ATC, CSCS

Chapter 9   Injuries to the Thoracic Region 131
               Michael A. Prybicien, MA, ATC, CSCS, CES, PES

Chapter 10   Abdominal and Pelvic Injuries 143
               David A. Middlemas, EdD, ATC

Chapter 11   Fractures and Soft Tissue Injuries 161
               Michael A. Prybicien, MA, ATC, CSCS, CES, PES and
               Louis Rizio, MD

Chapter 12   General Medical Emergencies 181
              John L. Davis, MS, ATC

Chapter 13   Environmental Emergencies 195
              Rebecca M. Lopez, PhD, ATC, CSCS

Chapter 14   Managing Mental Health Emergencies...................................... 211
              Eileen Lubeck, PsyD

Chapter 15   Emergency Care Considerations for the Pediatric and Youth Athlete........ 221
              Jeff G. Konin, PhD, ATC, PT, FACSM, FNATA and
              Rebecca M. Lopez, PhD, ATC, CSCS

Financial Disclosures *239*
Index...*241*

ACKNOWLEDGMENTS

Developing *Sports Emergency Care: A Team Approach, Second Edition* was just that ... a team approach. There are several people who were instrumental in the development of this book that I wish to thank. Without their help, this book would never have been written.

To the contributing authors:

Mike Prybicien, my colleague and longtime friend. We have come a long way from those early days in our careers. Thanks for being involved in this project and for helping out in so many ways.

Casey Christy, you have a passion for this subject, and I'm glad we got you involved in this project. You are a true professional and a good friend.

John Davis (the original "cover boy" for the book), you are a friend, colleague, and role model. It meant a lot to have you involved in this project. Thanks for everything.

Jeff Konin, I am honored to have you involved in this project. Thanks for your contribution to this book, as well as for your mentorship and friendship. You make this stuff look easy.

Dave Middlemas, this book is better because of your involvement. Thanks for your contribution, your friendship, and also for your help with the photo shoot.

Jaclyn Norberg, for assisting in the development of this book and the instructor materials. I know I can always count on you to come through.

Eileen Lubeck, for filling a critical need in this book, and for being a great example of inter-profession collaboration. Your addition to this book makes it stronger.

Rebecca Lopez, for contributing great content on such an important topic. You were wonderful to work with.

Lou Rizio, for finding the time in your busy schedule to contribute to this project. Your contributions were invaluable.

Joelle Rehberg, for illustrating much of the line art that appears in this book, countless hours of manuscript review, and simply for putting up with me in the process.

Thanks also to the athletic training faculty and staff at William Paterson University: Linda Gazzillo Diaz, Toby Barboza, Alison Bewalder, and Dondi Boyd, for their never-ending assistance in getting this book off the ground. Thanks also to the athletic training students of William Paterson University, especially Matthew Bergh and Tedd Rossillo (who served as models), and the athletic training students and EMS staff at Montclair State University for participating in the photo shoot for this book.

Special thanks to the staff at SLACK Incorporated, especially John Bond, Brien Cummings, April Billick, and especially to Carrie Kotlar for believing in this book and finally making it happen.

ABOUT THE AUTHOR

Robb S. Rehberg, PhD, ATC, CSCS, NREMT is an Associate Professor and Coordinator of Athletic Training Clinical Education at William Paterson University in Wayne, New Jersey. He is also a partner of The Rehberg Konin Group and serves as co-founder and Executive Director of Sport Safety International. Dr. Rehberg previously served as the Director and Chief of Emergency Services at Montclair State University in Montclair, New Jersey. Prior to teaching at William Paterson, Dr. Rehberg spent 13 years as the head athletic trainer at Westwood Regional High School in Westwood, New Jersey.

Dr. Rehberg earned his PhD in Health Science from Touro University International in 2003, a master of sport science degree from the United States Sports Academy in 1999, and a bachelor of science in Athletic Training from West Chester University in 1991.

Dr. Rehberg has spent his career working in both the athletic training and emergency services fields and has published and spoken frequently at state and national meetings on sports emergency care. Dr. Rehberg served as a member of the medical staff for athletics (track and field) at the 1996 Olympic Games in Atlanta, Georgia. He has been active on both state and national levels, having served on the National Athletic Trainers' Association (NATA) Inter-Association Task Force for the Appropriate Care of the Spine-Injured Athlete, the Task Force on Appropriate Medical Coverage for the Secondary School-Aged Athlete, and the NATA Hall of Fame Subcommittee. Dr. Rehberg is a past-president of the Athletic Trainers' Society of New Jersey. He has also served as the Chair of the National Safety Council Emergency Care Advisory Committee since 1992 and was a member of the American Heart Association Task Force that developed the first-ever international guidelines for first aid in 2000. He was a charter member of the New Jersey Disaster Medical Assistance Team. Dr. Rehberg is a member of the New Jersey Scholastic Coaches Association Hall of Fame, Athletic Trainers' Society of New Jersey Hall of Fame, and is the recipient of the Ordo Honoris medal from the Kappa Delta Rho National Fraternity.

Dr. Rehberg and his wife, Dr. Joelle Rehberg, are the authors of *Cram Session in General Medical Conditions: A Handbook for Students & Clinicians*, a textbook available from SLACK Incorporated.

Contributing Authors

Casey Christy, MA, ATC, CSCS (Chapter 8)
Head Athletic Trainer
Eastern High School
Voorhees, New Jersey
Adjunct Instructor
Athletic Training Education Program
Rowan University
Glassboro, New Jersey

Ron Courson, ATC, PT, NREMT-I, CSCS (Foreword)
Associate Athletic Director—Sports Medicine
University of Georgia
Athens, Georgia

John L. Davis, MS, ATC (Chapter 12)
Coordinator of Athletic Training and Sports Medicine
Montclair State University
Montclair, New Jersey

Jeff G. Konin, PhD, ATC, PT, FACSM, FNATA (Chapter 15)
Director of Intercollegiate Athletics
Eastern Connecticut State University
Willimantic, Connecticut
Partner
The Rehberg Konin Group
Wayne, New Jersey

Rebecca M. Lopez, PhD, ATC, CSCS (Chapters 13 and 15)
Assistant Professor and Director
Post-Professional Graduate Athletic Training Program
Department of Orthopaedics & Sports Medicine
University of South Florida
Tampa, Florida

Eileen Lubeck, PsyD (Chapter 14)
Director of Counseling, Health & Wellness
William Paterson University
Wayne, New Jersey

David A. Middlemas, EdD, ATC (Chapters 7 and 10)
Professor and Athletic Training Education Program Director
Montclair State University
Montclair, New Jersey

Michael A. Prybicien, MA, ATC, CSCS, CES, PES (Chapters 9 and 11)
Athletic Trainer
Passaic Board of Education
Passaic, New Jersey

Louis Rizio, MD (Chapter 11)
Director
Sports Medicine & Orthopaedic Center
Livingston, New Jersey
Clinical Assistant Professor of Orthopaedics
NYU-Hospital for Joint Diseases
New York, New York

PREFACE

There have been illnesses and injuries related to sports for as long as there have been organized sports. Some of these conditions can be life and limb threatening and are considered emergencies. While life-threatening injuries and illnesses do not occur often, proper management of these conditions is arguably the most important job that members of the sports emergency care team will ever face.

Sports Emergency Care: A Team Approach, Second Edition was primarily designed to fill the void that has traditionally existed in athletic training education on the subject of emergency care.

Traditionally, athletic training educators have had to resort to developing courses based on existing first aid materials or developing materials on their own in order to meet the needs of the athletic training student. This book, which was the first of its kind, contains all the necessary information needed to prepare athletic training students beyond traditional first aid training.

This book was also designed to provide specific information on emergency situations in sports for emergency medical services (EMS) professionals. To date, no such text has ever addressed sports emergency care for EMS providers. While this book was written with athletic trainers, athletic training students, and EMS personnel in mind, all health care providers who play a role on the sports emergency care team will find this book useful in preparing for emergency situations in sports.

This book can be used in several different ways. It can be used in athletic training education programs as a core textbook as part of a sports emergency care course. It can also be used as a supplemental text in several courses that address immediate care within an athletic training education curriculum. EMS educators may also find this book useful in developing continuing education programs for prehospital providers. An added feature that instructors will find helpful is the *Sports Emergency Care: A Team Approach, Second Edition, Instructor's Manual*, which was developed to guide instructors in the delivery of course content. Complete with lecture outlines, test questions, and lab activities, the *Instructor's Manual* is a valuable tool that can be used in developing a sports emergency care course.

Finally, this book is also designed to be used as a reference and field guide for all health care providers who serve as members of the sports emergency care team, including athletic trainers, emergency medical technicians and paramedics, and physicians.

Regardless of discipline, it is important for all health care providers charged with caring for ill or injured athletes to be knowledgeable and proficient in managing sports emergencies. This ability can only be achieved through preparation and practice. Health care providers who utilize this book to enhance their emergency care skills and practice together as a team will ultimately be prepared to provide the best care possible in emergency situations.

FOREWORD TO THE FIRST EDITION

Although most injuries in athletics are relatively minor, life- or limb-threatening injuries are unpredictable and can occur without warning. Due to the relatively low incidence rate of catastrophic injuries, health care providers may develop a false sense of security. Catastrophic injuries can occur during any physical activity and at any level of participation. When this happens, there is typically heightened public awareness associated with the nature and management of the emergency situation. Medical-legal interests may lead to questions regarding qualifications of the health care personnel involved, the preparedness of the athletic organization, and actions taken.

In an emergency situation, proper management of life- and limb-threatening injuries is critical. Ideally, properly trained medical and allied health personnel should handle emergencies. Preparation should include education and training in emergency evaluation and management of injuries and illnesses, emergency procedures, selection and maintenance of emergency equipment and supplies, appropriate use of emergency personnel, and formation and implementation of an emergency action plan.

Emergencies are rarely predictable. When they occur, a rapid but controlled response is indicated. All personnel involved with the organization or sponsorship of athletic activities share a professional responsibility to provide for the emergency care of an injured person. The goal of the sports medicine team is delivery of the highest possible quality of health care to the athlete. Accordingly, the sports medicine team must work together as an efficient unit to accomplish these goals. By sharing information, training, and skills between team members, the injured or ill athlete may receive the highest quality emergency care. The importance of being prepared when emergencies occur cannot be stressed enough. Survival may hinge on how well trained and prepared athletic health care providers are.

Sports Emergency Care: A Team Approach is a valuable educational tool in the area of athletic emergencies. By reading and reviewing in the area of emergency medicine, the health care provider better prepares to manage athletic emergencies. Vince Dooley, head football coach for the University of Georgia, was often quoted as saying, "Proper preparation prevents poor performance." This is particularly true in the area of emergency medicine. Be well prepared in all of your endeavors!

—*Ron Courson, ATC, PT, NREMT-I, CSCS*
Associate Athletic Director—Sports Medicine
University of Georgia
Athens, Georgia

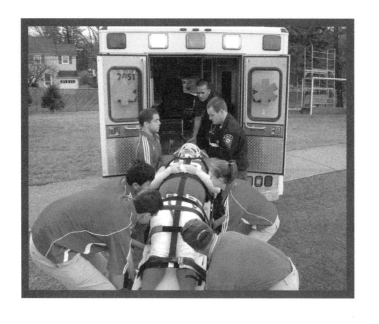

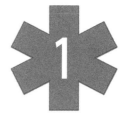

Introduction to Sports Emergency Care

Robb S. Rehberg, PhD, ATC, CSCS, NREMT

A 14-year-old male high school cross country athlete suddenly collapses after finishing a 5-mile practice run...

A 14-year-old female high school basketball player collapses on the bench during a game...

An 18-year-old high school wrestler injures his neck during a match. He cannot move his arms or legs...

A high school baseball player is hit in the neck by a line-drive–batted ball while pitching batting practice. The athlete collapses and is unconscious...

An 18-year-old male track athlete was impaled by a javelin during track practice...

A high school football player is injured during a game after tackling with his head down, resulting in helmet-to-helmet contact. He lies motionless on the turf...

These types of emergencies occur every season on the courts and fields; at the professional, college, high school, and youth levels; and in organized and informal activities. Are you prepared to handle these emergencies?

Health care professionals who are entrusted with the health and safety of athletes must ask themselves this question every day. The possibility of serious injury or sudden illness exists in all sports, regardless of the level or type of play. The examples above are based on real situations in

Rehberg RS.
Sports Emergency Care: A Team Approach,
Second Edition (pp 1-4).
© 2013 SLACK Incorporated.

which an athlete died or became permanently disabled.[1] It is not enough for health care professionals to renew their cardiopulmonary resuscitation (CPR) certification every 2 years and hope for the best. Health care professionals who work with athletes must have a unique understanding of the potential emergency situations that can arise and must possess the skills and knowledge to manage such emergencies. They must be proficient in sports emergency care.

WHAT IS SPORTS EMERGENCY CARE?

Emergency care is defined as the immediate care given to an injured or suddenly ill person. Practitioners of emergency care must be proficient in the recognition of sudden illness and injury, as well as possess skills necessary to manage the condition until more definitive medical care is available. Emergency care usually goes beyond first aid treatment and may involve more advanced skills and specialized equipment. Keeping this definition in mind, *sports emergency care* can be defined as the immediate care given to an injured or suddenly ill sports participant. Sports emergency care is an area of specialization that is necessary for health care providers who are involved in caring for physically active individuals.

WHY IS SPORTS EMERGENCY CARE NEEDED?

There is an inherent risk of injury in sports. In more physically demanding sports, athletes compete at full speed, with great intensity, and in some cases, at the expense of bodily injury. While the incidence of catastrophic injury in sports is relatively low, immediate recognition of emergencies and appropriate care is crucial in order to provide the athlete with the best chance of survival. Health care professionals covering sports must be prepared for injuries and illnesses that are a direct result of sports participation (such as spinal injuries, head injuries, and fractures), as well as indirect causes (such as congenital heart abnormalities and other medical emergencies). The needs of sports participants with these types of injuries and illnesses go far beyond first aid care. Specialized knowledge of such situations and their unique relationship to sports participation is necessary to provide the best care possible.

SPORTS EMERGENCY CARE: A TEAM APPROACH

Preparing for and managing sports emergencies must be a team effort. Each member of the team must understand, respect, and appreciate the capabilities and specialized skills possessed by the other members of the team. Historically, there have been situations in which athletic trainers and emergency medical technicians (EMTs) have differed in their approach to managing emergency situations in sports. (The issue of athletic helmet removal has traditionally been at the center of this controversy.) Oftentimes, this difference in approach can lead to on-field confrontation at the scene of an emergency. It is not hard to see why athletic trainers and EMTs may, at times, differ in their approach to managing a specific injury or illness. After all, the background, training, and areas of specialization differ for each discipline. However, prior planning and dialogue among all health care professionals involved in managing sports emergencies can yield a competent sports emergency care team that is prepared to work together efficiently.

The sports emergency care team is a subset of the sports medicine team that includes individuals with specialized training in emergency care. Naturally, the athletic trainer will be a key player in the sports emergency care team. Other important members of the team include, but are not limited to, EMTs, advanced EMTs, paramedics, emergency medical responders (EMRs), emergency nurses, and physicians. The sports emergency care team should highlight each member's strengths. For instance, EMTs may have more experience in the packaging of cervical-spine injuries than any other team member. Conversely, the athletic trainer may be more familiar with the equipment worn by the athlete (ie, helmet, shoulder pads) and have a deeper knowledge of neurological function and assessment. The physician, if present, may have an even deeper understanding of the pathophysiology of the injury and possible complications. Understanding the strengths of each team member and learning how to best put each team member's strengths to use comes only through practice and is essential for providing quality emergency care to the injured athlete.

HOW TO USE THIS BOOK

It is the author's vision that members of the sports emergency care team—athletic trainers, EMTs, physicians, and others—will utilize this book to further their knowledge and skills in the management of sports emergencies. However, just reading this text is not enough. Sports emergency care must be a team approach. Health care professionals must practice together often to refine skills, stimulate discussion, foster teamwork, and identify deficiencies in the emergency plan. Ultimately, patient care in the field relies on sound judgment, planning, and teamwork.

In addition to practicing sports emergency care, all members of the sports emergency care team should maintain current certification in CPR at the professional rescuer level, in addition to maintaining continuing education requirements necessary to maintain their respective credentials.

There may be skills and techniques presented in this book that fall outside the scope of practice for some health care professionals. Readers should always act within their scope of practice. Moreover, local protocols may differ from information presented. Sports emergency care personnel should always follow local protocol.

ATHLETIC TRAINERS

In most cases, it is the athletic trainer who will be at the center of the sports emergency care team. Most often, it is the athletic trainer who works with the athlete on a daily basis and knows the athlete's history well. Additionally, athletic trainers have a strong background in anatomy and physiology and extensive knowledge of athletic injuries and illnesses. However, while athletic trainers routinely handle musculoskeletal injuries and other conditions, they rarely handle emergencies. Therefore, it is important for athletic trainers, regardless of the setting, to develop a sports emergency care team to ensure the proper care for the athletes they serve. The information contained in this book will provide the athletic trainer with a deeper understanding of the types of emergencies that can occur in sports. Athletic trainers are urged to strive to learn as much as possible about emergency care and the emergency medical services (EMS) system that responds to their place of employment. Athletic trainers might consider riding along with the local EMS unit to gain a better understanding of the EMS system and the training and background of EMTs and paramedics. Athletic trainers may also consider enrolling in an EMT or medical first responder course to increase their depth of knowledge of emergency care.

EMERGENCY MEDICAL SERVICES PROFESSIONALS

The National EMS Education Standards,[2] from which training for EMRs, EMTs, advanced EMTs, and paramedics is based, provides a foundation for the management of a number of medical and trauma situations. However, EMT training cannot and does not cover every conceivable emergency. While EMTs handle medical emergencies more frequently than athletic trainers, most EMTs are largely unfamiliar with the unique nature of sports injury and illness, mechanisms of sports injury, and equipment used in certain sports. It is important for the practicing EMT to seek continuing education to strengthen his or her knowledge in areas in which he or she will ultimately be involved. There are a number of continuing education programs available for EMTs, from hazardous materials to incident command. EMTs who are involved in the coverage of sporting events should be familiar with the types of illness and injury germane to the sports environment, as well as an understanding of mechanism of injury, equipment used, and unique situations that can present in an emergency. EMTs should also consider working with a local athletic trainer and observing day-to-day activities in order to obtain a better understanding of athletic injuries and illnesses, as well as a better understanding of the field of athletic training.

EDUCATORS

Athletic training education programs have undergone a major transformation in the past decade. Clinical proficiencies and competencies on immediate care of athletic injury and illness are a critical part of an athletic training student's education. However, content on sports emergencies is often piecemeal, and courses used to cover immediate care competencies and proficiencies usually consist of first aid courses being "retrofitted" to cover emergencies. However, sports emergency care goes beyond typical first aid training. This text can be used in athletic training education programs as a stand-alone course or in several athletic training courses to cover information in the immediate care of sports emergencies. Athletic training educators are also encouraged to involve the local EMS agencies in their education program to further strengthen the bond between athletic training and EMS.

EMS educators may want to consider developing a continuing education course focusing on sports emergency care. Specialized continuing education training programs are widely available on topics such as trauma, pediatrics, geriatrics, and farm injuries. The types of injuries and illnesses related to sports participation also warrant specialized education, especially for those EMS professionals who cover sporting events. EMS educators could benefit from collaborating with athletic trainers in the development and implementation of such programs.

Train. Train often. Train together. The athletes you serve are depending on you!

REVIEW QUESTIONS

1. What is sports emergency care?
2. Why is sports emergency care needed?
3. What are the advantages of a team approach to sports emergency care?

REFERENCES

1. Mueller FO, Cantu RC. National Center for Catastrophic Sports Injury Research: 25th annual report: fall 1982–spring 2007. http://www.unc.edu/depts/nccsi/AllSport.htm. Accessed September 29, 2012.
2. National Highway Traffic Safety Administration. EMS education standards. http://www.ems.gov/pdf/811077a.pdf. Published January 2009. Accessed October 12, 2011.

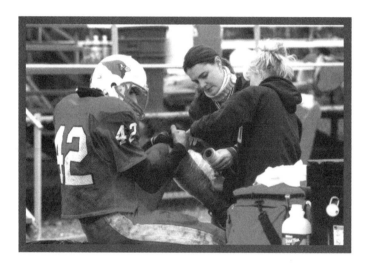

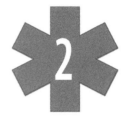

Preparing for
Sports Emergencies

Robb S. Rehberg, PhD, ATC, CSCS, NREMT

> *You are covering a wrestling tournament. As you watch the last match of the night, one of the wrestlers is thrown to the mat by his opponent, violently striking his head. He lies motionless on the mat, and the referee stops the match. You rush to the side of the athlete. Are you prepared? Are there other personnel on site to assist you? Is an ambulance needed, and if so, who will call? Do you know what EMS professionals will be responding to the scene? And are you all in agreement with the procedures to follow in order to provide the best care for the athlete?*

Proper management of emergencies in sports does not happen by accident. Preparation is the key to ensuring that the appropriate resources and procedures exist to ensure the best care possible. Preparation for sports emergencies is a dynamic process, and planning should begin well in advance of the injury, game, or even the season.

There are many factors that should be considered when preparing for sports emergencies. In order to address each of these factors, the acronym PREPARE can be used. PREPARE emphasizes the critical elements of emergency planning: personnel, rules, equipment, planning, arena, rehearsal, and evaluate and educate. Each of these critical elements must be addressed when developing an emergency action plan (EAP) for sports emergencies.

PERSONNEL

Who are the members of your sports emergency care team? This question may be answered differently depending on the level of play and the size of the institution. For instance, a sports emergency care team in the National Football League may have more members than a small high school. All personnel must be identified and included in the preparation and planning process regardless of the size of the venue or the number of members of the team. It is important that each member of the team understands the qualifications, expertise, and limitations of the other

Rehberg RS.
Sports Emergency Care: A Team Approach,
Second Edition (pp 7-17).
© 2013 SLACK Incorporated.

members. It is equally important for all team members to be comfortable with the capabilities and roles of each team member. Some of the personnel that should be included in the sports emergency care team include athletic trainers, emergency medical services (EMS) personnel, physicians, hospital staff, coaching staff, athletic training students, athletics staff, athletes, and other personnel.

ATHLETIC TRAINERS

Athletic trainers are health care professionals who collaborate with physicians to optimize activity and participation of patients and clients. Athletic trainers are experts in injury prevention, diagnosis, and intervention of emergency, acute, and chronic medical conditions involving impairment, functional limitations, and disabilities.[1] Athletic trainers are certified by the Board of Certification, Inc (www.BOCATC.org), and the practice of athletic training is regulated in 48 states. Athletic trainers have been recognized by the American Medical Association as health care professionals since 1990. In order to be eligible for certification, athletic trainers must graduate from an accredited undergraduate or graduate athletic training curriculum, which consists of coursework and clinical experience in several areas, including assessment and evaluation, acute care, general medical conditions and disabilities, and pathology of injury and illness. Athletic trainers must hold a minimum of a bachelor's degree, although nearly three-quarters of all certified athletic trainers hold a master's degree or higher. In addition to certification, nearly all states regulate the athletic training profession through licensure, registration, or certification.

In most situations, the athletic trainer will serve as the "captain" of the sports emergency care team. The athletic trainer is often responsible for assembling the sports emergency care team, developing site-specific EAPs, ordering necessary equipment, ensuring that the members of the team are informed of the plan, and conducting regular training and drills.

EMERGENCY MEDICAL SERVICES PERSONNEL

EMS personnel are important members of the sports emergency care team. Ultimately, it will be the EMS personnel who will assume responsibility for packaging and transporting the injured athlete to the hospital. There are 4 distinct levels of emergency care providers: emergency medical responders (EMRs, formerly called *first responders*), emergency medical technicians (EMTs), advanced emergency medical technicians (AEMTs), and paramedics. Each level of training represents a different level of expertise in the continuum of emergency medical care. EMS education in most states follows the National Emergency Medical Services Education Standards,[2] developed by the National Highway Traffic Safety Administration. EMRs are the most basic level of EMS training, and are trained to assess and stabilize ill and injured patients until additional EMS assistance arrives. EMRs complete approximately 40 hours of training in the areas of assessment, airway management, management of medical and trauma emergencies, and emergency childbirth. Police officers, firefighters, and lifeguards are often trained at the EMR level.

EMTs are the next level in the continuum of EMS training. EMTs (also known in some states as *EMT-Basic*, *EMT-Intermediate* [EMT-I], *EMT-Ambulance*, or *EMT-Defibrillator*) undergo approximately 110 to 120 hours of training in patient assessment, airway management, management of respiratory and cardiac emergencies, management of medical and trauma emergencies, bleeding, fractures, and emergency childbirth. EMTs can usually administer or assist in the administration of oxygen, epinephrine (for allergic reactions), nitroglycerin, and metered dose inhalers depending on state or local protocols. Although discontinued in the most recent EMS education standards document, EMT-Is still exist in some states. EMT-Is require a higher level of training (approximately 200 to 400 hours), and in addition to the regular functions of an EMT, EMT-Is can also administer intravenous fluids and certain medications, depending on state or local protocol.

While possessing the same basic life support qualifications as an EMT, AEMTs (sometimes called *EMT-Is* in some jurisdictions) are also trained to provide limited advanced emergency medical care.

Paramedics (sometimes known as *EMT-P*) are allied health professionals who provide emergency medical care to critically ill or injured patients. Paramedic education, which is accredited by the Committee on Accreditation of Educational Programs for the Emergency Medical Services Professions, is the highest level of EMS education, typically consisting of more than 1000 hours of training and a minimum of an associate's degree. Paramedics can perform advanced procedures and administer a wider array of medications.

It is worth noting that while the EMS levels described here are defined in the National EMS Education Standards, some states recognize and credential other EMS providers (such as pre-hospital registered nurses and medical intensive care nurses).

Members of the sports emergency care team should be familiar with the EMS system in their state or jurisdiction, as well as the professionals who will be responding to a sports emergency, and understand the varying levels of care that they provide. In some jurisdictions, EMS is constructed as a 2-tiered system: basic life support and advanced life support. In a 2-tiered system, EMTs respond to all emergency calls, while paramedic units only respond to calls that are determined to need ALS (eg, respiratory or cardiac emergencies, unconscious persons). In some jurisdictions, ambulances are staffed with paramedics, while others may only utilize EMTs with paramedics responding only when needed. Additionally, there are still some jurisdictions where EMT-level training is not required to serve as an EMS responder on an ambulance. Never assume what the capabilities of the responding EMS squad may be.

PHYSICIANS

Physicians are important members of the sports emergency care team. Athletic trainers work under the supervision of a physician, so close collaboration regarding the implementation between the physician and the athletic trainer is essential. Typically, team physicians are most involved with the development of the sports emergency care team. Team physicians have varying degrees of experience in handling sports emergencies, depending on medical specialty and additional training.

HOSPITAL STAFF

Although it is important to work closely with team physicians to develop the sports emergency care team, other physicians, such as emergency department (ED) physicians, should also be considered when developing the emergency plan. Ultimately, the ED physicians and nurses will play a key role in the management of the ill or injured athlete upon arrival at the hospital, so it is important to include the ED physician and staff in developing the EAP as well as training exercises.

COACHING STAFF

At the very least, coaches should be trained in first aid and cardiopulmonary resuscitation (CPR) in order to assist an athlete until further help arrives. They can also assist the sports emergency care team in the prevention of athletic injuries by promoting proper techniques and practices to the athletes they coach. However, coaches can also play a greater role as a member of the sports emergency care team, especially in situations when there are fewer human resources (such as in a small high school). Coaches can be included in the emergency plan and trained to assist the athletic trainer in techniques such as CPR, splinting, and management of spine-injured athletes. Since coaches have a personal relationship with their athletes, they may also be valuable in helping to keep the injured athlete calm in an emergency.

Figure 2-1. Team members working together.

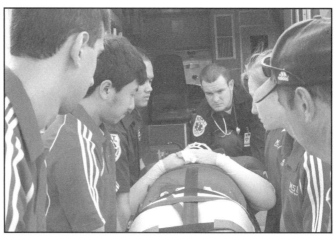

ATHLETIC TRAINING STUDENTS

Students in athletic training education programs who are at the scene of an emergency can play an important role in managing an emergency. They should be familiar with emergency supplies and equipment, and be ready to retrieve such equipment and assist in its use. Athletic training students should be trained in first aid and professional rescuer CPR.

ATHLETICS STAFF

Other nonmedical staff and support personnel play essential roles in the overall management of emergencies in sports. Athletics staff, site managers, grounds crew members, and others can assist in tasks such as ensuring scene safety, crowd control, and allowing access and guiding EMS to the location of the emergency.

ATHLETES

Athletes should not be excluded when developing the EAP. They can loosely be considered a member of the sports emergency care team by knowing what to do and what not to do when a teammate is injured. Athletes should know never to move an injured athlete because doing so can cause further injury. Athletes should also be taught to report all injuries and not ignore symptoms no matter how insignificant they may seem. In some cases, medical emergencies such as concussion or intracranial bleeding often present first with mild symptoms.

OTHER PERSONNEL

EAPs should be specifically tailored for each venue. Therefore, there is no limit to the number or type of personnel who are involved in the management of a sports emergency. While the most common members of the sports emergency care team are listed here, it is by all means not intended to be a complete list (Figure 2-1).

RULES

What rules will be followed when managing an emergency? Is every team member on the same page with regard to protocol? Who is in charge? Will the helmet be removed? These are all questions that must be addressed well in advance of any emergency. The time to argue about protocol

---

Examples of Members of the Sports Emergency Care Team

Athletic trainers
Emergency medical services personnel
Emergency medical responders
Emergency medical technicians
Advanced emergency medical technicians
Paramedics
Physicians
Hospital staff
Coaching staff
Athletic training students
Athletics staff
Athletes

---

for management of an athlete should never take place during an emergency situation. Each member should be included in the development of the EAP to ensure that he or she is comfortable with the protocol that will be used as well as his or her role in the management of an emergency.

Determining how to manage a spine-injured athlete wearing a helmet is of particular importance. While it would appear on paper that athletic trainers, physicians, and EMS personnel are in agreement as to what circumstances warrant helmet removal versus nonremoval, oftentimes local protocols (or even lack of protocols) can be a source of conflict between providers. In 1998, the Inter-Association Task Force for Appropriate Care of the Spine-Injured Athlete published recommendations for management of spinal injuries in athletes wearing protective equipment.[3] The task force consisted of representatives from more than 40 professional organizations in the fields of athletic training, emergency sports care, and EMS. These recommendations, which are widely used in sports medicine, agree with the most recent EMT-Basic: National Standard Curriculum[4] (the document that preceded the National EMS Education Standards). These and other procedural issues must be discussed and agreed upon by members of the team in advance of the start of the season.

Other elements that may seem less critical but are still important include answers to some of the following questions: Who will call 911? Where is the emergency equipment located? Who will retrieve the equipment? Who will guide the ambulance to the scene? Who will notify the athlete's family? Where will the athlete be transported? Of course, this is not a complete list of questions that must be addressed; rather, they are suggestions that should prompt the sports emergency care team to think about as many aspects of responding to an emergency as possible in order to develop a comprehensive EAP.

EQUIPMENT

Sometimes, the immediate care given to an ill or injured athlete is dependent upon the equipment available at the time of the emergency (Figure 2-2). The sports emergency care team should assess what equipment is needed and what will be available at the venue they are covering. Moreover, all members of the team should be familiar with the location of the equipment, as well as their application and operation. In addition to the usual athletic training supplies, additional emergency equipment should be considered.

Figure 2-2. Emergency equipment.

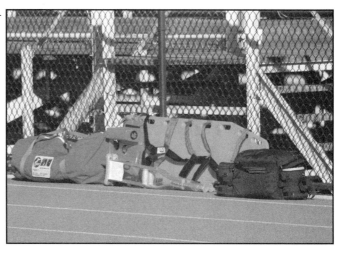

AIRWAY ADJUNCTS

Airway adjuncts are devices that help establish and maintain an open airway, and include equipment such as a CPR mask, bag-valve mask, oropharyngeal and nasopharyngeal airways, and an advanced airway device (such as a CombiTube [Tyco Healthcare Group, Mansfield, MA] or a laryngeal mask airway).

BACKBOARDS

Although backboards are standard equipment on an ambulance, the sports emergency care team should consider having a backboard available at venues where there is a higher risk of spinal injury. The team should also take into consideration what size is most suitable, as well as the fastening system (seat belt-style straps versus Velcro [Velcro USA Inc, Manchester, NH]). Some larger athletes, especially football players wearing protective equipment, may be too large for a standard-sized backboard. Oversize backboards, which are wider, taller, and able to accommodate heavier patients, are available and may be a better choice for larger athletes. One drawback, however, is that oversized backboards may not fit well in some smaller ambulances, and they cannot be used in many medical evacuation helicopters. The sports emergency care team should ensure that equipment that will be used is compatible before the beginning of the season.

SPLINTS

There are several types of commercially available splints, including padded board splints, SAM splints (SAM Medical Products, Wilsonville, OR), air splints, traction splints, and vacuum splints. Each splinting system has its own advantages and disadvantages. Regardless of the type of splint used, all members of the sports emergency care team should know how to use the splinting system that will be available at the time of an emergency.

COMMUNICATIONS EQUIPMENT

Clear communication is crucial in any emergency situation. In some cases, such as in a high school, athletic trainers may not be able to be present at every activity. In these cases, coaches must be able to communicate with athletic trainers if an emergency occurs. While the use of cellular telephones may be suitable in some areas, they may be unreliable in others due to weak cellular signals and should not be relied upon as the only means of communication. The use of portable radios may be a more effective means of communication between coaches and athletic training staff, depending on terrain and area covered. Sports emergency care personnel should know the locations of land line telephones for calling 911. In some cases, EMS systems may consider issuing a portable radio to the athletic training staff for communication in an emergency.

TRANSPORTATION DEVICES

Depending on the severity of the injury or illness, one of a number of different transportation methods may be necessary to move the patient. Crutches, a wheelchair or "sports chair" (a wheelchair designed for use in athletic fields), or a motorized cart may be necessary for minor emergencies. Transportation by ambulance may be necessary in more serious emergencies. Sports emergency care personnel should ensure that these devices or vehicles are available and in working order.

Evacuation via a medical evacuation helicopter may be another option for serious injuries or illnesses that occur in remote locations where transportation times by ground may be excessive or in situations in which the ill or injured athlete requires specialized care that can only be received at a hospital farther away from the scene (such as a trauma or burn center). Sports emergency care personnel should consult with local EMS providers to find out if there is a predesignated landing zone in the area, or to determine an appropriate area near the venue that can serve as a landing zone.

RESUSCITATION EQUIPMENT

Resuscitation equipment, including an automated external defibrillator (AED) and oxygen, should be available in the event of respiratory or cardiac emergencies. Although ambulances are equipped with AEDs, sports emergency care personnel should ensure that an AED is on hand during athletic events. According to the American Heart Association, chances of survival from cardiac arrest decrease 7% to 10% for every minute a shock from a defibrillator is delayed for a victim with a shockable rhythm.[5] If an AED is not available on the field or court, waiting for the ambulance to arrive with an AED can significantly decrease the athlete's chances of survival.

FACEMASK REMOVAL TOOLS

Facemask removal tools should be available at venues where athletes will be wearing helmets with removable facemasks, such as football, lacrosse, and hockey. A universal facemask removal tool, such as a cordless screwdriver or specialized facemask extraction tool, can aid in facemask removal. Regardless of what facemask removal system is used, sports emergency care personnel must practice frequently with their tool of choice in order to be proficient in its use.

DIAGNOSTIC TOOLS

Assessing an acute injury or illness with diagnostic tools can help provide a more accurate picture of the athlete's condition. Examples of diagnostic tools that should be available include a stethoscope, penlight (to assess pupillary reaction), thermometer, a blood pressure cuff set (including large, regular, and pediatric sizes), and a pulse oximeter.

LIFESAVING MEDICATIONS

In some cases, athletes may carry prescribed lifesaving medications, such as metered dose inhalers, insulin, glucagon, or EpiPens (Dey Pharma, L.P., Napa, CA). These medications should be readily accessible on the sideline in the event the athlete needs them. A spare prescription dose and a copy of the prescription should be kept by the athletic trainer if possible and if permitted by local policy.

PLANNING

Developing the EAP must take all the other PREPARE components into account: what personnel will be involved, what rules will be followed, what equipment will be available, what the arena for the event will be, when the plan will be rehearsed, how will it be evaluated, and what the educational process will be in terms of informing sports emergency care providers, coaches, athletes, and others. The person in charge of developing the EAP should ensure that all stakeholders (eg, administrators, coaches, EMS providers) are part of the planning process. The EAP should be distributed to all members of the sports emergency care team and athletics staff and should also be posted at each venue. Visiting teams should also be provided with a copy of the EAP.

The EAP need not be a lengthy document. However, it should provide detailed instructions as to who will act, what actions will be taken, and how and where they will be taken (Table 2-1). A separate venue-specific EAP should be developed for each venue, complete with detailed instructions and information including but not limited to the address of the venue, a description of the location of emergency equipment, telephone locations, a list of emergency phone numbers, a list of emergency hand signals (for use on the field), and detailed instructions for staff and sports emergency care personnel.[6,7]

ARENA

A separate EAP must be designed for each venue, or "arena," because each arena is unique. Sports emergency care personnel must be familiar with the arena in which the athletic event will occur. Sports emergency care personnel should identify the following prior to any event:

* Condition of the court or field (to identify any potential hazards)
* Location of emergency exits and other routes of egress
* Location of ambulance (if present) or entrance where ambulance or EMS personnel will arrive
* Location of emergency equipment

Consideration must be given as to how an athlete will be transported from the field of play. It may be possible at some outdoor venues for the ambulance to drive on the field. However, sports emergency care personnel must assess the field conditions prior to the game to ensure vehicles will not become stuck if the field is wet. Other venues, such as an ice rink, may present hazardous conditions for rescuers. Rescuers must prepare for extrication from the field of play in advance and work to minimize any hazards (Figure 2-3).

REHEARSAL

An EAP is only useful if it is rehearsed. Frequent practice with all members of the sports emergency care team must occur in order for the plan to work effectively (Figure 2-4). The only way to improve response to emergencies and to detect deficiencies in a plan is to identify them through practice. Rehearsing a number of different types of situations will help prepare the team for emergencies. At a minimum, rehearsal should occur before the season begins and should incorporate as many scenarios as possible. Rehearsing scenarios that involve as many members of the sports emergency care team as possible will allow the members of the team to become more comfortable working together and increase the likelihood of a smooth working relationship at the time of an emergency, which ultimately provides for better patient care.

Table 2-1
SAMPLE EMERGENCY ACTION PLAN

_____ *University Sports Medicine*
Football Emergency Protocol

1. Call 911 or other emergency number consistent with organizational policies.
2. Instruct emergency medical services (EMS) personnel to "report to _____ and meet _____ at _____ as we have an injured student-athlete in need of emergency medical treatment."
    University Football Practice Complex: _____ Street entrance
    (gate across street from _____), cross street: _____ Street
    University Stadium: Gate _____ entrance off _____ Road
3. Provide necessary information to EMS personnel:
    *   Name, address, telephone number of caller
    *   Number of victims, condition of victims
    *   First aid treatment initiated
    *   Specific directions as needed to locate scene
    *   Other information as requested by dispatcher
4. Provide appropriate emergency care until arrival of EMS personnel. On arrival of EMS personnel, provide pertinent information (method of injury, vital signs, treatment rendered, medical history) and assist with emergency care as needed.

Note
*   Sports medicine staff member should accompany student-athlete to hospital
*   Notify other sports medicine staff immediately
*   Parents should be contacted by sports medicine staff
*   Inform coach(es) and administration
*   Obtain medical history and insurance information
*   Appropriate injury reports should be completed

Emergency Telephone Numbers
Hospital   _____
Emergency Department _____
University Health Center _____
Campus Police   _____

Emergency Signals
*   Physician: arm extended overhead with clenched fist
*   Paramedics: point to location in end zone by home locker and wave onto field
*   Spine board: arms held horizontally
*   Stretcher: supinated hands in front of body or waist level
*   Splints: hand to lower leg or thigh

Reprinted with permission of National Athletic Trainers' Association.

Figure 2-3. The location of the ambulance near the field is important.

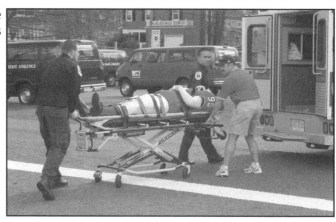

Figure 2-4. Practicing together is crucial in planning for sports emergencies.

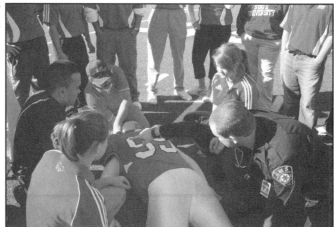

EVALUATE AND EDUCATE

After rehearsing emergency scenarios, and after every actual emergency, the sports emergency care team should evaluate the event to determine how well the EAP worked, how well the team performed, and what unforeseen factors affected the incident. An after-action report should be completed by the athletic trainer and shared with all members of the team. In some situations, it may be appropriate to have a debriefing after the incident, so that all members of the team can discuss how the incident was handled and how patient care can be improved in the future. The conclusions from the after-action report, as well as the recommendations from the debriefing, should be considered when updating the EAP.

The EAP should be a living document; it should be evaluated throughout the year and updated whenever necessary. Changes to the venue, changes to telephone numbers, and procedural changes may happen over time. It is critical that the EAP incorporates these changes when they happen.

SUMMARY OF KEY POINTS

➡ All sports emergency care providers should be familiar with each other prior to any emergency.
➡ Athletic trainers often serve as the "captain" of the sports emergency care team and must be prepared for sports emergencies.

➡ The EMS Educational Standards now delineate 4 levels of EMS education:
  1. EMR
  2. EMT
  3. AEMT
  4. Paramedic

➡ Other personnel, such as physicians, hospital staff, coaching staff, athletic training students, and athletics staff, are all potential members of the sports emergency care team.

➡ Know the rules, policies, and procedures you will follow before the emergency occurs. The time to argue about protocol for management of an athlete should never take place during an emergency situation.

➡ All sports venues must have a site-specific EAP, and the plan must be disseminated and understood by all members of the sports emergency care team.

➡ EAPs must be rehearsed on a regular basis by the members of the sports emergency care team.

➡ After rehearsing emergency scenarios, and after every actual emergency, the sports emergency care team should evaluate the event to determine how well the EAP worked, how well the team performed, and what unforeseen factors affected the incident.

REVIEW QUESTIONS

1. Who are the members of the sports emergency care team?
2. What are the different levels of training in the EMS system?
3. What does the PREPARE acronym stand for?
4. Describe in detail what must be included in the EAP?
5. What are the advantages of rehearsing the EAP?

REFERENCES

1. Board of Certification. Defining athletic training. http://www.bocatc.org//index.php?option=com_ content&view =article&id=31&Itemid=33. Accessed July 13, 2011
2. National Highway Traffic Safety Administration. EMS education standards. http://www.ems.gov/pdf/811077a. pdf. Published January 2009. Accessed October 12, 2011.
3. Kleiner DM, Almquist JL, Bailes J, et al. *Prehospital Care of the Spine-Injured Athlete: A Document From the Inter-Association Task Force for Appropriate Care of the Spine-Injured Athlete.* Dallas, TX: National Athletic Trainers' Association; 2001.
4. National Highway Traffic Safety Administration. Emergency medication technician-basic: national standard curriculum. http://www.nhtsa.dot.gov/people/injury/ems/pub/emtbnsc.pdf. Accessed November 2, 2006.
5. Cummins RO, Ornato JP, Thies WH, Pepe PE. Improving survival from sudden cardiac arrest: the "chain of survival" concept. A statement for health professionals from the Advanced Cardiac Life Support Subcommittee and the Emergency Cardiac Care Committee, American Heart Association. *Circulation.* 1991;83(5):1832-1847.
6. Anderson JC, Courson RW, Kleiner DM, McLoda TA. National Athletic Trainers' Association position statement: emergency planning in athletics. *J Athl Train.* 2002;37(1):99-104.
7. Casa DJ, Guskiewicz KM, Anderson SA, et al. National Athletic Trainers' Association position statement: preventing sudden death in sports. *J Athl Train.* 2012;47(1):96-118.

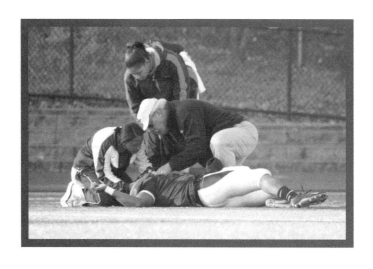

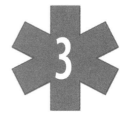

Assessment of
Sports Emergencies

Robb S. Rehberg, PhD, ATC, CSCS, NREMT

> *You are summoned by a frantic coach to the basketball court.*
> *The team had been practicing, and during a water break, one of the players*
> *suddenly collapsed. By the time you arrive, she is conscious and alert.*
> *How will you assess the athlete? What questions will you ask?*
> *What signs will you look for?*

Proper assessment of sports injury and illness is an essential skill for health care providers covering sporting events. Rapid assessment on the field can speed appropriate care and mean the difference between life and death in some cases. Assessment of an injury immediately following the traumatic event often reveals clinical indicators that may not be present if proper assessment is delayed due to factors such as swelling, muscle guarding, etc. Moreover, rapid assessment facilitates proper and immediate treatment. A delay in treatment can often complicate an injury (as in a dislocation with muscle spasm) or even decrease chances of survival (as in cardiac arrest).

Various assessment methods will be introduced in this chapter. Many of these assessment tools are designed to uncover signs and symptoms that will be useful in determining the nature of the illness or injury. It is important to note that regardless of the injury or illness, signs and symptoms are like different colors in a detailed painting. The more colors used to paint a picture, the more detailed the painting becomes and the easier it is for the viewer to understand what the painting depicts. The same is true when assessing an ill or injured victim. Usually, one symptom is not enough to determine the condition. It usually takes several signs and symptoms to clearly paint the picture and illustrate the condition.

MECHANISM OF INJURY

In many cases, proper assessment of an athletic injury does not begin when the athletic trainer reaches the athlete. Rather, it begins before athlete contact, at the moment the injury occurs.

Rehberg RS.
Sports Emergency Care: A Team Approach,
Second Edition (pp 19-34).
© 2013 SLACK Incorporated.

Figure 3-1. Trailing the action provides a better view of the field of play.

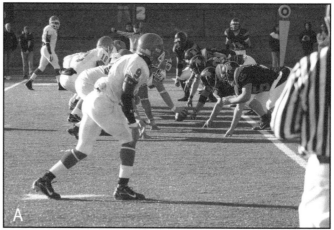

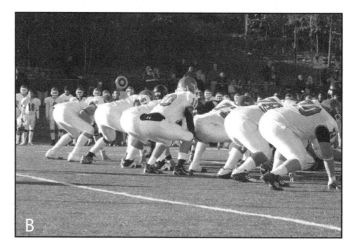

When covering an athletic event, athletic trainers, emergency medical services (EMS) personnel, physicians, and other on-field medical staff are in a unique position to actually see the injury occur, a luxury that most health care professionals do not have. We will discuss in this chapter the importance of interviewing the injured athlete about how the injury occurred; however, oftentimes a witnessed mechanism of injury can be just as valuable. In cases in which an athlete is unconscious, a witnessed mechanism of injury by sports emergency care personnel can be invaluable in determining the injury. It is not enough for sports emergency care personnel to merely be present at an athletic event. They must have an understanding of the game, know what to look for, and pay close attention to the field of play. Sports emergency care personnel should always position themselves where they have an optimum view of the field of play and can view as many athletes as possible. This is especially true in football. Athletic trainers should resist the urge to stand at the line of scrimmage or in a crowd. Instead, the athletic trainer should trail the team he or she is covering to ensure that he or she can visualize every player on the field (Figure 3-1).

APPROACHING THE ATHLETE: FIRST STEPS

Prior to assessing any athlete, the sports emergency care personnel should ensure that he or she has taken proper precautions to protect him- or herself from harm and from disease. Rescuers should approach any injured person with open eyes, paying attention not only to

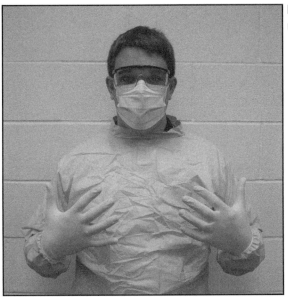

Figure 3-2. Personal protective equipment.

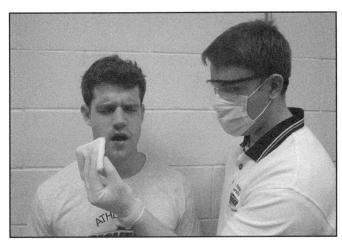

Figure 3-3. Stand to the side when treating a mouth injury.

the patient but also to the environment surrounding the patient. An athletic event is usually a controlled environment; however, certain conditions can create a harmful situation for both the injured athlete and the athletic trainer. Athletic trainers should survey the scene and pay particular attention to hazards such as weather conditions, unstable surfaces, and uncontrolled crowds. Always remember that while it is important to provide rapid intervention in an emergency situation, rescuers must always place their own safety first.

It is a given that athletic trainers have disposable examination gloves readily available. However, in situations where there is a reasonable anticipation of exposure to potentially infectious material such as blood or body fluids containing blood, athletic trainers may require additional personal protective equipment. In addition to gloves, items such as face shields, gowns, and masks may be necessary (Figure 3-2). Athletic trainers should always minimize their exposure to blood or other potentially infectious materials by following the Occupational Safety and Health Administration's Bloodborne Pathogens Standard (29 CFR 1910.1030).[1] Likewise, athletic trainers must be aware of the potential risk of airborne pathogens and take precautions to minimize exposure. This is especially true when assessing or treating an injury around the mouth and nose (Figure 3-3).

Table 3-1
ASSESSING LEVEL OF CONSCIOUSNESS: THE AVPU SCALE

- Alert: Victim is alert and oriented
- Verbal: Victim responds to verbal stimuli
- Painful: Victim responds to painful stimuli
- Unresponsive

Try to determine the mechanism of injury as you approach the victim. If you did not witness the mechanism of injury, you may need to rely on bystanders and the victim's recollection of the event. If the victim is suffering from an illness, try to determine the nature of the illness.

INITIAL ASSESSMENT

Regardless of the mechanism of injury, the athletic trainer should always assess immediate life threats first. Immediate life threats are symptoms that must be addressed immediately to sustain life. Assessing for immediate life threats begins with checking the athlete's mental status. A victim's mental status is determined by using the following AVPU scale (Table 3-1):

* A—Alert: If a victim is alert, assess whether he or she is oriented to time (what time is it?), place (where is he or she?), person (who is he or she?), and event (what is he or she doing?). This is often documented as being conscious, alert, and oriented times 4 (often documented as CAOx4). The inability of a victim to recognize time, place, person, and/or event may be an indication of a brain injury.

* V—Verbal: The victim responds to verbal stimuli only. This means that the victim is unresponsive, but responds when the rescuer speaks to him or her. In this case, the victim may appear to be unconscious but does respond to questions when asked by the rescuer.

* P—Painful: The victim is unresponsive and does not respond to questions asked by the rescuer but does respond when a painful stimulus is applied. An example of a painful stimulus might be rubbing the sternum or pinching the nail bed of the victim's thumb.

* U—Unresponsive: The victim is unconscious and unresponsive to verbal or painful stimuli.

Once the victim's mental status is determined, the athletic trainer should continue the initial assessment by checking for and correcting immediate life threats. All health care providers are familiar with the initial assessment of circulation, airway, and breathing (CAB), and some health care providers follow an assessment algorithm that adds deformity (D) and exposure (E). Because of the unique nature of the types of emergencies common to sports, a variation of the CAB algorithm is recommended. The CAB Sx3 (CAB, S times 3) algorithm (Table 3-2) adds 3 important components to the initial assessment: checking for and treating severe bleeding, shock, and spinal injury. Using the CAB Sx3 algorithm allows the athletic trainer to quickly identify and treat immediate life threats in order of severity.

CIRCULATION

Assess the victim's pulse at the carotid artery. If there is no pulse, begin cardiopulmonary resuscitation (CPR) and if equipped, use an automated external defibrillator (AED) as per the most recent guidelines for CPR and emergency cardiovascular care. If a pulse is present, note the rate and quality of the pulse (ie, rapid and weak, slow and strong). There is some evidence in the

---

Table 3-2

THE ABCS OF SPORTS EMERGENCY CARE: CAB Sx3

- Circulation
- Airway
- Breathing
- Severe bleeding
- Shock
- Spinal injury

---

literature that suggests the presence of a palpable pulse at the carotid artery is an indication of a systolic blood pressure of at least 80 mm Hg.[2]

AIRWAY

If the patient is found to be alert, the athletic trainer knows that the athlete has an airway, is breathing, and has a pulse. A quick scan of the body for severe bleeding, a visual inspection of the skin temperature and condition, assessing capillary refill, and a cursory motor/sensory assessment can also rule out other immediate life threats. However, if a victim is unresponsive, the athletic trainer must ensure the victim has a patent airway. Open the airway by using either a head-tilt chin-lift or a jaw thrust if a spinal injury is suspected (Figure 3-4). Rescuers may consider using airway adjuncts to keep the airway open. This will be discussed further in Chapter 4. The airway must be protected at all times regardless of the nature of the injury or illness.

BREATHING

Once the airway is open, rescuers should assess for breathing. If breathing is absent, rescue breathing should be performed as per the most current guidelines for CPR and emergency cardiovascular care. If the victim is breathing, the athletic trainer should note the rate and quality of breathing. Breathing rates of less than 8 and greater than 30 require ventilatory support. This will be discussed further in Chapter 4.

SEVERE BLEEDING

Quickly assess for severe bleeding, and control bleeding by using direct pressure. Quickly limiting severe blood loss can increase the patient's chances of survival. When assessing for severe bleeding, it is important to assess the entire body.

SHOCK

In addition to assessing pulse and breathing rate and quality, there are several key signs of shock that rescuers should assess, including skin color, skin temperature and condition, and capillary refill. These quick assessments will help the rescuer form a general impression of how adequately the victim is perfusing oxygenated blood throughout the body. Changes in normal skin complexion, such as pale, cyanotic, flushed, red, or jaundice skin, may be an indication of shock. Skin temperature and moisture (eg, hot and dry or cool and clammy) may also be indicators of shock.

Figure 3-4. (A) Head-tilt chin-lift. (B) Modified jaw thrust.

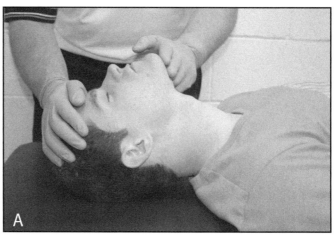

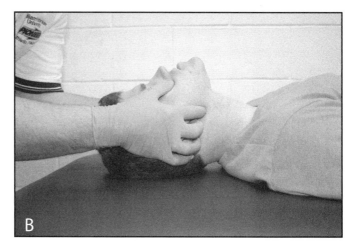

Spinal Injury

A cursory assessment of motor and sensory function in the extremities should be performed next. While a more detailed neurological examination will be discussed later, a brief assessment of sensory and motor function in the extremities, combined with the mechanism of injury and the victim's chief complaint, will help determine whether or not spinal precautions will be necessary. A spinal injury should be suspected in all traumatic injuries until proven otherwise.

Assess for sensory nerve function by brushing or gently pinching the victim's hands and feet. The athletic trainer should ask the victim to squeeze his or her fingers with his or her hands and plantar flex his or her ankle against resistance to assess motor function. The absence of sensory and/or motor function does not conclusively indicate a spinal injury. Nonetheless, spinal precautions must be taken in any situation where a sensory or motor deficit is present. Conversely, although a victim's ability to feel sensation and provide resistance indicates that a spinal injury is not likely, it does not rule out a spinal fracture that may endanger the spinal cord if managed poorly. The sports emergency care team must complete a thorough assessment and take appropriate precautions based on their findings. Additional information on management of spinal injuries is found in Chapter 6.

Table 3-3
SAMPLE HISTORY

- Signs/symptoms
- Allergies
- Medications (including over-the-counter medications, vitamins, supplements, etc)
- Past medical history
- Last oral intake (including food, drink, smoking, inhalation, medications)
- Events leading to the injury/illness

FOCUSED HISTORY AND PHYSICAL EXAMINATION/RAPID ASSESSMENT

Once immediate life threats are assessed, the sports emergency care team member should focus on the injury or illness. If the injury or illness is obvious, the athletic trainer can perform a focused history and physical examination by obtaining a SAMPLE history (signs/symptoms, allergies, medications, past medical history, last oral intake, events leading to the injury/illness) (Table 3-3); examining the injured area (including performing any necessary special tests); and obtaining a set of baseline vital signs (including but not limited to pulse, respiratory rate, and blood pressure). Since most traumatic injuries in sports are not multiple systems trauma in nature (meaning several body systems are involved), it is usually easy to quickly identify the injured area and move directly to the focused history and physical examination. However, there may be situations in which more than one body system is injured or the victim is unable to verbalize the location of the injury. In these situations, a rapid trauma assessment consisting of a head-to-toe examination and baseline vital signs should be performed. The athletic trainer should keep in mind that this algorithm for assessment is designed for emergencies. Other serious but nonemergent conditions (such as a shoulder dislocation or an anterior cruciate ligament [ACL] sprain) may not require a comprehensive assessment as described here.

SAMPLE HISTORY

If the injury or illness is obvious, begin the focused history and assessment by asking the athlete about his or her chief complaint (what hurts?) and beginning an examination of the injured area and a SAMPLE history. The SAMPLE acronym can help rescuers systematically obtain necessary medical information in an emergency situation. EMS professionals have used the SAMPLE history for several years. Athletic trainers who obtain a SAMPLE history and are able to convey these findings during the transfer of care will present the necessary information in a format that is familiar to EMS personnel. Oftentimes, it takes a degree of "detective work" when interviewing a patient about his or her medical history, and thus, it is important to be thorough and to ask the right questions in order to receive the complete picture. For instance, "Do you take any medications?" may not be enough to ask a victim. While that question may prompt some victims to provide a very thorough answer, others may not consider over-the-counter medications and supplements worth mentioning. Rescuers should choose their words carefully and pay close attention to the victim's responses when obtaining a medical history from a victim. Taking a SAMPLE history includes the following information:

✳ Signs/symptoms: Signs (something the rescuer can see) will be uncovered by performing a quick visual inspection. Further assessment of signs will occur during the detailed assessment. The patient will reveal symptoms (something the victim tells you) during the interview.

✳ Allergies: Ask the victim if he or she has any known allergies. Allergies to penicillin-based or sulfa-based medications will be significant to note because this may be a cause of the illness. This information may also impact the patient's care so as not to administer medication to which the patient may be allergic. Food allergies such as to shellfish or nuts may be relevant to uncovering the nature of the illness. Seasonal allergies should also be noted because they could also be a contributing factor. Allergies to fabrics and other synthetic materials should also be noted. (Rubber is a material to be aware of with the prevalence of synthetic turf fields, many of which contain rubber.) Awareness of latex allergies is important as well. Sports emergency care providers should be sure to have nonlatex examination gloves readily available.

✳ Medications: Ask the victim what medications he or she is taking, including prescription and over-the-counter medications, vitamins, supplements, and herbal remedies. Note the last time the victim ingested a medication as well as the amount taken. This information is important for several reasons because the victim may require additional medication or surgery, the victim may be directed to take a medication but has missed one or more doses, or the medication may be a contributing factor to the present illness.

✳ Past medical history: Any significant past medical history, including major or chronic illnesses, surgeries, or hospitalization, should be noted. While obtaining a thorough history is of value to the medical staff at the receiving hospital, past medical history may provide important clues as to the nature of the present illness.

✳ Last oral intake: When was the last time the patient ate, drank, smoked, chewed tobacco, or placed any substance in his or her mouth? Note the time and quantity of each. Once again, this information may provide clues as to the history of the present illness. It will also be valuable to the receiving medical staff in the event surgery is necessary.

✳ Events leading to the injury/illness: Asking the victim if he or she remembers the events leading to the injury or illness can prove valuable in determining the cause. While information from bystanders regarding the incident can also be valuable, it is important to determine whether the victim can remember the events by him- or herself. After the victim provides information, ask him or her, "Is that what you remember happening, or is that what others told you?" The inability to remember the events leading to the injury or illness may be a significant clinical indicator. Moreover, a thorough history must include questions regarding the event in order to ascertain the exact cause. For instance, if you find a victim with a head injury having seizures, did the victim have a seizure and subsequently hit his or her head or did an injury to the head cause the seizure?

OBTAINING ADDITIONAL INFORMATION: OPQRST

In some situations, obtaining information on the characteristics of the pain experienced by the injured athlete may assist the athletic trainer during the assessment process. OPQRST (onset, provocation/palliation, quality, region/radiation, severity, time) is another commonly used acronym by EMS professionals that is useful in assessing pain characteristics The OPQRST assessment includes the following:

✳ Onset: What time did the pain begin? Did the pain begin suddenly, or did it come gradually?

✳ Provocation/palliation: What was the victim doing when the pain began? Did the victim do something to cause the pain? Is there anything that makes the pain worse? Is there anything that relieves the pain?

	Table 3-4
	HEAD-TO-TOE ASSESSMENT
Body Area	**Assess for**
Head	DCAP-BTLS plus pupillary response, drainage or bleeding from ears or nose, and crepitation
Eyes	DCAP-BTLS plus foreign bodies and blood in anterior chamber (hyphema)
Mouth	DCAP-BTLS plus dislodged teeth, airway obstructions, swollen or lacerated tongue, odors, and discoloration
Neck	DCAP-BTLS plus jugular vein distension and crepitation
Chest	DCAP-BTLS plus paradoxical motion, crepitation, and breath sounds (presence, absence, equality)
Abdomen	DCAP-BTLS plus note firmness, softness, and distension
Pelvis	DCAP-BTLS plus check for pelvic stability
Extremities	DCAP-BTLS plus assess distal pulse, sensation, motor function, and medic alert tags

* Quality: What does the pain feel like? Oftentimes, pain is characterized as sharp, dull, aching, throbbing, stabbing, shooting, or intermittent. Understanding the type of pain may hold clues to the condition producing the pain.
* Region/radiation: Where is the pain? Where does the pain begin? Is it localized or diffuse? Does it radiate to another part of the body?
* Severity: How severe is the pain? How does it compare to previous injuries? Often, a scale of 1 to 10 is used to assess pain. (While this scale is useful to determine whether pain increases or decreases, it is subjective in nature and thus, not reliable as an indicator to the type of injury/illness.)
* Time: When did the pain begin? How long does the pain last?

RAPID TRAUMA ASSESSMENT

If the injury or illness is not immediately known, a rapid trauma assessment should be performed. Beginning at the head and working toward the toes, the athletic trainer should visually inspect and palpate for abnormalities (Table 3-4). During the assessment, the athletic trainer should look for deformities, contusions, abrasions, punctures/penetrations, burns, tenderness, lacerations, and swelling (DCAP-BTLS).[3] Assessment for other body-area specific conditions should also be performed.

OBTAINING VITAL SIGNS

Vital signs such as pulse, respirations, and blood pressure can be key in determining how efficiently the body is functioning. Vital signs that fall outside normal range limits may be an indication of severe or acute injury or illness. A set of baseline vital signs, including but not limited to pulse, respirations, and blood pressure, should be taken. Continuous reassessment of vital signs should be performed throughout treatment and transportation to the hospital. Table 3-5 lists the

Table 3-5
NORMAL VITAL SIGN VALUES IN HEALTHY INDIVIDUALS

	Adult	Adolescent (11 Years to 14 Years)	Child (6 Years to 10 Years)
Pulse (per minute)	60 to 100	60 to 105	70 to 110
Respirations (per minute)	12 to 20	12 to 20	15 to 30
Systolic blood pressure (mm Hg)	90 to 140	88 to 140	80 to 122
Diastolic blood pressure (mm Hg)	60 to 90	Approximately two-thirds of systolic pressure in adolescents and children	
Temperature	~ 98.6°F for all ages		
Capillary refill	<3 seconds for all ages		
Pulse oximetry (for all ages)	95% to 100% Normal 91% to 94% Mild hypoxia 86% to 90% Moderate hypoxia <85% Severe hypoxia		

Vital Sign Changes With Exercise

Vital Sign	Exercising Person
Pulse	Faster and stronger
Respirations	Faster and deeper
Blood pressure (systolic)	Elevated
Blood pressure (diastolic)	About the same
Skin color	Flushed if warm and sweating, grey or whitish if cold
Skin temperature	Cool with sweat or hypothermia, warm to hot if flushed or heat stroke
Sweating	Present, could be significant

normal range limits for vital signs in healthy individuals. However, the athletic trainer should be reminded that normal resting vital signs in elite athletes might be lower than that of the average person. Conversely, athletes who were actively participating in their sport just prior to assessment may present with vital signs that are higher than the normal limits.

PULSE

While the presence of a pulse was assessed during the initial assessment by palpating the carotid artery, assessing for a pulse at the radial artery is a useful diagnostic tool (Figure 3-5A). As mentioned earlier, presence of a radial pulse represents a systolic blood pressure of at least

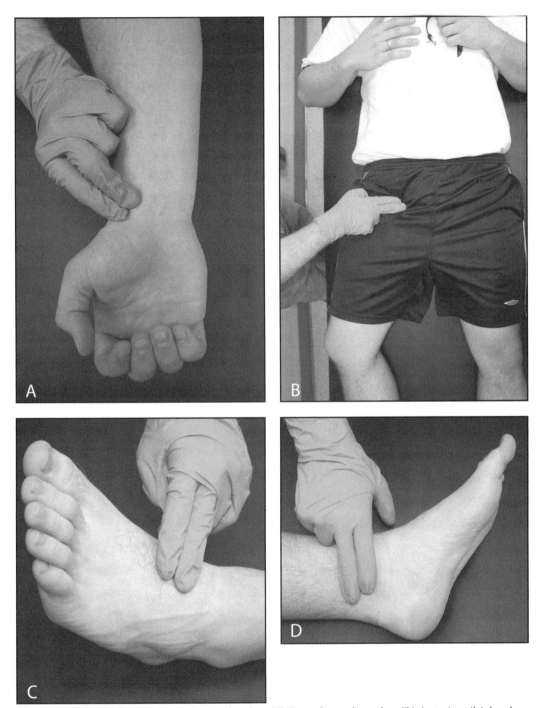

Figure 3-5. (A) Radial pulse. (B) Femoral pulse. (C) Dorsalis pedis pulse. (D) Anterior tibial pulse.

80 mm Hg. Note the rate and quality of the pulse felt when assessing a radial pulse. The rate should be determined by counting the number of beats for 15 seconds and multiplying by 4 to determine the number of beats per minute. Also note the strength of the pulse. Is the pulse bounding (strong) or thready (weak)? If a radial pulse cannot be felt, assess for a pulse at the femoral artery (Figure 3-5B). For severe injuries to the lower extremity, presence of a pulse at the dorsalis pedis (Figure 3-5C) or anterior tibial location (Figure 3-5D) may be necessary.

RESPIRATIONS

Assess respirations by watching the athlete's chest rise and fall. In some instances, it may be helpful to place a hand on the athlete's chest to aid in assessing respirations. Assess breathing for 15 seconds and multiply by 4 to determine breaths per minute. While assessing respirations, note whether or not the chest expands symmetrically on both sides. Also note the quality of breaths (eg, normal versus labored, deep versus shallow, regular versus irregular). Assessment of lung sounds via auscultation will be discussed in Chapter 4.

BLOOD PRESSURE

Blood pressure is the key diagnostic test that determines a victim's condition in an emergency. Assessment of blood pressure can be performed using 2 different methods: auscultation (preferred) or palpation. Assessing blood pressure by auscultation is preferred because it provides a more accurate reading, and both the systolic and diastolic values can be obtained. Assessing blood pressure by palpation only produces a systolic value and may be less accurate. While auscultation is the preferred method of blood pressure assessment, assessing blood pressure by palpation does offer advantages in situations where noise from a crowded stadium or arena may prevent an accurate auscultative reading. Although assessment by palpation does not produce a diastolic value, it is the systolic value that is of greater importance in emergency situations.

It is important that the correct cuff size is used when performing a blood pressure assessment. Standard size blood cuffs should not be used in patients with an upper arm circumference of more than 34 cm.[4] Sports emergency care providers should be prepared for any size athlete and should have access to different cuff sizes, including pediatric, regular, and large cuffs.

Blood Pressure by Auscultation

Place the sphygmomanometer cuff around the upper arm and just above the elbow. Follow the directions on the cuff for proper placement, if present. Secure the cuff snugly around the arm. Place the earpieces of the stethoscope in your ears and place the bell of the stethoscope over the brachial artery at the medial aspect of the antecubital space (Figure 3-6A). Next, close the valve and inflate the cuff. As the cuff inflates, a pulse will be audible. Continue to inflate the cuff until the audible pulse disappears, then continue to inflate the cuff at least 30 mm Hg further. Slowly release air from the valve at a rate of about 5 to 10 mm Hg per second. Note the reading at which the first audible pulse is heard. This is the systolic value. Continue to steadily release air from the bladder until the audible pulse disappears and note the reading when it does. This is the diastolic value.

Blood Pressure by Palpation

Place the sphygmomanometer in the same manner described above. Next, palpate the radial pulse (Figure 3-6B). Once the radial pulse is felt, inflate the cuff until you can no longer feel the radial pulse. Then, inflate the cuff an additional 30 to 40 mm Hg past that point. Finally, while still keeping your fingers in place to palpate the radial pulse, slowly begin releasing air from the cuff at a rate of about 5 to 10 mm Hg per second. Note the pressure at which the radial pulse returns. This is the systolic value. For instance, if the pulse returns at 140 mm Hg, the blood pressure is 140 by palpation, or 140/p.

OTHER SIGNIFICANT DIAGNOSTIC SIGNS

There are other diagnostic signs that are useful in determining the athlete's overall condition (see Table 3-5).

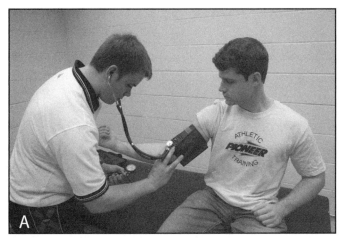

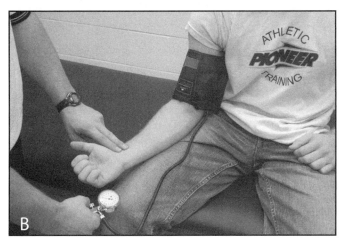

Figure 3-6. (A) Assessing blood pressure by auscultation. (B) Assessing blood pressure by palpation.

Skin Assessment

Assessing the skin for color (pallor), temperature, and moisture can be of particular importance. Pale skin (or loss of normal skin complexion in darker skinned individuals) may be an indication of shock. Flushed, red skin may be an indication of heat illness, anaphylaxis, hypertension, or emotional distress. Clammy or moist skin may indicate shock as well. Hot skin may indicate heat illness or fever, cool skin may indicate shock, and cold skin may indicate prolonged cold exposure.

Pulse Oximetry

Use of a pulse oximeter is helpful in determining how adequately oxygen is perfusing throughout the body. The pulse oximeter is a device that measures oxygen saturation using a photoelectric sensor that attaches to the athlete's finger or ear. There are several types of pulse oximeters available that range in price and size. Sports emergency care providers should consider having a pulse oximeter as standard equipment.

Capillary Refill

If a pulse oximeter is not present, the capillary refill test can be used as a method to assess perfusion of oxygenated blood to the extremities. When a victim is in shock, the body shunts

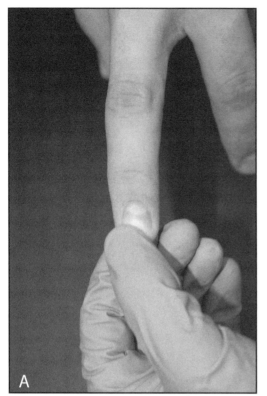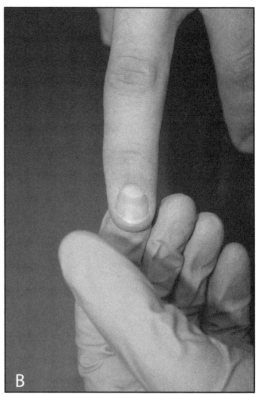

Figure 3-7. Assessing capillary refill.

blood away from the skin. The capillary refill test, also known as the blanch test, is performed by pressing on the nail bed until it turns white (Figure 3-7A). This forces oxygenated blood out of the tissues being depressed. In victims with adequate perfusion, blood should return to the underlying tissue and the nail bed should return to its normal pink color within 2 seconds (Figure 3-7B). A capillary refill time greater than 2 seconds is a sign of inadequate perfusion and may be an indication of shock, dehydration, hypothermia, or a peripheral vascular disease.

TEMPERATURE

Temperature should be assessed whenever fever or environmental emergencies such as heat illness or hypothermia are suspected. In the field, temperature should be assessed orally or with the use of a tympanic thermometer. If using a tympanic thermometer, the rescuer should be properly trained and proficient in its use. While there are conflicting studies regarding the reliability of tympanic thermometers, improper use of tympanic thermometers will contribute to faulty readings. Serial temperature measurements should be obtained in order to ensure an accurate reading.

VITAL SIGN TRENDING: THE RULE OF 100

As stated earlier, signs and symptoms aid in painting a picture of the victim's condition. Each vital sign can be likened to a color in a detailed painting. The more colors used in the painting, the more detail is seen and the picture becomes clearer. The same is true for vital signs. The Rule of 100 pays particular attention to 3 vital signs in predicting the severity of injury or illness. Specifically, the assessment of pulse, systolic blood pressure, and temperature can be useful in determining serious cardiopulmonary conditions. The Rule of 100 states that if the systolic blood pressure is greater than 100, and the pulse and temperature are less than 100, significant injury is unlikely. Conversely, a systolic blood pressure of less than 100, and/or a pulse and temperature greater than 100 may indicate a serious injury or illness requiring further medical evaluation. A series of vital sign assessments at intervals of 10 minutes or less and over at least a 30-minute period should be obtained in order to determine trends in the readings obtained.[5]

SUMMARY OF KEY POINTS

➡ Proper assessment of sports injury and illness is an essential skill for health care providers covering sporting events.

➡ When covering an athletic event, athletic trainers, EMS personnel, physicians, and other on-field medical staff are in a unique position to actually see the injury occur, a luxury that most health care professionals do not have.

➡ Sports emergency care personnel must have an understanding of the game, know what to look for, and pay close attention to the field of play.

➡ Prior to assessing any athlete, the sports emergency care personnel should ensure that he or she has taken proper precautions to protect him- or herself from harm and from disease, and must always place his or her own safety first.

➡ A victim's mental status is determined by using the AVPU scale.

➡ Once the victim's mental status is determined, the athletic trainer should continue the initial assessment by checking for and correcting immediate life threats using the CAB Sx3.

➡ The SAMPLE acronym can help rescuers systematically obtain necessary medical information in an emergency situation.

➡ In some situations, obtaining information on the characteristics of the pain experienced by the injured athlete may assist the athletic trainer during the assessment process. OPQRST is another commonly used acronym by EMS professionals that is useful in assessing pain characteristics.

➡ If the injury or illness is not immediately known, a rapid trauma assessment should be performed. The athletic trainer should look for DCAP-BTLS.

➡ Vital signs such as pulse, respirations, blood pressure, skin assessment, pulse oximetry, capillary refill, and temperature can be key in determining how efficiently the body is functioning.

➡ Through the use of the Rule of 100, the assessment of pulse, systolic blood pressure, and temperature can be useful in determining serious cardiopulmonary conditions.

REVIEW QUESTIONS

1. What are the components of an initial assessment?
2. In CAB Sx3, what do the 3 S's stand for?
3. What does the acronym SAMPLE stand for?
4. Describe the Rule of 100.
5. Aside from pulse, respirations, and blood pressure, what are some other vital signs that should be assessed?

REFERENCES

1. United States Department of Labor, Occupational Safety and Health Administration. CFR 1910.1030 (Bloodborne pathogens standard). http://www.osha.gov/pls/oshaweb/owadisp.show_document?p_table=standards&p_id=10051. Accessed September 29, 2012.
2. American College of Surgeons. *Advanced Trauma Life Support for Doctors*. 6th ed. Chicago, IL: Author; 1997.
3. National Highway Traffic Safety Administration. Emergency medical technician-basic: national standard curriculum. http://www.nhtsa.dot.gov/people/injury/ems/pub/emtbnsc.pdf. Accessed September 29, 2012.
4. American Academy of Family Physicians. Medical care for obese patients: advice for health care professionals. *Am Fam Physician*. 2002;65(1):81-88.
5. Kyle J, Leaman J, Courson R, Rehberg R, McGrady T. Sports trauma "red bag" vital sign trending. http://www.sportsafetyinternational.org/content/vst. Accessed July 12, 2011.

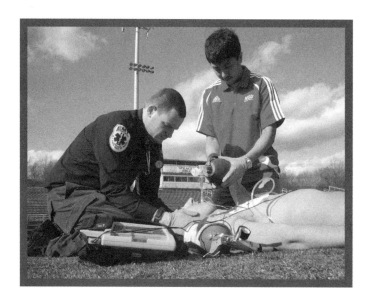

Author's Note: While Chapter 4 covers important aspects of airway and breathing management, it does not address cardiopulmonary resuscitation (CPR), and is not intended to serve as a substitute for training in CPR. All members of the sports emergency care team should maintain current certification in CPR and emergency cardiac care from a recognized authority, such as the American Heart Association, American Red Cross, or National Safety Council.

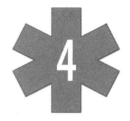

Airway Management
and Breathing

Robb S. Rehberg, PhD, ATC, CSCS, NREMT

> *While covering an ice hockey game, one of your players is checked
> into the boards and lies motionless on the ice.
> When you arrive at the athlete's side, you notice he is not breathing.
> What would you do?*

Establishing and maintaining a patent airway are perhaps the most important tasks with which sports emergency care providers are faced. Breathing cannot occur without an airway, and if breathing ceases, so does circulation, and death is the result. There are a multitude of injuries and illnesses that can contribute to respiratory compromise and difficulty breathing, many of which will be covered throughout this book. The sports emergency care team must anticipate that trauma related to sports participation may result in airway and breathing compromise and must have appropriate plans in place to manage such emergencies. This chapter will address methods of establishing and maintaining an airway, as well as the management of respiratory emergencies.

All sports emergency care personnel should be trained and current in professional rescuer basic life support. Professional-level basic life support courses cover content including adult, infant, and child rescue breathing and cardiopulmonary resuscitation (CPR); foreign body airway obstruction; 2-rescuer resuscitation; and use of adjunctive equipment such as a CPR mask and bag-valve mask. While airway management and breathing are covered in this chapter, it is not intended to be a substitute for skills covered in a professional-level CPR course.

REVIEW OF CLINICALLY RELEVANT ANATOMY

In order to successfully manage a patient's airway, sports emergency care providers must have an understanding of the anatomical features of the upper and lower airway (Figure 4-1). Air enters the upper airway via the nose or mouth. The palate separates both airway openings. Behind the

Rehberg RS.
Sports Emergency Care: A Team Approach,
Second Edition (pp 37-49).
© 2013 SLACK Incorporated.

Figure 4-1. Upper and lower airways. (Illustration by Joelle Rehberg, DO.)

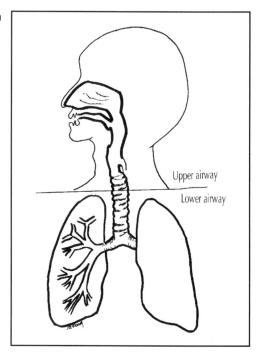

Upper airway

Lower airway

nose and above the palate is the nasal floor, which gives rise to the nasopharynx. In the mouth (below the palate), the oropharynx runs posteriorly, and both the nasopharynx and the oropharynx join at the posterior aspect of the airway, called the pharynx. The pharynx descends behind the tongue where the epiglottis separates the pharynx and the larynx. The larynx extends past the lower pharynx to the trachea.

The lower airway consists of the right and left main bronchi. Each of the main bronchi branch off to each of the lobes of the lungs (2 on the left and 3 on the right). In the lungs, the bronchi branch off into smaller bronchioles, and finally to alveolar ducts, which are lined with alveoli. The alveoli are small air sacs where gas exchange occurs.

ESTABLISHING AN AIRWAY

Assessing and establishing a patent airway is the first priority in any emergency. Most conscious victims are able to maintain a patent airway without assistance. If an athlete is able to verbalize any response, we know the airway is open. However, unconscious victims and victims with an altered mental status may need assistance in keeping the airway open. The procedures for airway evaluation (ie, opening the airway and artificial ventilation) should be performed with the patient lying supine. The primary method of establishing an open airway is the head-tilt chin-lift. The head-tilt chin-lift is accomplished by placing one hand on the forehead, grasping the bony aspect of the chin with the other hand, and tilting the head and lifting the chin simultaneously (Figure 4-2). The rescuer should be sure to tilt the head so that the jaw is near perpendicular to the ground.

If a spinal injury is suspected, the rescuer should instead use the jaw thrust maneuver. To perform the jaw thrust, place the thumbs on the cheeks, and the index and middle fingers behind the angle of the jaw, and slide the jaw forward like a drawer (Figure 4-3).

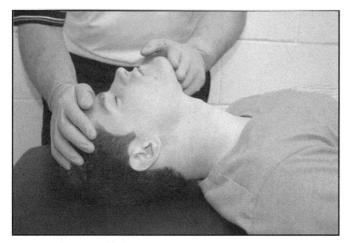

Figure 4-2. Head-tilt chin-lift.

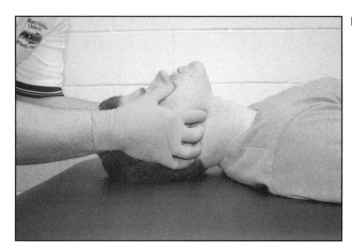

Figure 4-3. Jaw thrust.

USE OF AIRWAY ADJUNCTS

In some cases, it is difficult to maintain an open airway by using manual methods alone. If a victim requires ventilation, the use of airway adjuncts or advanced airway devices can aid in ensuring a patent airway during resuscitation.

Oropharyngeal Airway

Oropharyngeal airways are effective in maintaining a patent airway in victims who are unconscious and do not have a gag reflex. Oropharyngeal airways should not be used in patients who are conscious or who have a gag reflex because they may cause the victim to vomit. Oropharyngeal airways come in assorted sizes, and the correct size is selected by measuring the distance between the tip of the ear and the corner of the mouth (Figure 4-4A). Once the correct size is selected, the following steps should be taken:

* Place the patient in the supine position with the head in a neutral position.

* Perform a crossed-finger technique. Cross the thumb and forefinger of one hand and place them on the upper and lower teeth at the corner of the athlete's mouth. Spread your fingers apart to open the athlete's mouth.

* Position the airway so that its tip is pointing toward the roof of the patient's mouth.

Figure 4-4. (A, B) Oropharyngeal airway insertion. (C) A properly inserted oropharyngeal airway.

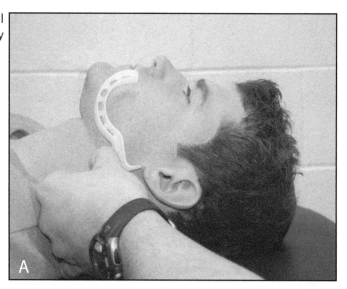

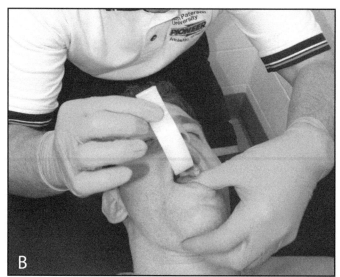

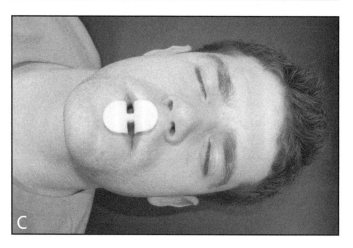

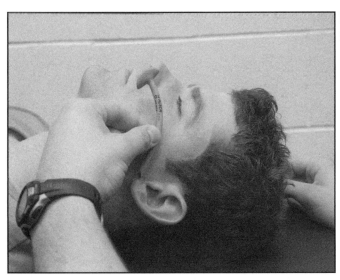

Figure 4-5. Measuring a naso-pharyngeal airway.

* Insert the airway and slide it along the roof of the mouth, past the soft tissue hanging down the back or until you meet resistance against the back of the soft palate.

* Gently rotate the airway 180 degrees so that the tip is pointing down into the patient's pharynx (Figure 4-4B).

* Once properly inserted, the end of the oropharyngeal airway will rest just above the lips (Figure 4-4C).

Nasopharyngeal Airway

A nasopharyngeal airway is another mechanical airway device that can be used for maintaining a patent airway. Unlike oropharyngeal airways, nasopharyngeal airways are usually better tolerated because they are less likely to produce a gag reflex. Nasopharyngeal airways are measured by selecting an airway with a diameter similar to that of the nasal passage. This can usually be measured by comparing the airway diameter to that of the patient's fifth finger. Measure the length by measuring from the athlete's nostril to the earlobe or to the angle of the jaw (Figure 4-5). Choosing the correct length also helps ensure the appropriate diameter. Once the correct size has been selected, the following steps should be taken:

* Lubricate the airway with a water-soluble lubricant.

* Keep the patient's head in a neutral position.

* Gently push the tip of the nose upward.

* Insert the airway into the nostril (use the right nostril when possible) with the bevel of the airway toward the septum.

* Nasopharyngeal airways should not be used on patients with severe head trauma or where a basal skull fracture may be present.

Advanced Airway Devices

Advanced airway devices such as a laryngeal mask airway (LMA), CombiTube (Tyco Healthcare Group, Mansfield, MA; Figure 4-6), or an endotracheal (ET) tube are more reliable means of airway management than oropharyngeal and nasopharyngeal airways and are often used by prehospital care personnel in the field. The use of these devices may be restricted depending on state or local regulations. Sports emergency care providers should follow local protocol before

Figure 4-6. CombiTube.

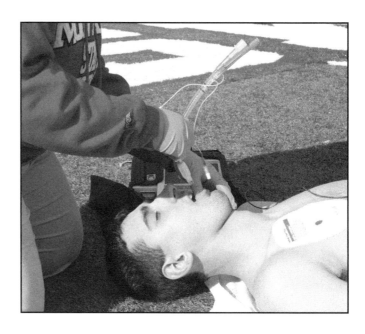

considering the use of advanced airway devices for sports emergencies. The LMA and CombiTube are designed for blind insertion unlike an ET tube, which requires the use of a laryngoscope for proper placement. In the prehospital setting, ET tubes are typically inserted by advanced life support personnel, such as paramedics. However, depending on local or state regulations, basic life support personnel (and possibly athletic trainers) may be permitted to insert an LMA or CombiTube with proper training.

Sports emergency care personnel should be prepared to clear the airway in the event the patient vomits. Aspiration of vomitus into the airway is a serious complication that can hamper resuscitation efforts and cause further injury to the patient. In the event a patient vomits, suction may be necessary to clear the airway. Suction devices should be readily available for use. There are 3 different types of suction units that are typically used in the prehospital setting. Battery-powered suction units are often carried by emergency medical services (EMS) units and operate using a pump that is powered by a rechargeable battery (Figure 4-7A). Oxygen-powered suction units create suction from the flow of oxygen and do not rely on batteries or electricity for power. Manual suction units (Figure 4-7B) are compact and inexpensive and can easily be kept in a medical kit.

There are different types of suction catheters that can be used for suctioning. The most common types are flexible (also known as *French*) and rigid (also known as *Yankauer*).

Indications for suctioning include vomiting in an unresponsive patient, in a patient with an altered mental status, or in a patient who has been secured to a spine board. Before suctioning begins, the maximum depth that the suction catheter is to be inserted should be measured using the distance from the corner of the mouth to the earlobe. The suction catheter should not be inserted deeper than this measurement. Suctioning should then be performed by inserting the catheter and using a figure-8 motion. For powered suction units, inserting the catheter in sterile water before and after suctioning is recommended in order to clean the catheter and decrease the chances of blockage. Do not suction for more than 10 seconds at a time.

ASSESSING BREATHING

When assessing for the presence of breathing, rescuers look for chest rise and listen and feel for breathing. However, once the primary assessment has been completed, and airway, breathing, and

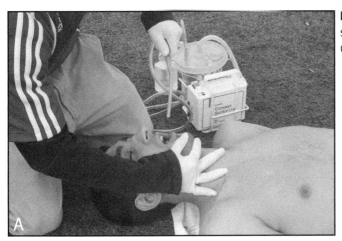

Figure 4-7. (A) Battery-powered suction unit. (B) Manual suction unit.

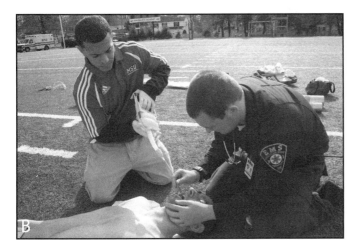

Table 4-1

RESTING RESPIRATORY RATES (PER MINUTE)

Adult	12 to 20
Adolescent	12 to 20
Child <10 years old	15 to 30

circulation are confirmed, a more detailed assessment of breathing will be necessary. Specifically, assessment of breathing rate and quality is usually performed during a detailed physical examination. Table 4-1 lists normal respiratory rates by age; however, it is important to realize that athletes who have been participating in physical activity may present with higher respiratory rates. The respiratory rate can be assessed by counting the number of times the chest rises and falls in a 15-second period and multiplying it by 4. Additionally, sports emergency care personnel may choose to use a stethoscope to determine respiratory rate.

In addition to respiratory rate, respiratory quality should be assessed by observing the patient and by listening to breath sounds. Patients in respiratory distress may exhibit visual signs such as nasal flaring, intercostal retractions, and cyanosis. Sports emergency care personnel should assess

Figure 4-8. Assessing breath sounds.

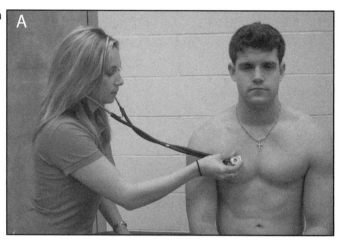

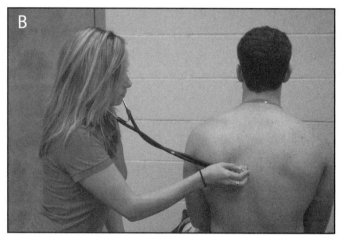

breath sounds over both the anterior and posterior aspects of the chest (Figure 4-8). Breath sounds in a healthy person should be clear and equal over both lungs. Breath sounds should always be assessed before and after insertion of an advanced airway to ensure proper placement.

Absent, diminished, or abnormal breath sounds may indicate respiratory compromise. Common abnormal breath sounds that may be present include the following:

❋ Rales (wet crackling noises) are a sign of fluid in the lungs. Rales are often heard in patients with pneumonia.

❋ Rhonchi are coarse rattling or snoring sounds, indicative of inflammation or secretions in the bronchial tubes.

❋ Stridor is a high-pitched wheezing sound indicating narrowed airway passages. Stridor is typically heard during inhalation and exhalation.

While the presence of abnormal breath sounds alone may not be sufficient to form a clinical impression, they do serve as valuable clues when combined with other symptoms. Sports emergency care personnel should note respiratory rate and quality, and reassess every 5 minutes.

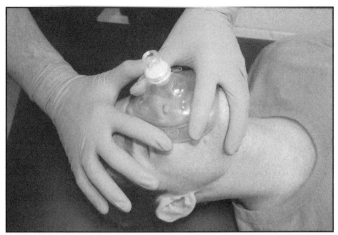

Figure 4-9. CPR mask.

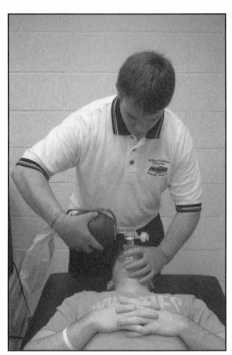

Figure 4-10. Bag-valve mask.

BREATHING SUPPORT

The primary assessment begins with assessing circulation, airway, and breathing.[1] If breathing is absent, or if breathing and pulse are both absent, rescue breathing or CPR will be required. Rescue breathing or CPR should be administered per the most recent CPR guidelines and should be delivered using either a CPR mask (Figure 4-9) or a bag-valve mask (Figure 4-10).

If breathing is present, the rate, quality, and equality of breathing should be assessed. Patients whose respiratory rate is less than 8 breaths per minute may need supplemental ventilation. Patients whose respiratory rate is greater than 20 breaths per minute may need assistance in regaining control of breathing. This can be accomplished by reassuring the victim, instructing him or her in deep diaphragmatic breathing, and breathing in through the nose and out through the mouth. Breathing into a paper bag is not recommended because it can decrease oxygen levels and lead to hypoxia. Additional support for breathing includes placing the patient in a position of comfort

---

Table 4-2
MANAGEMENT OF BREATHING EMERGENCIES

- Assess CAB. If breathing and/or pulse is absent, begin rescue breathing or CPR.
- If breathing is present, assess rate, quality, and equality.
- Place the patient in a comfortable position.
- Obtain a SAMPLE history.
- Assist with metered dose inhaler if indicated and permitted by local protocol.
- Provide supplemental oxygen if trained.
- Reassess breathing every 5 minutes.
- Be prepared to provide rescue breathing.

---

and loosening any restrictive clothing. Patients who are experiencing difficulty breathing may feel most comfortable in the tripod position (seated forward with elbows on knees). The sports emergency care provider should continue to perform a detailed physical examination, as well as obtain a SAMPLE history (signs/symptoms, allergies, medications, past medical history, last oral intake, events leading to the injury/illness; refer to Chapter 3 for details). If the patient has a prescription for medication to assist breathing (such as for asthma), assist him or her in administering the medication if local protocol allows (Table 4-2).

OXYGEN ADMINISTRATION

The use of oxygen in emergency situations can be beneficial because it increases the concentration of oxygen inhaled and aids in the prevention and management of hypoxia and shock. For emergency medical technicians and paramedics, the use of supplemental oxygen is standard practice for treatment of suddenly ill or injured victims. However, while the use of oxygen is a skill routinely performed by EMS professionals, there has been some debate as to whether athletic trainers can administer oxygen. Athletic trainers can, in fact, administer oxygen in emergency situations.

The Food and Drug Administration classifies oxygen as a drug, and as such containers used to store oxygen (the oxygen tank) are subject to specific regulations.[2] Oxygen equipment is divided into 2 categories: therapeutic oxygen and emergency oxygen (Figure 4-11). In both categories, the gas is the same; it is the method of delivery that differs.

Therapeutic oxygen systems such as those commonly found in hospitals and ambulances may only be operated by allied health and medical personnel licensed to do so and only if authorized by a prescription from a licensed physician. Therapeutic oxygen delivery systems must include a container suitable for holding medical grade oxygen, a pressure-reducing system (often called a *regulator*), a contents indicator such as a gauge, and some means of delivering oxygen to the patient such as through the use of a mask or cannula. Therapeutic oxygen delivery systems are able to deliver oxygen at a flow rate of less than 6 liters per minute (LPM) and last less than 15 minutes.

Like therapeutic oxygen delivery systems, emergency oxygen delivery systems include a container, pressure-reducing system, gauge, and a patient delivery system (mask). However, there are 2 main differences between emergency and therapeutic oxygen systems (Table 4-3). Emergency oxygen delivery systems must be capable of delivering oxygen at a minimum flow rate of 6 LPM for at least 15 minutes. Furthermore, emergency oxygen delivery systems are available over the

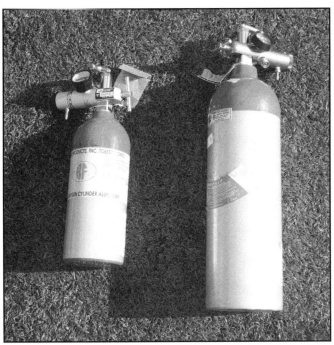

Figure 4-11. Oxygen delivery systems.

Table 4-3	
DIFFERENCES BETWEEN THERAPEUTIC AND EMERGENCY OXYGEN SYSTEMS	
Therapeutic Oxygen	*Emergency Oxygen*
Has a container holding medical grade oxygen Has a pressure-reducing system Has a contents indicator (gauge) Uses a mask or other means to deliver oxygen	
Able to deliver oxygen at a flow rate of <6 LPM or lasts <15 minutes	Delivers oxygen at a flow rate of at least 6 LPM for at least 15 minutes
Delivers oxygen via an adjustable flow regulator	Delivers oxygen at a fixed flow rate
Prescription required for use	Available over the counter without prescription

counter and may be obtained without prescription. Anyone who has received proper training in the use of emergency oxygen—including athletic trainers—may use it when providing emergency care to an ill or injured person.

CONCLUSION

Establishing and maintaining a patent airway should always be the primary concern when treating a suddenly ill or injured athlete. Regardless of the nature of the injury or illness, the lack of a patent airway can lead to respiratory compromise, respiratory arrest, and even death. Sports emergency care personnel should be proficient in airway management and the use of airway adjuncts, as well as possess the ability to recognize and treat breathing emergencies.

SUMMARY OF KEY POINTS

➡ All members of the sports emergency care team should be trained and maintain current certification in health care provider-level CPR.

➡ Assessing and establishing a patent airway is the first priority in any emergency.

➡ If a victim requires ventilation, the use of airway adjuncts or advanced airway devices can aid in ensuring a patent airway during resuscitation.

➡ Oropharyngeal and nasopharyngeal airways are both effective means of maintaining a patent airway in victims who are unconscious.

➡ Advanced airway devices are more reliable means of airway management and are often used by prehospital care personnel in the field. The use of these devices may be restricted depending on state or local regulations.

➡ Sports emergency care providers should follow local protocol before considering the use of advanced airway devices for sports emergencies.

➡ Suction devices should be readily available for use.

➡ When assessing for the presence of breathing, rescuers look for chest rise and listen and feel for breathing. Assessment of respiratory rate and quality should be assessed as well.

➡ Absent, diminished, or abnormal breath sounds, such as rales, rhonchi, or stridor, may indicate respiratory compromise.

➡ Patients whose respiratory rate is less than 8 breaths per minute may need supplemental ventilation. Patients whose respiratory rate is greater than 20 breaths per minute may need assistance in regaining control of breathing.

➡ The use of oxygen in emergency situations can be beneficial because it increases the concentration of oxygen inhaled and aids in the prevention and management of hypoxia and shock. Anyone who has received proper training in the use of emergency oxygen—including athletic trainers—may use it when providing emergency care to an ill or injured person.

REVIEW QUESTIONS

1. What are the major advantages/disadvantages of oropharyngeal and nasoparyngeal airways?
2. Name the 3 common abnormal breath sounds and what the presence of each sound indicates.
3. Are athletic trainers permitted to administer emergency oxygen? Explain your answer.
4. Name the 3 types of suction devices commonly used in emergency care.
5. In what situations might a patient require supplemental ventilation?

REFERENCES

1. Field JM, Hazinski MF, Sayre MR, et al. Part 1: executive summary: 2010 American Heart Association Guidelines for Cardiopulmonary Resuscitation and Emergency Cardiovascular Care. *Circulation.* 2010;122:S640-S656.
2. U.S. Department of Health and Human Services, Food and Drug Administration. *Review guidelines for oxygen generators and oxygen equipment for emergency use.* http://www.fda.gov/downloads/MedicalDevices/ DeviceRegulationandGuidance/GuidanceDocuments/UCM081735.pdf. Accessed June 1, 2011.

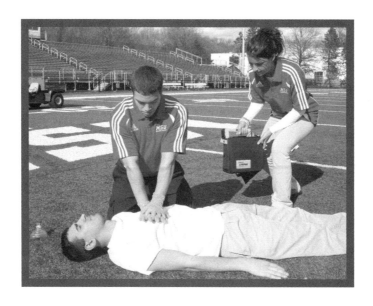

Author's Note: While Chapter 5 covers important aspects of airway and breathing management, it does not address car-diopulmonary resuscitation (CPR), and is not intended to serve as a substitute for training in CPR. All members of the sports emergency care team should maintain current certification in CPR and emergency cardiac care from a recognized authority, such as the American Heart Association, American Red Cross, or National Safety Council.

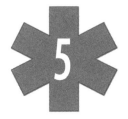

Cardiovascular Emergencies

Robb S. Rehberg, PhD, ATC, CSCS, NREMT

> *While covering a track meet, you witness one of your team's*
> *best distance runners suddenly slow down and stop running during her event.*
> *As you approach her, she takes a few steps off of the track and collapses.*
> *When you reach the athlete, you realize that she has no pulse.*

Of all the possible injuries and illnesses with which sports emergency care personnel are faced, cardiovascular emergencies can be the most challenging. Prompt recognition of signs and symptoms of cardiovascular emergencies followed by rapid intervention can mean the difference between life and death. While most athletes are generally healthy and do not fit the profile of individuals at risk for cardiovascular disease and related conditions such as heart attack and stroke, they are not immune to these types of conditions. Moreover, other cardiovascular conditions such as underlying congenital heart defects, trauma, and other cardiovascular disorders do occur in sports.

Sports emergency care personnel must anticipate cardiovascular emergencies and be prepared to quickly manage these conditions. All sports emergency care personnel should be trained in cardiopulmonary resuscitation (CPR) for health care professionals and be proficient in resuscitative skills.

REVIEW OF CLINICALLY RELEVANT ANATOMY

The heart is the central organ in the cardiovascular system. It is positioned centrally in the thoracic cavity. It lies obliquely between the lungs. One-third of the heart is posterior to the sternum; the remainder lies to the left of the sternum.

The heart is a muscular organ composed of 4 chambers and is enclosed by the pericardium. The upper chambers are the 2 atria; the lower chambers are the 2 ventricles. The atria are separated by a partition called the interatrial septum. The ventricles are separated by the interventricular

Rehberg RS.
Sports Emergency Care: A Team Approach,
Second Edition (pp 51-57).
© 2013 SLACK Incorporated.

Table 5-1
COMMON CAUSES OF CHEST PAIN

Cardiac	*Noncardiac*
Myocardial infarction	Gastroesophageal reflux disease
Angina	Esophagitis
Hypertrophic cardiomyopathy	Esophageal spasm
Aortic stenosis	Ulcers
Cardiac tamponade	Asthma
Cardiac contusion	Gastritis
Coronary artery disorders	Pneumothorax
Valve disorders	Pulmonary embolism
Aortic dissection	Pleuritis
	Bronchitis
	Costochondral injury
	Rib fracture
	Herpes zoster

septum. There are 4 valves in the heart to ensure proper flow of blood through the 4 chambers of the heart and connecting great vessels. The blood supply to the heart muscle itself is supplied by the coronary arteries.

The flow of blood through the heart starts in the right atrium. The right atrium receives deoxygenated blood from the superior vena cava, the inferior vena cava, and the coronary sinus. From the right atrium, blood flows through the tricuspid valve, into the right ventricle. The right ventricle pumps blood into the right and left pulmonary arteries, which carries blood to the lungs, where it is oxygenated. Blood returns to the heart via the pulmonary veins, which empty into the left atrium. From the left atrium, blood flows through the mitral valve into the left ventricle. The left ventricle pumps blood out of the heart through the aortic valve into the ascending aorta. The ascending aorta becomes the arch of the aorta, then the thoracic aorta, and then the abdominal aorta. These vessels supply blood to the rest of the body.

ASSESSMENT OF CHEST PAIN

Sports emergency care personnel must pay particular attention to the athlete who presents with chest pain or chest discomfort. While chest pain is often considered a cardinal sign of a cardiac-related event, chest pain can present as a result of several factors, some cardiac related and others of noncardiac origin. Any athlete who presents with chest pain, regardless of age or fitness level, should be assessed thoroughly to rule out a cardiac-related illness. Additionally, while chest "pain" is the most common descriptor of the sensation in the chest as a result of a cardiac-related event, some patients experiencing a cardiac-related event may use other descriptors such as discomfort, pressure, ache, burning, or fullness rather than pain.[1] Therefore, sports emergency care personnel should treat chest discomfort that is unrelated to trauma as a cardiac-related event until proven otherwise. Noncardiac-related chest pain can often be explained due to obvious injury, mechanism of injury, or recent illness. Other causes may be more difficult to determine. Table 5-1 lists examples of cardiac- versus noncardiac-related chest pain.

SUDDEN CARDIAC ARREST IN SPORTS

Sudden cardiac arrest (SCA), also known as *sudden cardiac death*, is defined as the sudden, abrupt loss of heart function in a person who may or may not have diagnosed heart disease.[2] It is the leading cause of death in young athletes.[3] Loss of heart function can occur as a result of many factors, both atraumatic, including hypertrophic cardiomyopathy and other congenital heart abnormalities, and traumatic, as in the case of commotio cordis.

HYPERTROPHIC CARDIOMYOPATHY

Hypertrophic cardiomyopathy is the leading cause of sudden cardiac death among young athletes. According to a study by Maron et al,[3] hypertrophic cardiomyopathy and cases suspected to be hypertrophic cardiomyopathy account for nearly half of all cases of sudden cardiac death. Hypertrophic cardiomyopathy is a congenital heart defect characterized by an abnormal enlargement or thickening of the left ventricular wall of the heart in the absence of a cardiac or systemic condition that produces left ventricular hypertrophy. It is estimated that hypertrophic cardiomyopathy affects 1 in 500 people.[4] Many athletes with hypertrophic cardiomyopathy are often asymptomatic, with the first presenting sign being SCA. Therefore, sports emergency care personnel must be prepared to provide resuscitation at any time. Some athletes may present with cardiac-related symptoms on exertion, such as chest discomfort, shortness of breath, and syncope, so it is important that sports emergency care personnel conduct a thorough assessment on any athlete presenting with signs and symptoms that may be of cardiac origin.

COMMOTIO CORDIS

Commotio cordis, sometimes referred to as a concussion of the heart is defined as a sudden cardiac death that occurs as a result of a blow to the chest, caused when a blow to the chest occurs during the vulnerable repolarization phase of the cardiac electrical cycle (15 to 30 milliseconds prior to the T wave on an electrocardiogram).[5] Commotio cordis occurs most often in children, due to chest wall pliability. Although the occurrence of sudden cardiac death due to commotio cordis is relatively low, researchers speculate that this cause of death may be underreported.

Commotio cordis can be caused by a direct blow to the chest by an object such as a baseball or hockey puck, or a direct blow to the chest by an opponent through physical contact, as in martial arts. When commotio cordis occurs, the athlete usually collapses within seconds of the strike, although a brief moment of continued activity may be observed prior to the collapse. The athlete will present as unresponsive, apneic, and pulseless. The survival rate for victims of commotio cordis is approximately 15%.[6] Victims of commotio cordis have the best chance of survival when CPR and defibrillation are administered immediately.

MANAGEMENT OF SUDDEN CARDIAC ARREST

In August 2006, the National Athletic Trainers' Association convened an Inter-Association Task Force for Emergency Preparedness and Management of Sudden Cardiac Arrest in High School and College Athletic Programs. This multidisciplinary group consisted of representatives from 15 national professional organizations. The task force recommends the following steps be taken for the management of SCA[7,8]:

* Management begins with appropriate emergency preparedness, CPR, and automated external defibrillator (AED) training for all likely first responders and access to early defibrillation.
* Essential components of SCA management include early activation of emergency medical services (EMS), early CPR, early defibrillation, and rapid transition to advanced cardiac life support.

* High suspicion of SCA should be maintained for any collapsed and unresponsive athlete.

* SCA in athletes can be mistaken for other causes of collapse. Rescuers should be trained to recognize SCA in athletes with special focus on potential barriers to recognizing SCA, including inaccurate rescuer assessment of pulse or respirations, occasional or agonal gasping, and myoclonic or seizure-like activity.

* Young athletes who collapse shortly after being struck in the chest by a firm projectile or by contact with another player should be suspected of having SCA from commotio cordis.

* Any collapsed and unresponsive athlete should be managed as a SCA with application of an AED as soon as possible for rhythm analysis and defibrillation, if indicated.

* CPR should be provided while waiting for an AED.

* Interruptions in chest compressions should be minimized and CPR stopped only for rhythm analysis and shock.

* CPR should be resumed immediately after the first shock, beginning with chest compressions, with repeat rhythm analysis following 2 minutes or 5 cycles of CPR, or until advanced life support providers take over or the victim starts to move.

* Rapid access to the SCA victim should be facilitated for EMS personnel.

OTHER COMMON CARDIOVASCULAR EMERGENCIES

MYOCARDIAL INFARCTION

Myocardial infarction, otherwise known as a *heart attack*, can occur in any athletic setting. Although athletic trainers often work with athletes in generally good health, sports emergency care personnel must be prepared to manage myocardial infarction in athletes, coaches, officials, and others. Myocardial infarction occurs when there is a decrease in oxygenated blood flow to the heart muscle due to a blockage of a coronary artery. Signs and symptoms of myocardial infarction may be overt, with classic chest pain and associated signs and symptoms including profuse sweating (diaphoresis), difficulty breathing, respiratory difficulty, nausea, and dizziness. Pain may also radiate to the neck, jaw, arms (the left arm is more common), and back. Some patients may not complain of pain but of pressure or ache; thus, it is important for the sports emergency care personnel to perform a thorough assessment.

Sports emergency care personnel should manage an individual experiencing signs and symptoms of myocardial infarction by performing a thorough assessment, placing the victim in a position of comfort (usually in a reclining position), and loosening any restrictive clothing. High-flow oxygen should be administered if available, and EMS should be activated immediately. Sports emergency care personnel should continuously monitor vital signs and be prepared to provide resuscitation or defibrillation if the victim's condition deteriorates to cardiac arrest.

ANGINA PECTORIS

Angina pectoris is a transient chest pain that results when the heart's demand for oxygenated blood exceeds supply from the coronary arteries. This decrease in oxygenated blood supply is usually caused by coronary artery spasm. Signs and symptoms of angina pectoris are similar to that of myocardial infarction. The main difference in the sports setting is that most athletes who present with angina pectoris will have already been diagnosed with the condition. Patients diagnosed with angina pectoris are often prescribed nitroglycerin to be used when symptoms occur. If permitted by local protocol and properly trained, sports emergency care personnel should assist patients in the administration of their prescribed nitroglycerin medication as directed. If symptoms do not resolve with medication or if symptoms become worse, provide similar care for that of a patient presenting with a myocardial infarction.

STROKE

Incidence of stroke is rare in sports. Stroke (also known as *cerebrovascular accident*) is defined as a decrease in oxygenated blood flow to the brain. Stroke is commonly classified by the cause of the decrease in oxygenated blood. Ischemic stroke, the most common form, occurs when an artery carrying blood to the brain is blocked. Causes of blockage include a narrowing of the arteries (atherosclerosis) and a blood clot (thrombus or embolus). Hemorrhagic stroke occurs when an artery carrying blood to the brain ruptures, either due to traumatic injury or as a result of an aneurysm that has ruptured.

Signs and symptoms of stroke include sudden numbness; decrease or loss of function of the face, arm, or leg, usually affecting only one side of the body; sudden severe headache; vision disturbances; unequal pupils; loss of balance or coordination; mental confusion; difficulty speaking or swallowing; and loss of bowel and bladder control.

Sports emergency care personnel should provide immediate care for the stroke patient by protecting the airway, assessing vital signs, performing a detailed history and physical exam, and administering high-flow oxygen, if trained. Patients exhibiting signs and symptoms of stroke should be transported by EMS to the nearest hospital immediately. Recent advances in the treatment of ischemic stroke can often provide the patient with a favorable prognosis if treatment is initiated immediately.

CARDIAC TAMPONADE

Cardiac tamponade is a compression of the heart caused by a collection of blood or fluid in the pericardial sac. The pericardial sac is an inelastic membrane that surrounds the heart. If blood collects rapidly between the heart and pericardium from a cardiac injury, the ventricles are compressed. It is most often associated with penetrating chest trauma and is rare in sports. Cardiac tamponade can be fatal if not recognized and treated immediately. Even a small amount of pericardial blood may compromise cardiac function. As the compression of the ventricles increases, the heart is less able to refill and cardiac output decreases.

Clinical presentation of cardiac tamponade includes signs and symptoms of shock, as well as hypotension, jugular vein distention, and muffled heart sounds. Muffled heart sounds may be difficult to hear at some sports venues due to the noise level. The athlete may have a paradoxical pulse. If the athlete loses his or her peripheral pulse during inspiration, this is suggestive of a paradoxical pulse and the presence of cardiac tamponade. The major differential diagnosis in the field is tension pneumothorax. However, unlike a pneumothorax, the patient with cardiac tamponade will present with a midline trachea (as opposed to tracheal deviation) and equal breath sounds unless there is an associated pneumothorax or hemothorax.

TRAUMATIC AORTIC RUPTURE

Traumatic aortic rupture is a very rare injury in sports and is most common in motor vehicle accidents and falls from great heights. The vast majority of patients die immediately. For those who survive, fast proper diagnosis is essential because emergency surgery is necessary for survival. Traumatic thoracic aortic tears are usually due to deceleration injury with the heart and aortic arch moving suddenly anteriorly, transecting the aorta. In the patients who do not exsanguinate quickly, the surrounding tissue may temporarily contain the aortic tear and limit bleeding.

The diagnosis of a contained thoracic aortic laceration is extremely difficult, especially in the field. Sports emergency care providers should consider mechanism of injury since victims of aortic lacerations often show no outward signs of chest trauma. In rare cases, the athlete may present with upper extremity hypertension and diminished pulses in the lower extremity.

MYOCARDIAL CONTUSION

Myocardial contusion is a potentially life-threatening injury that can occur in contact sports from a blunt trauma chest injury. Blunt injury to the anterior chest is transmitted via the sternum to the heart, which lies immediately posterior. Cardiac injuries from this mechanism may also include valve rupture, pericardial tamponade, or cardiac rupture. Due to the position of the heart, contusions to the right atrium and right ventricle occur more commonly than those to the left atrium and left ventricle. A victim with a myocardial contusion will present with similar signs and symptoms as in an acute myocardial infarction, including chest pain, dysrhythmia, or cardiogenic shock. In the field, cardiogenic shock may not be distinguishable from cardiac tamponade. Chest pain may be difficult to differentiate from the associated musculoskeletal discomfort (sternal contusion or rib contusion/fracture) that the athlete may suffer as a result of the injury.

CARDIAC ARRHYTHMIAS

Abnormal heart electrophysiology can produce arrhythmias (abnormal heart rhythms) that have the potential to cause cardiovascular emergencies. They can reduce cardiac output, impairing perfusion of the myocardium or the brain and causing myocardial infarction or a syncopal or near-syncopal episode. Cardiac arrhythmias can sometimes be detected during preparticipation physical examination; however, they are often detected only after signs and symptoms of a cardiac event have occurred.

There are many types of arrhythmias and treatment plans will vary, as will clearance for level of physical activity. While arrhythmias among young athletes are usually benign, they raise concern due to the heightened awareness of sudden death that has been attributed to cardiac conditions. Many common arrhythmias such as Wolff-Parkinson-White and Long QT syndromes may not be symptomatic. When symptomatic, signs and symptoms of a cardiac arrhythmia may include palpitations, syncope, near syncope, dizziness, fatigue, or sudden death.

MYOCARDITIS

Myocarditis is an inflammation of the myocardium caused by infection. Common signs and symptoms of myocarditis can include cough, shortness of breath, and chest pain, all of which intensify with exercise. Athletes with myocarditis will likely exhibit flu-like symptoms, including body ache, joint pain, headache, sore throat, fever, and diarrhea. Myocarditis may be difficult to detect in the field due to the accompanying flu-like symptoms. Athletes with myocarditis risk developing a fatal arrhythmia upon exertion, further reinforcing the need for careful medical evaluation for any athlete exhibiting possible signs of cardiac nature.

SYNCOPE

Syncope is a loss of consciousness, usually caused by a decrease of oxygenated blood to the brain. This condition can be benign, such as syncope due to emotional distress or orthostatic hypotension. However, syncope can also be an indicator of cardiac insufficiency. Sports emergency care personnel should conduct a thorough assessment on any athlete who loses consciousness and consider all possible causes. Additional information on syncope is included in Chapter 7.

VALVE AND BLOOD VESSEL DISORDERS

Other conditions related to valve defects such as aortic stenosis, aortic regurgitation, mitral valve stenosis, and mitral valve regurgitation have the potential to produce a cardiac event upon exertion. Additionally, blood vessel disorders such as aortic aneurysm and aortic dissection can cause SCA upon exertion. These conditions may be difficult, if not impossible, to detect in the field unless revealed by the patient while obtaining medical history.

CONCLUSION

There are many cardiovascular conditions that affect athletes. Some conditions are benign and do not pose a threat while participating in physical activity. Others can be fatal if untreated or undetected. Still other traumatic events can cause sudden cardiac death in athletes. While there can be many causes of chest pain and sudden cardiac death in athletes, sports emergency care personnel must take great care in recognizing potential cardiac-related events and must be prepared to provide resuscitative efforts at any time.

SUMMARY OF KEY POINTS

➡ Any athlete who presents with chest pain, regardless of age or fitness level, should be assessed thoroughly to rule out a cardiac-related illness.

➡ Although "pain" is the most common descriptor of the sensation in the chest as a result of a cardiac-related event, some patients experiencing a cardiac-related event may use other descriptors such as discomfort, pressure, ache, burning, or fullness rather than pain.

➡ SCA is the leading cause of death in young athletes and can occur as a result of both atraumatic and traumatic pathology.

➡ Management of cardiac emergencies begins with appropriate emergency preparedness, CPR and AED training for all likely first responders, and access to early defibrillation.

➡ Although athletic trainers often work with athletes in generally good health, sports emergency care personnel must be prepared to manage conditions such as myocardial infarction, stroke, arrhythmias, and other cardiac conditions in athletes, coaches, officials, or others.

REVIEW QUESTIONS

1. Why is hypertrophic cardiomyopathy a major concern in sports?
2. Explain what happens to the heart when a patient experiences commotio cordis.
3. Describe the differences between myocardial infarction and angina pectoris.
4. How could a case of syncope be related to a cardiac event?
5. Name 2 cardiac arrhythmias that can cause a cardiac emergency in sports.

REFERENCES

1. Bahr RD, Christenson RH, Farin H, Hand F, Long JM. Prodromal symptoms of acute myocardial infarction: overview of evidence. *Md Med*. 2001;Spring(suppl):49-59.
2. American Heart Association. About cardiac arrest. http://www.heart.org/HEARTORG/Conditions/More/CardiacArrest/About-Cardiac-Arrest_UCM_307905_Article.jsp. Accessed September 29, 2012.
3. Maron BJ, Shirani J, Poliac LC, Mathenge R, Roberts WC, Mueller FO. Sudden death in young competitive athletes: clinical, demographic, and pathological profiles. *JAMA*. 1996;276(3):199-204.
4. Maron BJ. Hypertrophic cardiomyopathy: a systematic review. *JAMA*. 2002;287:1308-1320.
5. Link MS, Wang PJ, Pandian NG, et al. An experimental model of sudden death due to low energy chest-wall impact. *N Engl J Med*. 1998;338:180-181.
6. Maron BJ, Gohman TE, Kyle SB, Estes NA, Link MS. Clinical profile and spectrum of commotio cordis. *JAMA*. 2002;287:1142-1146.
7. Courson RW, Drezner J. Consensus statement: inter-association task force recommendations on emergency preparedness and management of sudden cardiac arrest in high school and college athletic programs. http://www.nata.org/sites/default/files/preventingsuddendeath-consensusstatement.pdf. Accessed September 29, 2012.
8. Casa DJ, Guskiewicz KM, Anderson SA, et al. National Athletic Trainers' Association position statement: preventing sudden death in sports. *J Athl Train*. 2012;47(1):96-118.

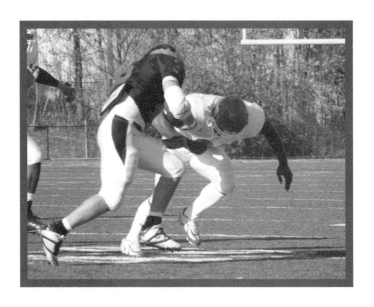

Management of Spinal Injuries

Robb S. Rehberg, PhD, ATC, CSCS, NREMT

> *During the kickoff of first game of the season, the kick returner catches the ball and begins running. He breaks free of a few tackles, and looks as if he could go all the way. With only one player to beat, he lowers his head and tries to run straight through him. Both players fall to the ground; however, only one gets up. The kick returner lies face-down on the ground and is not moving.*
> *What do you do?*

There is no way for anyone who has not experienced a medical emergency first hand to express the range of emotions that will be experienced when one is confronted with a critically injured athlete. In a single instant, an athlete is transformed from a competitive participant into a critically injured person—a critically injured person who is someone's child. It is at this instant that a sports health care professional will first see ultimate fear in an injured person's eyes and will feel this ultimate fear in the hearts of the injured athlete's family, friends, and teammates. It is at this moment that a sports emergency care professional realizes that only preparation, practice, and mental rehearsal can mean the difference between a living or dying person, between walking away from a serious injury or living a life with a devastating disability. It is only at this exact moment that a sports health care professional will truly come to realize what it means to be responsible for the care and management of athletic injuries and how vital it is to be able to rely on psychomotor skills and an emergency action plan (EAP) that have been practiced so frequently that they have become second nature.

This chapter is a pragmatic discussion regarding the emergency management objectives and psychomotor skills that every sports emergency care team must be able to demonstrate during the care and management of the athlete with a potential cervical spine injury (CSI). Injuries to the thoracic and lumbar spine also occur in athletics and require use of proper spine injury precautions during management. However, the focus of this chapter will be on injuries involving the cervical spine as they are the most prevalent and devastating spinal injuries in athletics. Additionally, this chapter will provide a brief overview of mechanisms of injury and neurophysiology as a basis for

Rehberg RS.
Sports Emergency Care: A Team Approach,
Second Edition (pp 59-92).
© 2013 SLACK Incorporated.

understanding the practical discussion regarding acute assessment of an athlete with a CSI. Also addressed will be the proper transfer of an athlete with a potential CSI to a rigid immobilization device and proper preparation of the immobilized athlete for transport to an appropriate medical facility. Finally, emergency department management, including initial radiographic assessment of the potentially spine-injured athlete, will also be discussed.

Spinal injuries can result from participation in any sport. However, this chapter's emphasis is on equipment-intensive sports such as football, lacrosse, and hockey due to the unique challenges that this protective equipment presents to sports emergency care team members during injury management. Regardless of the sport and type of protective equipment in use, the single most effective strategy for successful injury management begins with a sound EAP based on a sports emergency care team approach.

In 2009, the National Athletic Trainers' Association (NATA)[1] published its position statement on acute management of the cervical spine-injured athlete. This statement offers recommendations in all areas of acute management of CSIs, including prevention, planning and rehearsal, assessment, stabilization, airway management, and transfer and immobilization. Additional recommendations for management of equipment-laden athletes is also included. These recommendations serve as the basis for the information provided in this chapter.

MECHANISM OF INJURY

When caring for an athlete with a potential CSI, the foremost sign or symptom that warrants a conservative on-field assessment by the effective sports emergency care team is the mechanism of injury. Consideration of the mechanism of injury is an important first step in the on-field assessment of any athletic injury; however, perhaps in no other injury situation is initial determination of the mechanism of injury as vital as in the care of an athlete with a potential CSI. Failure to identify the mechanism of injury associated with a CSI could lead to major disability or death resulting from improper acute care. An athlete having suffered a significant CSI may not immediately present with the obvious neurological signs and symptoms so often associated with CSI, though more subtle signs and symptoms of underlying spinal trauma will be present. Therefore, the mechanism of injury alone indicates the need to carefully assess an athlete with a potential CSI for the presence of the obvious and more subtle signs and symptoms in order to render appropriate acute care for the athlete. The axial loading mechanism of injury is the most widely publicized mechanism of CSI in athletics.[2]

AXIAL LOADING

The axial loading mechanism of injury accounts for between 8 and 13 catastrophic CSIs annually in football.[3] The most disturbing aspect of CSI resulting from axial loading is that they are often avoidable. Too frequently, these injuries are brought about by a conscious effort to use the crown of the head as the initial point of contact or as a result of improper technique. Equally disturbing is that some are still inclined to present these injuries as freak accidents.[4,5] The physics of axial loading and its relationship to CSI is well documented. There is no such thing as a "freak" CSI. Athletes who place themselves in CSI-associated positions run a higher risk of CSI and paralysis. Covering these injuries with the freak-accident blanket only minimizes the importance of coaching and using proper technique.[6] The freak-accident blanket also allows others to play under the false pretense that these injuries are totally random occurrences. Sports health care professionals must understand axial loading in order to be able to recognize it on-field and to be able to clearly demonstrate to others that, in the majority of cases, intentional or unintentional head-down contact results in CSI in football.[7]

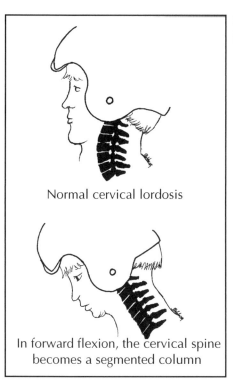

Figure 6-1. Axial loading. (Illustration by Joelle Rehberg, DO.)

Normal cervical lordosis

In forward flexion, the cervical spine becomes a segmented column

The cervical spine possesses a natural lordotic curve when erect. When in a head-down position the normal lordotic curve of the cervical spine is lost, resulting in a straight segmented vertebral column (Figure 6-1). The normal cervical lordotic curve is vital in helping the surrounding soft tissue absorb and dissipate energy through deformation and bending. When in a head-down position the vertebral column is in the straight segmented position. Contact with the top of the head when the cervical spine in a straight segmented position results in kinetic energy being transferred to the vertebral column as strain energy. When strain energy exceeds the absorbing capabilities of the column, the result is failure in the form of intervertebral disk space injury, vertebral body fracture, disruption of ligamentous and other soft tissues, or posterior element fracture. The location at which vertebral failure occurs becomes the most unstable segment in the column. Further compressive force produces a large angulation or hyperflexion as a means of releasing the additional strain energy. Hyperflexion at the failed vertebral level produces dislocation of the unstable segment, resulting in major neurological damage.

The compressive load limits or energy required to produce failure of a vertebral segment are between 3340 and 4450 newtons (N). These limits are easily reached when the head is lowered and used as the initial point of contact.[8] In fact, when contact is made at the apex or anterior to the apex of the helmet while in a head-down position, the compressive load limits of the cervical vertebral column are reached within 11 milliseconds of impact. The rapidness of which the compressive load limits of the cervical vertebral column are reached has 2 major implications for injury to the cervical spine. First, at the same time that compressive load limits within the cervical vertebra are being reached, the compressive force being applied to the cervical spine is continuing to increase due to the athlete's torso continuing to accelerate forward after the head decelerated upon impact. The continued force applied by the torso results in the cervical spine being exposed to compressive forces that cause hyperflexion, resulting in dislocation of unstable vertebral segments. A second important implication, resulting from the rapidness at which compressive load limits are reached in the cervical spine, is that 11 milliseconds is not enough time for reflex mediated muscle contraction. Reflex mediated muscle contraction occurs at 60 milliseconds, which is not enough time for the musculature of the neck to provide any resistance to the hyperflexion caused by continued force from the oncoming torso.[2,9]

In 1976, the National Collegiate Athletic Association (NCAA) and the National Federation of High Schools[10] instituted rule changes regarding the use of the head as the initial point of contact (also called *spearing*) based on the understanding of the axial loading mechanism. Proper technique and adherence to the revised rules could prevent many of the CSIs in football—whether intentional or unintentional. Still, it appears that spearing is as prevalent now as it was prior to the 1976 rule changes. Sports health care professionals should be educating players, coaches, and officials that head-down contact—whether intentional or unintentional—increases the likelihood of suffering a CSI in football. Coaches should increase the time athletes spend practicing proper techniques that keep the head out of contact, while officials should strive to enforce rules regarding involvement of the head in contact. The education of athletes, prudent coaching, and rule enforcement could reduce the incidence of head-down contact, thus reducing the possibility of axial loading and catastrophic CSI in football.[7]

Although axial loading accounts for 52% of the CSIs in football, 48% result from some other mechanism of injury.[11,12] CSI occurs in sports other than football as well. To discuss only axial loading in football suggests that CSIs only occur as a result of axial loading during football season. Discussing only axial loading would also suggest that only those signs and symptoms associated with major neurological complications resulting from fracture and dislocation of cervical vertebral segments during an axial load would compose a sufficient on-field assessment. CSIs happen in all sports and result from other mechanisms of injury that may or may not present with immediate signs and symptoms associated with major neurological complications. In fact, movement of the head and neck in any plane could be a mechanism of injury, particularly when the movement is excessive or rapid in nature.[9] Therefore, the sports emergency care team must be prepared to conduct a thorough on-field assessment with CSI precautions any time a possible injury to the cervical spine involves hyperflexion, hyperextension, lateral bending, or rotation.

NEUROPHYSIOLOGY

CSI resulting in severe neurological deficit may not be associated with injury to the vertebral column. In fact, in most spinal cord injury cases, the neural tissues remain intact.[13] Within 30 to 60 minutes after trauma, an autodestructive process referred to as *spinal shock* is initiated within the spinal cord. Spinal shock is characterized by mechanical, biochemical, and hemodynamic changes that bring about an ischemic or hypoxic state within the cells of neural tissues. Once initiated, these changes facilitate one another, leading to a worsening progression that has been reported to lead to necrosis involving up to 40% of the cross-sectional gray matter area within 4 hours of insult.[14,15]

Spinal shock has profound and lasting effects on all body systems. An understanding of spinal shock and its role in determining the extent of injury is an important aspect of acute spinal cord injury care and recovery. The importance of the sports emergency care team approach to acute prehospital care is emphasized throughout this text. Considering that the effects of spinal shock can take hold in as little as 30 minutes and can lead to significant neural tissue loss within 4 hours, the sports emergency care team must operate efficiently. In most instances, assessment, immobilization, and transfer of the athlete with a potential CSI to an emergency department is not a time-consuming process. However, injured neural tissue requires very specific acute care. This care is not readily available in any hospital emergency department; therefore, it is important for the sports emergency care team to work efficiently in assessing, immobilizing, and transporting the athlete to the hospital and to include local emergency department personnel.

This arrangement will give the athlete the best chance for proper initial on-field management, timely diagnosis, and quick transfer to a neural trauma center.

SPINAL SHOCK CASCADE

Spinal shock affects the spinal cord and neural tissues in 2 stages, identified as a primary and secondary phase of injury.

The primary injury phase of spinal shock involves actual structural damage to the neural tissues.[16] This injury is due to a mechanical insult, such as a vertebral fracture, subluxation, dislocation, intervertebral disk disruption, or pressure gradient changes. Within the spinal cord the initial response to a mechanical insult is hemorrhage, vacuolation, and swelling of capillary endothelium.[15] The extent of neural tissue injury is proportional to the force associated with the mechanical insult, affecting an area referred to as the *zone of injury*. The zone of injury can increase in less than 30 minutes due to the cascading complications of spinal shock typical in the secondary injury phase.[14,16] In order to restrict the zone of injury to the area of initial mechanical insult, the sports emergency care team must be able to recognize the subtle signs and symptoms indicating the presence of spinal shock and effectively care for the acutely injured athlete during the primary injury phase. Signs and symptoms indicating the presence of spinal shock may be immediately identified by the presence of hypotension, bradycardia, and loss of reflexes.[14]

The secondary injury phase has been characterized as a pathophysiologic cascade of injury initiated shortly after the primary injury. Ischemia is the dominant component of this phase, resulting from a decrease in the autoregulatory response of neural vasculature that can result in a significant reduction in blood flow to the spinal cord within 2 hours. In addition to ischemia, the progression of edema and an autodestructive biochemical process are serious complications associated with the secondary injury phase. Edema may first be observed at the injury site during the primary injury phase, but quickly spreads during the secondary injury phase. The net result of the secondary injury phase can be an autodestructive cascade of events that result in ischemia, cell death, and permanent neurological damage.[14,16]

PREVENTION

Of course, prevention of injuries is always the best medicine, and this is especially true with spinal injuries. According to the NATA position statement,[1] prevention of CSIs in sports should include the following:

* Familiarity with sport-specific causes of and acute physiological response to CSI

* Familiarity with and enforcement of safety rules designed to prevent CSIs

* Familiarity with manufacturer's recommendations and specifications for proper fit and maintenance of protective equipment

* Education by sports emergency care providers to coaches and athletes about mechanism of CSI, the dangers of head-down contact, and safety rules designed to prevent CSIs

PREPARE

As discussed in Chapter 2, an EAP is only useful if it is rehearsed. Frequent practice with all members of the sports emergency care team must occur in order for the plan to work effectively. This is especially true in preparing for CSIs, as an actual response will often involve several members of the sports emergency care team, and require skill in working with varying types of protective equipment, airway access equipment, facemask removal tools, and spinal immobilization equipment. It is imperative that these skills are practiced together as a team. The only way to improve response to emergencies and to detect deficiencies in a plan is to identify them through practice. At a minimum, rehearsal should occur before the season begins and should incorporate as many scenarios as possible.

ACUTE MANAGEMENT

Acute on-field management can have a significant impact on the extent of secondary injury suffered by athletes with spinal injuries.[17,18] Improved equipment, better safety techniques, and a more efficient emergency medical system decrease the time required to transfer spine-injured athletes to spinal cord trauma facilities and decrease the extent of neurological deficit at admission.[19] Thus, a team approach that incorporates the best equipment, techniques, and organized personnel provides the best chance for preventing secondary injury and can significantly improve a patient's prognosis for recovery.[19] The importance of sports health care professionals working together as part of an effective sports emergency care team, with effective on-field management of an athlete with a potential CSI, is undisputed.[14,20,21]

Acute on-field management of the athlete with a potential spine injury begins with the sports emergency care team conducting an initial assessment for immediate life-threatening injuries. A primary assessment is conducted to assess the athlete's circulation, airway, breathing, severe bleeding, shock, and spinal injury (CAB Sx3). Three unique considerations must be taken into account when conducting an initial survey on an athlete with a potential CSI.

First, upon determining a mechanism of injury that could involve the cervical spine, the sports emergency care team must immediately immobilize the athlete's head and neck in a neutral position to minimize spinal motion and to provide an optimal position for airway management.[22-26] If the spine is not already in a neutral position, it should be realigned to allow for optimal positioning for airway management and to reduce the chance of secondary injury.[24,25] However, sports emergency care providers should be aware of the following contraindications for repositioning the cervical spine into a neutral position[1]:

✳ Movement of the cervical spine causes pain, neurological symptoms, muscle spasm, and airway compromise

✳ Difficulty repositioning the cervical spine

✳ Resistance encountered when attempting to reposition the cervical spine

✳ Patient expresses apprehension

Immobilization of the head and neck is accomplished by the first team member to reach the athlete. The sports health care professional immobilizing the head and neck should place his or her hands such that the palms face each other. The hands are then slid alongside the athlete's head and neck until the web space of the thumb meets the base of the neck. The arms are then positioned on the lateral aspects of the head and neck so as to prevent as much motion as possible within the head and neck complex (Figure 6-2). It is important that the team member immobilizing the head and neck rests his or her forearms on his or her thighs, keeping a straight back posture, as the immobilization of the athlete's head and neck may have to be maintained for an extended period of time. Discomfort or injury to the sports health care provider due to poor ergonomics could result in unnecessary movement of the injured athlete when forced to reposition him- or herself or transfer immobilization of the injured athlete's head and neck.

A second unique consideration for the sports emergency care team to consider when planning the care of an athlete with a potential CSI is gaining immediate control over the injury scene, particularly being able to ensure that the athlete remains still and cooperative during the assessment process.

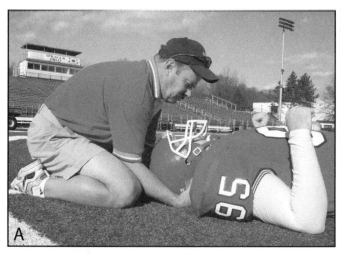

Figure 6-2. Spinal stabilization techniques.

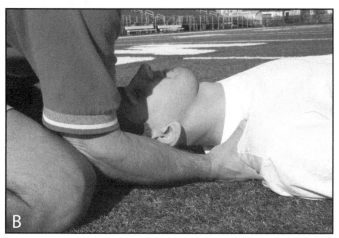

Finally, the sports emergency care team must be sensitive to subtle abnormalities when assessing an athlete's vital signs. Careful assessment and interpretation of the athlete's vital signs may provide important clues regarding the presence of spinal shock when more obvious signs and symptoms of spinal injury are not present. The following section details specific signs and symptoms of underlying spinal shock that can be observed when assessing the athlete's vital signs when conducting an initial assessment.

INITIAL ASSESSMENT

The initial injury assessment of an athlete with a potential CSI begins with an assessment of the athlete's circulation, airway, and breathing. The efficient sports emergency care team is able to render emergency care for an athlete's vital signs while taking precautions to protect the cervical spine. The following discussion will review assessment of an athlete with a potential CSI and spinal shock. Special consideration is given to athletes in protective equipment and spine injury precautions when relevant.

As discussed in Chapter 3, assessment of level of consciousness, circulation, airway, and breathing can be done simultaneously by attempting to communicate with the patient. If the patient is responsive, we know that circulation is present, as well as a patent airway and breathing. If there is no response, a quick assessment for response to verbal and painful stimulus is appropriate.

Circulation

Normal physiological function of the cardiovascular system ensures adequate blood flow throughout the body. This requires that the heart be functioning properly, an adequate amount of blood be circulating in the body, and that blood vessels are capable of properly adjusting blood flow. Disruption of neurological tissues may interrupt communications between the brainstem and sympathetic neurons. The result is failure of the cardiovascular system to maintain adequate blood flow throughout the body resulting in systemic vasodilatation and decreased cardiac function leading to vasomotor shock, postural hypotension, and edema in the lower extremities.[27] Other complications due to failure of the cardiovascular system include bradycardia, decreased myocardial contractility, hypothermia, and a predisposition to supraventricular tachycardia (SVT). Cardiac complications relating to neural damage typically arise due to 1 of 2 scenarios. One possible scenario involves immediate cardiac arrest resulting from damage at the C1 level. Management of immediate cardiac arrest would necessarily supersede specific care of the cervical spine. A second scenario involves injury to the cervical spine above the C4 level that affects the phrenic nerve, resulting in immediate or delayed decreased respiratory efforts due to loss of function of the diaphragm.

Circulation must be immediately assessed in an unresponsive patient. If circulation is not present, immediate management for cardiac arrest supersedes care for CSI. However, if the effects on the cardiovascular system are delayed, the sports emergency care team has an opportunity to assess and prepare for the possible onset of cardiac complications, possibly avoiding the onset altogether.[15] Further assessment of the cardiovascular system will be covered when assessing for shock.

Airway

The critical components of airway maintenance include immediately exposing the airway and ensuring an open and clear airway. The sports emergency care team should not rely on the conventional head-tilt chin lift technique as an initial means of opening a compromised airway because hyperextension within the cervical region associated with the head-tilt chin-lift maneuver could cause unstable vertebrae to intrude on the vertebral canal. As little as 1 mm of movement within the cervical vertebral column could increase the risk of further injury to the athlete.[20] The well-equipped and prepared sports emergency care team is prepared to avoid the head-tilt chin-lift maneuver by making use of alternative techniques such as the modified jaw thrust. The modified jaw thrust is performed by lifting the chin without tilting the head. If this technique is not successful in establishing an airway, an advanced airway should be used to avoid the dangers associated with the head-tilt chin-lift maneuver. For athletes wearing protective equipment such as a helmet, exposing the airway may require facemask removal. Facemask removal will be covered in detail when discussing breathing assessment and care.

The jaw thrust and advanced airway techniques are particularly challenging techniques to perform on an athlete in a protective helmet. Therefore, the sports emergency care team must practice these techniques on athletes in protective gear to ensure that personnel have the psychomotor skills required to perform these tasks in an emergency. Once the athlete's airway has been established, the sports emergency care team can assess the athlete's breathing status.

Breathing

During initial assessment of the athlete's breathing, the sports emergency care team will be confronted with one of the following situations: the athlete is breathing well enough on his or her own; the athlete is not breathing; or the rate and tidal volume of breathing is insufficient to support vital body function.

Breathing, or respiration, rates that are sufficient in the athlete with a potential CSI may be disrupted as a result of a somewhat likely chance that a CSI athlete will vomit. Therefore, suction should be available and immediately administered with the onset of vomiting to prevent disruption of the flow of oxygen.[28] Clearing the airway of vomit without suction will prove much more challenging, particularly following immobilization of the athlete to a rigid support.

In the absence of vomit or other foreign airway obstructions that are disrupting normal respiration, artificial ventilation should begin immediately if the athlete's respiration is ineffective or nonexistent. Insufficient respiration, or hypoventilation, is observed when the breathing rate is less than 10 or greater than 30 breaths per minute, indicating inadequate rate or volume, respectively. Insufficient respiration requires immediate care from the sports emergency care team in order to support central nervous and cardiovascular system function. Decreased respiration rates are associated with the onset of cardiac complications that will intensify a critical situation.[29,30] In addition, the spinal cord may suffer a 20% to 30% decline in oxygenation due to swelling and vascular compromise following injury.[18] The combined effect of declining oxygenation due to injury and decreased plasma oxygen concentrations resulting from insufficient respiration can significantly magnify the ischemic condition experienced by the spinal cord following injury.

If the athlete is breathing adequately, there is no immediate need to use manual or mechanical procedures to ensure the athlete is receiving ample oxygen.[30,31] However, if respiratory irregularities exist, the sports emergency care team must be prepared to act. Rendering care to an athlete with a potential CSI in protective athletic equipment may require the sports emergency care team to extract the facemask from a protective athletic football helmet. Unlike motorcycle helmets, when properly fit, football helmets can aid the sports emergency care team in maintaining immobilization of the head and neck during transfer and transport, thereby protecting the cervical spine from further injury. Additionally, extraction of the facemask from a football helmet is preferred to complete helmet removal because it is associated with significantly less extraneous movement of the head and neck. Therefore, leaving a football helmet in place while extracting the facemask to gain access to an athlete with a potential CSI's airway reduces the risk of secondary injury.[32]

The considerable attention given to facemask extraction throughout the years is testament to the necessity of possessing the psychomotor skills required to efficiently remove a facemask.[32-37] However, few sports health care professionals have an appreciation for just how difficult the task of facemask extraction really is. The sports emergency care team must undertake regular rehearsal to ensure that each member possess the psychomotor skills required to efficiently extract a facemask from an athletic helmet in an emergency. The effective sports emergency care team is able to accomplish this task in 30 to 60 seconds. When facemask extraction is required, complete extraction of the facemask from the helmet is preferred to retraction of the facemask. Complete extraction of the facemask results in less extraneous cervical spine movement compared to facemask retraction, while a retracted facemask could provide a lever through which torque could be applied to the cervical spine during the care and management process.[34] Additionally, there seems to be little time-saving benefit to retraction relative to extraction of a facemask since retraction of the facemask requires releasing the more difficult lateral facemask fasteners from the football helmet while leaving the relatively easy-to-release forehead fasteners in place. If there is any time savings of retraction versus extraction of a facemask, it is likely minimal and offset by the movement that would be applied to the injured cervical spine if contact were to be made with the retracted facemask while the sports emergency care team rendered care.

The equipment used to extract a facemask is a team decision. Advantages and disadvantages of all facemask extraction equipment must be carefully considered. The effectiveness of any facemask extraction tool is a product of time required for extraction and movement within the cervical spine during extraction.[33,34,36] There are various facemask fasteners used to secure facemasks to athletic helmets. A facemask removal tool must be evaluated by the sports emergency care team based on time and motions relative to all the various fasteners in use. Current recommendations involve using a combined tool approach[1,38-40] (ie, using a combination of one or more tools, such as cutting tool and a power screwdriver). Facemask removal techniques for the various facemask fasteners in use will be discussed later in the chapter.

Severe Bleeding, Shock, and Spinal Injury

In completing the CAB Sx3 primary assessment, the sports emergency care team should quickly assess the athlete for and control any major bleeding. Assessing and treating for shock should also be considered. An important consideration in treating any injured athlete for shock is temperature. Internal temperature regulation is dependent upon interrelations between the hypothalamus, autonomic nervous system (ANS), and the cardiovascular system. Disruption of the ANS affects the body's ability to react to changes in temperature through vasodilatation and vasoconstriction. The sweating mechanism may become disrupted leading it to react to stresses other than increasing temperature (ie, autonomic hyperreflexia).[41] In severe CSI, the diminished ability to react to increasing body temperature results in the body assuming the temperature of the surroundings (poikilothermia). Therefore, it is vital to avoid and render treatment for extreme temperatures. Characteristically, low body temperature presents with chills, chattering teeth, blue lips, goose bumps, and/or pale skin.[30]

Cardiovascular function should be assessed when treating for shock, and can be readily assessed by the sports emergency care team through conscientious monitoring of the injured athlete's pulse and respiration that provide clues as to the status of blood pressure and the overall status of the cardiovascular system. Normal resting pulse rate for adults ranges from 80 to 100 beats per minute. It should be noted that a trained athlete may have a significantly lower resting heart rate. Conversely, an athlete participating in physical activity may have a higher than normal heart rate that should begin to normalize shortly after cessation of activity. The presence of a strong, rapid pulse is to be expected in athletes during competition. A better indication of problems related to pulse and blood pressure is a delay in normalization. Normal systolic blood pressure for a 15- to 20-year-old male is 115 to 120 mm Hg. Normal diastolic pressure ranges from 75 to 80 mm Hg. The average pressure for a female in the same age range is generally 8 to 10 mm Hg lower than that of males.

In general, determination of a carotid pulse indicates a systolic pressure above 60 mm Hg. The presence of the femoral pulse indicates a systolic pressure of between 70 and 80 mm Hg. If the radial pulse is present, the systolic pressure is at least above 90 mm Hg, indicating a minimal blood pressure is present. A conscientious check of the athlete's nail beds and extremity temperature can also be used to grossly assess tissue perfusion, possibly indicating cardiovascular system failure. Although absence of the carotid pulse determines the need for cardiopulmonary resuscitation (CPR) or defibrillation, a weak or absent radial pulse, bradycardia, or perfusion abnormalities are significant indicators of hypotension and oncoming cardiac complications due to failure of the cardiovascular system.[23]

A radial pulse check provides the sports emergency care team with an immediate initial assessment of cardiovascular function that is vital to making primary assessment and care decisions for the spine-injured athlete. Hypotension leads to decreased cord perfusion and consequent worsening of deficit.[21] If proper cardiovascular function is not maintained, hypotension may facilitate the progression of spinal shock. As a result of decreased oxygen delivery to the neural tissues, even a complete lesion may be worsened by allowing associated necrosis to progress throughout the neural tissues.

When assessing and monitoring an athlete's vital signs, it is important for the sports emergency care team to realize that the measures discussed here are for the normal person at rest. An athlete's vital signs may vary from norms due to such factors as cardiovascular conditioning, body size, and physical exertion. Cardiovascular conditioning, body size, and exertion are factors that must be taken into account when determining if any variations from vital sign norms actually indicate bradycardia, hypoventilation, or cardiac complication that requires immediate care.

The last S, spinal injury, is the focus of this chapter. A simple gross motor and sensory test to determine any loss of strength or sensation should be used. Though upper and lower neurological screens are an effective means of determining the lesion site and involved neural tissue, this information is quite often much more than is needed to determine the immediate course of care. The most important aspect of this stage of care is the informed decision to transport and to ensure that no further injury results from the process. There are a number of signs and symptoms that are indicative of the need for conservative measures that will be greater influences on the decision to immobilize and transfer the athlete than the neurological screen. Unconsciousness and other general signs and symptoms may indicate the need for immobilization and transfer prior to the more involved neurological screening. Still, the upper and lower neurological screens are assessment skills the sports health care professional must possess in order to safely rule out neurological involvement during potential CSI situations that are not immediately recognizable.

Other injuries such as burners and stingers present with similar neurological presentations. The sports health care professional must be able to distinguish between other injuries involving neurological presentations. If spinal cord injury cannot be definitively ruled out, the athlete must be immobilized and transported. Some of the distinguishing characteristics that can be used to help determine whether an injury involves the cervical spine will be discussed later.

THE RULE OF 100

As previously stated, a conscientious primary assessment of an athlete with a possible spinal injury can yield vital clues that may indicate presence of significant injury in the absence of the more obvious gross neurological signs and symptoms most often associated with a spinal injury. An effective means of analyzing the information gathered during the acute initial assessment with regard to spinal shock is comparing the initial measure to the Rule of 100 associated with vital signs trending.

When any of these initial measures fall outside of the Rule of 100, action may be warranted. The Rule of 100 can be very helpful in determining possible cardiopulmonary conditions that can be subtle indicators of the underlying presence of spinal shock. According to the Rule of 100, if the pulse or temperature is less than 100 or the systolic blood pressure is greater than 100, significant injury is less likely; assuming there are no other indicators of significant injury.

Early in the primary assessment, indications of possible spinal injury will become evident, as will any need for CPR or defibrillation. Care for the spinal cord during administration of CPR and/or cardiac defibrillation is not the primary objective in light of respiratory or cardiac emergencies. However, sports emergency care team members must possess the skills necessary to protect the spine from further injury while caring for immediate medical emergencies. In athletics, caring for immediate life-threatening injuries in addition to spinal injuries may involve management of protective athletic equipment, including protective shoulder pads, athletic helmets, facemasks, and other protective equipment.

With proper preparation, most immediate life-threatening conditions identified during the primary assessment can be managed with little interference from protective athletic equipment. It has been demonstrated that proper airway evaluation, establishment, maintenance, and rescue breathing can be administered by removing the facemask from protective athletic helmets, while leaving the helmet and shoulder pads in place.[20,32,42,43] Cutting away of the athlete's jersey, shoulder pad strings, and any underclothing is sufficient for effective cardiac monitoring as long as the skin is dry.[30] It has also been demonstrated that CPR can be effectively administered with the shoulder pads in place by spreading the pads apart wide enough to expose the chest.[32] Incorporation of these techniques allows the majority of emergent situations to be effectively cared for while leaving the athlete's equipment in place, thus, protecting the spine from further injury due to excessive and unnecessary movement. All sports emergency care team members should possess the skills to effectively perform the techniques required for effective equipment management.

Complete equipment removal in order to expose the athlete for further assessment is unnecessary in caring for the spine-injured athlete. If the athlete complains of chest pain or shortness of breath, the chest must be exposed to allow for evaluation of lung sounds and cardiac monitoring. These evaluations can be accomplished without complete removal of the equipment. When exposing large portions of the body, steps must be taken to protect the athlete from hypothermia. This is especially true in cases of spinal cord injury when the body's thermoregulatory systems may be impaired.

As outlined previously, exposure of the chest can be accomplished by cutting away the jersey, the strings and straps securing the pads in place, and any clothing worn under the pads. The shoulder pads can then be carefully spread apart to allow further evaluation. When spreading the shoulder pads, be aware of the system used to secure the pads posteriorly. In some systems, spreading the anterior plates of more rigid pads may cause a bunching together of the straps or plates that may result in discomfort or undesired movement.

EQUIPMENT REMOVAL ON THE FIELD

For the athlete with protective football or hockey equipment, the combination of properly fitted shoulder pads and helmet serve the athlete and the sports emergency care team well in maintaining immobilization and axial alignment during transfer to a rigid immobilization system. Therefore, it is suggested that this equipment be left in place whenever possible, with the facemask removed for airway access.[32,44] However, if equipment does not fit properly (ie, the helmet is too loose), is partially dislodged, or if the facemask cannot be removed in a reasonable amount of time, the equipment may need to be removed. Equipment removal should be considered an all-or-nothing proposition; that is, if the helmet is removed, the shoulder pads should also be removed.

Lacrosse helmets can pose a unique challenge when managing CSIs. A properly fitted lacrosse helmet can provide immobilization; however, leaving the helmet in place may not provide neutral alignment of the spine, and facemask removal may be difficult on some models. As a result, lacrosse helmets may need to be removed in the field.

Every situation involving a potential CSI in an athlete wearing protective equipment is unique, and sports emergency care providers should be trained in removal of protective equipment in the field if the situation requires such action.

TRANSFER AND IMMOBILIZATION

Once EMS has been activated, the sports emergency care team must begin preparing the athlete for transport to a regional trauma center. This process is initiated with the transfer of the athlete to a rigid immobilization support such as a spine board. Prior to transfer to a rigid immobilization support, cervical spine immobilization in athletes not wearing protective football equipment should be completed by applying a rigid cervical collar.

Transfer of the spine-injured athlete is a technique that has received much attention. The most common technique for repositioning of the athlete is the log-roll.[45] However, 6-plus-person lift and lift-and-slide techniques have been shown to produce less head and cervical spine movement when transferring an injured athlete to a rigid support as compared to the log-roll.[46,47] Different situations may dictate the use of different techniques, and sports emergency care providers should be familiar and experienced in each technique.

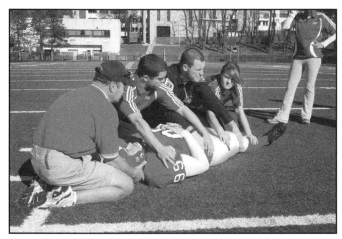

Figure 6-3. Log-roll procedure.

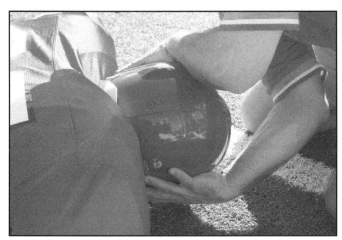

Figure 6-4. Hand position for log-roll maneuver.

LOG-ROLL TECHNIQUE

When using the log-roll technique, the team must pay particular attention to lumbar and thoracic as well as cervical movements that have been associated with this technique. This is especially true in the presence of protective sporting equipment. Team members who will roll the athlete should position themselves on the side to which the athlete will be rolled, and should overlap arms so as to minimize uneven movement during the log-roll maneuver (Figure 6-3). The team member responsible for stabilization of the head and neck during the log-roll maneuver should serve as the "captain" of the team and provide clear instructions on when to begin the log-roll. The team member stabilizing the head and neck can help ensure a smooth transition of the head and neck from the prone position to the supine by reversing his or her hands on the athlete's helmet prior to rolling the athlete (Figure 6-4). Also, if this individual assumes a position at the head of the immobilization device (where the athlete will end up when the log-roll is completed) while reaching with his or her arms and hands to stabilize (much like the position a baseball catcher uses to reach for a low and outside pitch), a much smoother transition will ensue. Prior to the log-roll, be sure the team is positioned such that the athlete is not log-rolled over the facemask. Log-rolling over the facemask will force the neck into extension.

During a log-roll, the sports emergency care team must be conscious of, and prepared to manage, a 1- to 2-inch space between the back of an athlete's head or helmet and the ground or rigid immobilization device following log-rolling an athlete to the supine position, even when

Figure 6-5. A towel can be used to fill the gap beneath the helmet and the ground.

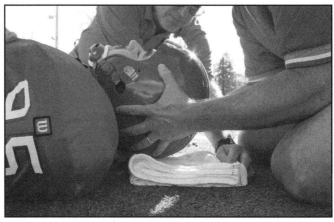

both the helmet and shoulder pads have been left in place. Failure to anticipate and account for the gap between the back of the athlete's head and the ground or rigid support will result in dangerous extension of the neck.[48] A simple solution is to pack and fill all voids using towels that can be folded and placed under the head or helmet as the athlete is log-rolled (Figure 6-5). Certain commercial rigid support devices that are equipped with padding may also be considered. Traditional backboards have been widely used to immobilize potential spinal cord injuries without much change in size since the 1960s; more recent models, which are longer, wider, and able to accommodate heavier patients, are also available. Vacuum mattresses are another type of rigid support device which can provide full-body immobilization. When combined with other immobilization devices, which may include straps, cervical collars, and head immobilization devices, the backboard is the standard rigid immobilization device most commonly used today.[46,49-51]

6-Plus-Person Lift Technique

The 6-plus-person lift technique is performed using 6 people (Figure 6-6). During the 6-plus-person lift, all rescuers should be positioned on their knees. One rescuer maintains manual, inline stabilization of the head, while 2 rescuers are positioned on either side of the patient's upper torso, placing one hand beneath the patient's shoulder and the other hand beneath the torso. Two rescuers are positioned at the hips and pelvis, placing one hand above and one below the pelvis. Finally, 2 rescuers are positioned at the knees and lower extremities, placing hands beneath the legs. The team member responsible for supporting the head directs the other team members to raise the injured athlete off the ground. As soon as the athlete is lifted off the ground, another rescuer slides the spine board beneath the athlete. Once the spine board is in place, the team member responsible for supporting the head instructs the team to gently bring the patient into place on a rigid support device.

Both the 6-plus-person lift and log-roll techniques can be effective means of transferring a spine-injured athlete to a rigid support device.[44,45] The sports emergency care team should evaluate both of these techniques for adoption into its protocol for transferring an athlete with a potential CSI to a rigid support. Regardless of the method employed, the sports emergency care team must make a conscious decision to rehearse transfer techniques regularly to ensure that the technique employed minimizes the chance for unwanted movement of the athlete. When reviewing the log-roll and slide methods for transferring an injured athlete, the sports emergency care team must also consider the rigid support that will be used to transfer the athlete. Regular-sized backboards may be too small for larger athletes. Oversized backboards, or sports boards, may be more appropriate for larger athletes, but may not fit in all ambulances and are too large for many medevac helicopters (Figure 6-7).

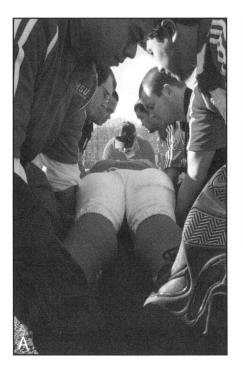

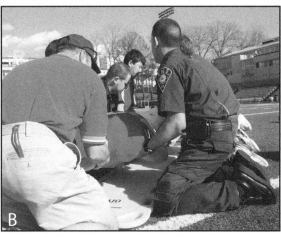

Figure 6-6. 6-plus-person technique.

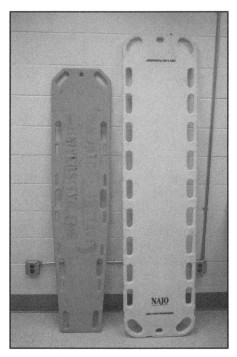

Figure 6-7. Backboards are available in different sizes.

Once the athlete is transferred to a rigid support device, stabilization of the head and neck is accomplished via the application of appropriate cervical immobilization devices and, in some instances, continued manual stabilization (Figure 6-8). Application of a cervical collar is not required when immobilizing an athlete in football shoulder pads and a protective helmet. In fact, the use of cervical immobilization collars may be contraindicated all together during immobilization of

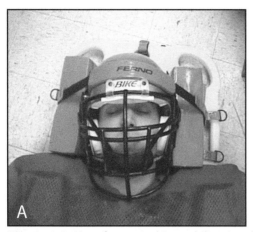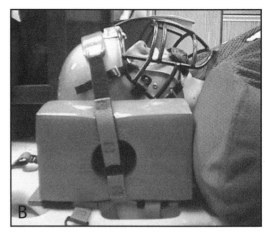

Figure 6-8. Use of a cervical immobilization device.

the injured football or hockey player. Since cervical immobilization collars are not designed for use with protective athletic equipment, the application of these collars results in significant and unnecessary movement of adjacent cervical vertebrae.[52] Additionally, the hands should be secured together using tape or a cravat.

In order to further reduce the risk of unnecessary movement, 2 precautionary measures should be taken prior to transferring and securing the athlete to a rigid immobilization device. First, regardless of the athlete's present condition, the facemask should be removed from the athlete's helmet upon determining the need to transport the athlete, and prior to transferring the athlete to a rigid support. Second, after the athlete has been transferred, the shoulder pads should be prepared. Shoulder pads are prepared by first cutting the athlete's jersey to expose the shoulder pads. Next, cut the shoulder pad lateral elastic straps followed by the breast plate laces (or breast plate) and any undergarments. Cutting the elastic straps prior to cutting the breast plate laces may reduce unwanted movement caused by the elastic straps pulling the breast plate apart when strings holding the breast plate together are cut. These measures will facilitate any emergency procedures that might be required should the athlete's condition worsen during transport by providing EMS with adequate access to the athlete without the movement and time associated with complete equipment removal.

FACEMASK REMOVAL

Removal of the athlete's facemask as a precautionary measure prior to transport significantly eases the work of EMS should breathing emergency arise during transport, by providing immediate airway access while avoiding the time delays and extraneous movement. With continual practice and rehearsal, the facemask of any helmet can quickly and safely be removed with minimal risk of extraneous movement of the cervical spine. Thus, it is suggested that the facemask be removed as a precautionary measure in every potential CSI.

The following section will cover several facemask fastening systems and hardware found on football helmets available at the time of this publication. As advancements in helmet technology continue, new and different types of fastening systems and hardware may become available. It is important for sports emergency care providers to be aware of the types of fastening systems and hardware they may encounter, and be proficient in their removal.

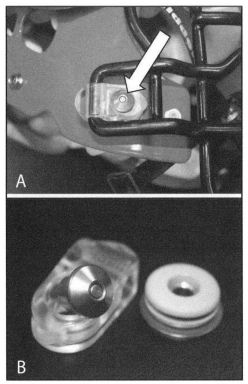

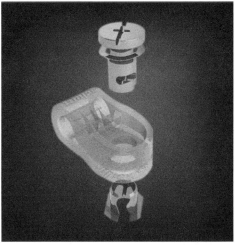

Figure 6-10. Schutt's Quarter Turn Release system.

Figure 6-9. Riddell's Quick Release system.

FACEMASK FASTENING SYSTEMS

Today there are several different facemask fastening systems that are used to secure facemasks to football helmets, including the standard loop strap, Shockblocker (Maxpro, Marietta, OH), Stabilizer (Innovative Co, Cleveland, OH), and Revolution (Riddell/Easton-Bell Sports, Van Nuys, CA). The various facemask fasteners presently in use are all widely available and all but the Revolution are easily retrofitted to any football helmet. Sports emergency care professionals responsible for the care of critically injured football players must be prepared to efficiently remove each of these facemask fasteners during care for an injured athlete. Although fasteners securing facemasks to lacrosse, hockey, and softball helmets may be similar to those securing facemasks to football helmets, the strength of the argument for facemask removal rather than protective helmet removal has yet to be determined for these protective athletic helmets.

FACEMASK HARDWARE

Advances in hardware that secures loop straps to the helmet have made the process of removing the facemask easier. Many helmets now come equipped with stainless steel screws and T-nuts, which help prevent rusting and allow easier removal when using a screwdriver. In addition, hardware such as Riddell's Quick Release (QR) system (Easton-Bell Sports) and Schutt's Quarter Turn Release (QTR) system (Schutt Sports, Litchfield, IL) make the task of removing the facemask even faster. The QR system hardware releases by pushing a springloaded pin (Figure 6-9), while the QTR system releases with a quarter turn of the screw using a screwdriver (Figure 6-10).

Figure 6-11. Chinstrap system looped through face-mask.

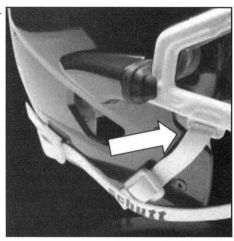

Figure 6-12. Xenith X1 helmet. Chinstrap is attached to bonnet system.

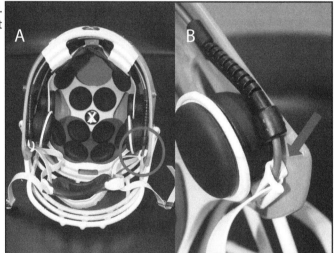

CHINSTRAPS

Another hardware feature that must be considered is the chinstrap. Some newer helmets have integrated systems in which the chinstrap is attached to more than one helmet component. For instance, in some helmets, such as the Schutt Ion (Figure 6-11), the chinstrap is looped through the facemask. When removing the facemask from a helmet that has a chinstrap looped through the facemask, the chinstraps must be cut prior to facemask removal. Other helmets, such as Xenith X1 ([Figure 6-12] Lowell, MA), integrate the chinstrap into the bonnet system. This type of system will not prevent facemask removal; however, prior to helmet removal, the chinstraps must be cut.

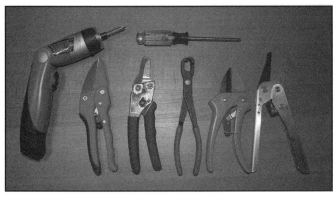

Figure 6-13. Facemask removal tools.

FACEMASK REMOVAL TOOLS

Historically, sports emergency care professionals have relied on power screwdrivers and cutting tools, such as the FMxtractor (Sports Medicine Concepts, Livonia, NY), anvil pruner, Trainer's Angel (Riverside, CA), and modified PVC pipe cutter (Figure 6-13), to remove the loop strap fasteners securing facemasks to protective athletic helmets. With the advances in fastening hardware, the use of a cordless screwdriver should be considered a primary means of facemask removal, as research has demonstrated greater efficiency and less movement of the head and cervical spine using a cordless screwdriver as opposed to other methods.[31,37,53] Rescuers who use a cordless screwdriver as a facemask removal tool should ensure that the battery is fully charged. As stated previously, a combined tool approach is recommended, and sports emergency care providers should carry (and be prepared to use) different tools for facemask removal.

The following section details specific techniques that sports emergency care team members may consider when evaluating different cutting tools and practicing facemask removal procedure.[54] It is difficult to fully demonstrate the various techniques used to cut through various facemask fasteners within the confines of a textbook. Therefore, it is strongly suggested that sports emergency care personnel acquire proper hands-on training in emergency facemask removal for a more thorough review of facemask removal techniques.

Loop Strap Fasteners

The forehead fasteners of every football helmet are similar, using a standard loop strap fastener consisting of a fixed screw end and a loop portion (Figure 6-14). The Revolution helmet uses slightly smaller versions of the standard loop strap fastener to secure the facemask to the forehead of the helmet. To release the forehead loop strap fasteners, position the cutting blade and opposing buttress of the cutting tool as depicted in Figure 6-15A. This will result in the fixed-screw portion of the loop strap remaining fixed to the helmet shell while the loop portion of the fastener remains on the facemask bar (Figure 6-15B). If the ends of the cutting device are not resting firmly against the helmet shell, the bottom portion of the loop strap is not likely to be completely transected, resulting in an inability to release the facemask bar from the loop strap.

Another option for cutting the loop strap when grip strength is an issue is to complete an initial cut as described previously, but cutting though only the top portion of the loop strap. Then, position the buttress of the cutting tool to make a second cut as depicted in Figure 6-16. This technique will release an area of plastic from the loop strap fastener sufficient to allow the facemask bar to be removed (Figure 6-17).

Figure 6-14. Standard loop strap face-mask fastener with screw and T-nut. (© Sports Medicine Concepts. Reproduced with permission.)

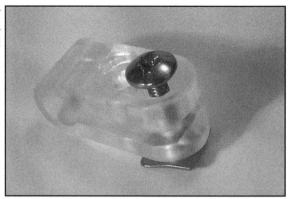

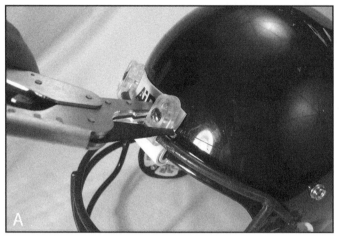

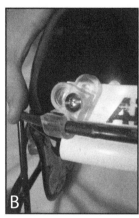

Figure 6-15. Technique for cutting standard forehead facemask fasteners results in the fastener being completely transected at its midsection. (© Sports Medicine Concepts. Reproduced with permission.)

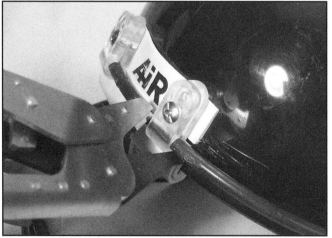

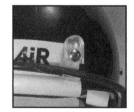

Figure 6-17. Standard side loop strap facemask fasteners after being cut using alternate method. (© Sports Medicine Concepts. Reproduced with permission.)

Figure 6-16. Second technique for cutting forehead standard loop strap facemask fasteners may require less grip strength to complete. (© Sports Medicine Concepts. Reproduced with permission.)

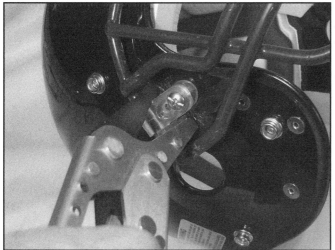

Figure 6-18. Technique for cutting standard loop strap facemask fasteners on the sides of football helmets. (© Sports Medicine Concepts. Reproduced with permission.)

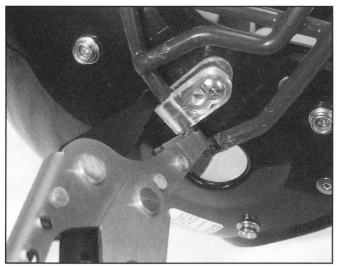

Figure 6-19. Second technique for cutting standard loop strap facemask fasteners on the sides of football helmets. (© Sports Medicine Concepts. Reproduced with permission.)

Loop strap fasteners along the sides of football helmet pose a significant challenge to emergent facemask removal. To facilitate removal of loop strap fasteners along the sides of the helmet, first observe how the loop strap is positioned relative to the facemask bars. If there is enough clearance between adjacent facemask bars and the loop strap, place the cutting tool over the loop strap fastener (Figure 6-18). If the approach detailed in Figure 6-18 does not successfully release the facemask bar from the loop strap after the first attempt, try repositioning the cutting device by placing the buttress of the cutting tool on the facemask bar as depicted in Figure 6-19. The result will be a gap in the loop strap that is wide enough for the facemask bar to be pulled out through.

If there is not ample room to position the cutting tool over the loop strap fastener within the confines of adjacent facemask bars, place the buttress of the cutting tool on the facemask bar at one side of the loop strap with the cutting blade positioned at the opposite side as depicted in Figure 6-19. Approximate the ends of the cutting tool to cut through the top half of the loop strap. Finally, leaving the buttress on the facemask bar, reposition the cutting blade parallel to the opposite side of the facemask bar and, again, cut the top half of the loop strap (see Figure 6-19). The result will be a gap in the loop strap that is wide enough for the facemask bar to be pulled out through.

Figure 6-20. A third technique for cutting standard side loop strap fasteners on football helmets. (© Sports Medicine Concepts. Reproduced with permission.)

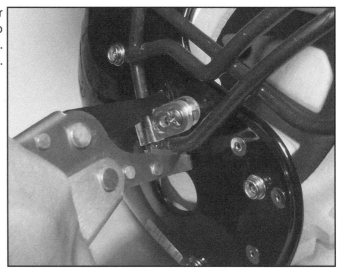

Figure 6-21. Shockblocker facemask fastener with screw and T-nut. (© Sports Medicine Concepts. Reproduced with permission.)

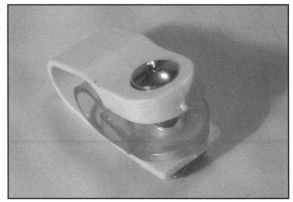

If the loop strap fastener is positioned off-center relative to adjacent facemask bars, it may be possible to rest the buttress of the cutting tool on the outside edge of the facemask bar with the cutting blade extended across the width of the loop strap fastener and resting firmly on the helmet shell (Figure 6-20). While in this position, approximate the ends of the cutting tool to transect the fastener at its midpoint. Often this technique results in a small remnant of plastic remaining uncut. To avoid the plastic remnant, end this cut by slightly rotating the approximated handles of the cutting tool around the facemask bar to allow the cutting blade to completely cut the loop strap. If the entire depth of the loop strap fastener is not completely transected, try repositioning as depicted Figure 6-19.

The same cutting options described for cutting standard loop strap fasteners can be applied to the other fastener variations. However, there are some considerations that can facilitate cutting these fasteners.

Shockblocker

The Shockblocker football helmet clip is designed with a hard outer plastic loop and a more pliable inner loop (Figure 6-21). The outer loop provides rigid support while the inner loop may provide some protection from concussion injury by absorbing some of the force from a blow to the facemask.

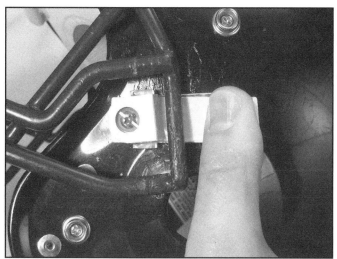

Figure 6-22. The Shockblocker may only require a single cut through both its inner and outer loops. (© Sports Medicine Concepts. Reproduced with permission.)

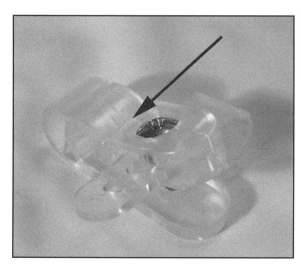

Figure 6-23. Position the cutting tool at the depression in the Stabilizer facemask fasteners. (© Sports Medicine Concepts. Reproduced with permission.)

To cut the Shockblocker, place the buttress and cutting blade over the fastener such that the top half of both the inner and outer loops can be cut simultaneously using one of the techniques outlined previously. Then simply push the inner and outer layer out of the way and pull the facemask bar out from the fastener (Figure 6-22).

Stabilizer

The Stabilizer loop straps come in thick and thin modes. Thick or thin fasteners are used depending on the circumference of the facemask bar being fixed to the football helmet shell. Stabilizer fasteners are also specifically designed for the right and left sides of the helmet. The Stabilizer fastener has a thin secondary plastic loop strap that may provide additional support and may help prevent concussion injury by absorbing some of the force due to a blow to the facemask. Look for the depression near the front of the loop portion of the fastener (Figure 6-23). This area of the Stabilizer has the least amount of plastic and may provide the least amount of resistance to cutting.

Figure 6-24. Position the cutting tool to cut the thin support loop before cutting the main body of the Stabilizer. (© Sports Medicine Concepts. Reproduced with permission.)

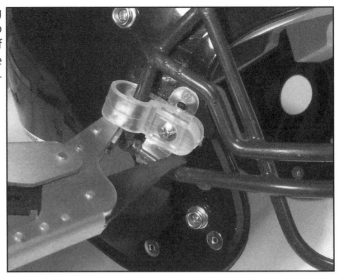

Figure 6-25. Cut the main body of the Stabilizer at the depression between the loop portion and fixed screw end. (© Sports Medicine Concepts. Reproduced with permission.)

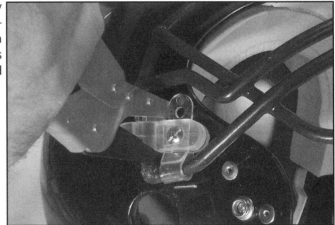

Begin cutting the Stabilizer fastener by first cutting the fastener's secondary loop strap (Figure 6-24). It is much more difficult to cut the secondary loop strap after the main body of the fastener has been cut. After cutting through the secondary loop strap, the main body of the Stabilizer can be cut by placing the buttress and blade of the cutting tool on either side of the fastener (Figures 6-25 through 6-27).

Revolution

The Revolution fastener is presently manufactured with 2 access slots to facilitate cutting the fastener. When the fastener is properly mounted on the helmet, the fore access slot is milled at approximately 12 to 15 degrees while the aft access slot is milled perpendicular to the helmet shell (Figure 6-28). According to Revolution manufacturer recommendations, the fore access slot should be cut first, followed by the aft. If your team is presently outfitted with Revolution helmets, be sure to check all helmets to ensure that the fasteners have access slots. Without access slots, facemask removal is limited to unscrewing the fastener hardware. If you find fasteners without access slots, replace the fasteners with those that do have access slots immediately.

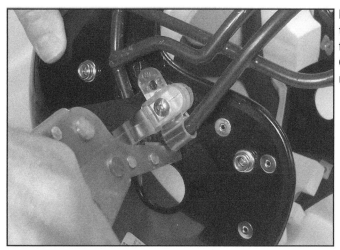

Figure 6-26. Alternate tool position to cut Stabilizer facemask fastener. (© Sports Medicine Concepts. Reproduced with permission.)

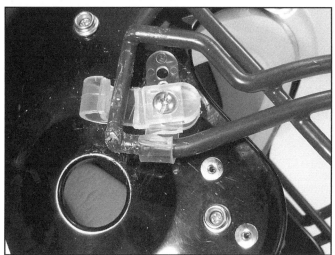

Figure 6-27. Stabilizer facemask fastener after using a 3-cut approach. This approach may require the least amount of grip strength to complete. (© Sports Medicine Concepts. Reproduced with permission.)

Many have come to prefer the screwdriver as the first option for removing the Revolution fastener (Figure 6-29). The screwdriver has been found to be a viable first option. However, due to the potential for hardware failure, a back-up cutting option is recommended.[38]

The Revolution manufacturer has specific instructions for cutting the Revolution fastener. These instructions must be followed precisely for the most effective and timely release of the fastener. To release the Revolution fastener, identify the fore access slot. Allow the cutting blade of the tool to fall into the access slot at 12 to 15 degrees, coming to rest on the helmet shell. Then, position the buttress of the cutting tool on the outside of the facemask bar (Figure 6-30). Approximate the ends of the cutting tool and ease the blade through the fastener. Reverse the position of the cutting tool and repeat the process to cut through the remaining portion of the fastener using the fore access slot (Figure 6-31). Next, repeat the process using the aft access slot. Keep in mind that the aft access slots are cut perpendicular to the helmet shell; therefore, the blade of the cutting tool should be directed straight into the access slot, not at a 12- to 15-degree angle. When initiating the cut, be sure that the blade is resting firmly against the helmet shell. Rotate the handles of the cutting tool slightly foreword after the blade contacts the facemask bar to complete the cut. When the Revolution fastener is properly fixed to the helmet and the cutting tool makes an efficient cut, each end of the Revolution fastener will fall away, exposing the facemask bars

Figure 6-28. Access slots for cutting the Revolution facemask fastener. (© Sports Medicine Concepts. Reproduced with permission.)

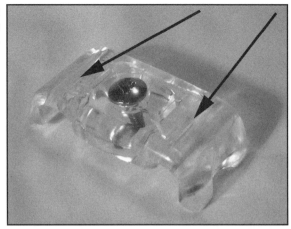

Figure 6-29. Using a screwdriver to release the Revolution facemask fastener. (© Sports Medicine Concepts. Reproduced with permission.)

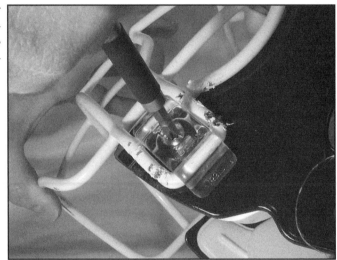

Figure 6-30. Manufacturer recommendations state to cut the fore access slots of the Revolution fastener first. (© Sports Medicine Concepts. Reproduced with permission.)

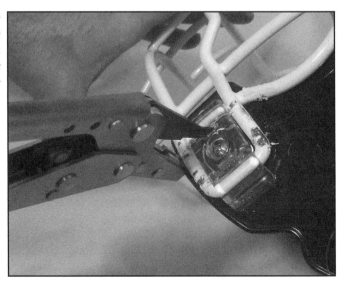

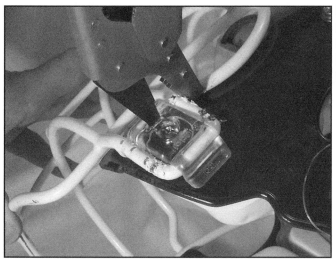

Figure 6-31. The Revolution fastener requires 4 cuts, 2 at both the fore and aft access slots. (© Sports Medicine Concepts. Reproduced with permission.)

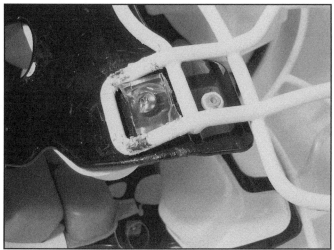

Figure 6-32. The midsection of the Revolution fastener will remain fixed to the helmet, but will permit the facemask to be lifted off the helmet. (© Sports Medicine Concepts. Reproduced with permission.)

(Figure 6-32). If the Revolution fastener remains in position after cutting, reposition the cutting tool to ensure that the fastener has been completely transected. In some cases, the Revolution fastener will remain in place even after completely transecting both ends. This is due to the pressure that the fastener is under. If this happens, simply ease the fastener off of the facemask bar. If this fails, use a screwdriver to unscrew the fastener from the helmet.

INITIAL EMERGENCY DEPARTMENT TRAUMA ASSESSMENT

Once the facemask has been removed and the shoulder pads properly prepared prior to transporting an athlete with a potential CSI, there is little chance that the helmet and shoulder pads will have to be removed from the athlete until after an initial emergency room trauma assessment has been completed.

In the absence of life-threatening conditions, initial emergency room assessment begins with a radiographic plain film trauma evaluation performed prior to removal of any equipment from the athlete. The initial emergency room radiographic film trauma series typically involves horizontal cross-table lateral (HL), anteroposterior (AP), oblique, and pillar films. Though HL films alone are not conclusive, they are generally sufficient to rule out gross instability in the cervical spine. Initial HL radiographic films provide the emergency room personnel with a general understanding of the osseous condition of the cervical vertebrae. The information provided on the HL views can be used by emergency room personnel in preparation for removing all protective equipment from the athlete in order to conduct a more thorough radiographic assessment. All protective equipment should be removed from the athlete using the spine injury precautions detailed below, regardless of what is depicted on the HL radiographic films.

Once protective equipment has been removed from the athlete, more extensive radiographic evaluation including AP and additional HL views using plain film are taken to further evaluate bony instability. Routine AP views are used to evaluate the integrity and alignment of the superior and inferior vertebral end plates, pedicles, and spinous processes of C3–C7. An open mouth AP view is necessary for evaluation of C1–C2. The open mouth AP is completed in order to observe the following:

❋ That the odontoid process is equidistant from the lateral masses of C1

❋ That C1 and C2 lateral masses are aligned

❋ The presence of a mach effect—a simulated fracture caused by C1 projecting over the dens

The additional HL views following protective equipment removal allow observation of the soft tissues, lordotic curve, disk space, posterior cortical margins of articular processes, spinolaminar lines, facets, intervertebral height, and interspinous distances of the spinous processes. Occasionally, C6–C7 and the odontoid process are obscured in the HL view by the shoulder girdle and mandible, respectively. If C6–C7 and the odontoid process are obscured, the swimmer's position may be used. To complete the initial radiographic plain film series, oblique and pillar views are completed to assess the interfacetal joints, laminae, intervertebral foramen, and lateral masses. If the athlete is unconscious or unstable, the complete radiographic plain film series may be contraindicated. If the complete initial radiographic plain film assessment is contraindicated, computed tomography (CT) may used to complete the initial trauma assessment. When indicated, CT and fluoroscopy can be used for more extensive evaluation of the vertebrae and canal while myelography may be combined with CT or magnetic resonance imaging (MRI) for evaluation of spinal cord and nerve root damage. Generally, fluoroscopy and CT are useful for specific views under direct control. CT is useful when vertebrae are superimposed or when it is necessary to observe a specific vertebral component, especially in evaluating the pedicle, lamina, cord, and canal.

Specific evaluation of the spinal cord and nerve roots requires myelography, CT, and/or MRI combined with contrast enhancement. Myelogram combined with a subarachnoid injection of contrast agent is used for observation of the subarachnoid space, cord, and nerve roots. MRI and CT following myelogram allows specific observation of the cord and canal contents.

Recent advances in CT and MRI have had important implications in the evaluation of alignment and integrity of bony structures, ligamentous stability, extradural mass effects resulting from osteophytes, herniated disks, fracture fragments and hematomas, and spinal cord status. MRI has been reported to be superior to CT for visualizing extradural mass effects and cord injury because of its sensitivity to subtle abnormalities, including syringomyelia. CT is unable to detect small areas of edema and swelling; therefore, only gross compression or altered cord contour is observable using CT. MRI has also been found to be more beneficial for analysis of disks because it is noninvasive and mulitplanar. However, MRI is limited in detecting fractures and dislocations, unless there is gross displacement and cord impingement. MRI is, generally, the modality of choice for soft tissue evaluation.[52]

Conversely, CT is especially sensitive to displacement of fracture fragments and the associated cord compromise. CT is particularly beneficial in observing the lateral mass and posterior elements that are often more difficult to read on plain radiographs due to overlap of normal structures and the patient positioning required to obtain these views. Visualization of horizontal fractures is a serious limitation of CT. CT is limited as a modality for follow-up of soft tissue injuries inferred from X-ray as well. If MRI is not available, postmyelogram CT with contrast agent is superior to normal CT for spinal canal analysis. Follow-up evaluation of fractures found on X-ray is enhanced with both the CT and MRI with the addition of a contrast agent.[54-56]

PROTECTIVE ATHLETIC EQUIPMENT REMOVAL

Regardless of the athlete's condition, sooner or later the protective equipment will need to be removed. It should be emphasized that the athlete's protective equipment should be left in place as long as possible. It is generally agreed upon that the emergency department (ED), with all the emergency equipment on hand, is preferred to the playing field when removing protective equipment from the potentially spine-injured athlete.[32,57,58] It is essential that prior planning and sports emergency care team development include educating ED staff regarding sports equipment and proper equipment removal protocol to ensure that the ED is, in fact, the safest place for removal of the athlete's protective equipment. Still, the type of protective equipment used and its specific characteristics may require on-field removal. Therefore, the efficient sports emergency care team is prepared with the proper psychomotor skills and equipment required to properly prepare an athlete for transport, including face-mask removal, preparation of the shoulder pads for proper transport, and complete equipment removal in the emergency room or on-field.

To date, research has centered on football equipment and the injured cervical spine, neglecting the unique challenges presented by protective equipment used in other sports. Hockey and lacrosse equipment, for example, are not associated with the same individual fitting guidelines associated with football.[50,59-61] Therefore, this often ill-fitting equipment may not afford the sports emergency care team the same luxuries relative to aided in-line immobilization during assessment and transfer procedures. When dealing with any type of protective equipment, the benefits of the presented equipment must be assessed by the sports emergency care team. If the protective equipment is aiding in-line stabilization and immobilization, the equipment should be left in place as long as possible. However, if the equipment is a liability during immobilization efforts, it must be removed. When left in place, an ill-fitting helmet may hamper immobilization efforts by allowing the athlete's head to move within the helmet during log-rolling or after the athlete has been immobilized on a rigid support. Ill-fitting helmets and shoulder pads only result in immobilization of the equipment, allowing dangerous movement of the athlete's body within.

Controversy surrounding removal of athletic equipment during emergency situations has centered on the criteria for removal rather than the removal technique.[62,63] With prior facemask removal and proper preparation for transport, there are few indications for complete removal of well-fitted equipment that aids in immobilization of the athlete without hindering acute management principles. However, unique situations, such as transferring an injured athlete following application of an AED, may require complete equipment removal because the equipment no longer aids in maintaining immobilization of the athlete during transfer to a rigid support. Indications for complete equipment removal are a protocol decision that must be made by individual sports emergency care teams. However, the guiding rule regarding removal of any piece of equipment should be whether or not the piece of equipment in question is assisting the team's primary objectives of maintaining the athlete's vital signs and maintaining in-line stabilization during transfer of the athlete to a rigid support. As long as the equipment does not hinder management of the sports emergency care team's primary objectives, it is best left in place in order to avoid unnecessary delays in transport and to minimize extraneous movement of the athlete.

Once again it must be emphasized that an athlete's helmet and shoulder pads should be left in place and only removed when emergently required or following initial radiographic assessment in the emergency room. With proper planning the sports emergency care team can all but eliminate any need to remove a protective helmet and shoulder pads from a potentially spine-injured athlete. This level of competency must be a primary objective of every sports emergency care team member. However, as is the case with any team approach or planning process, there are always unforeseen circumstances that are impossible to predict or plan for. Some of these might indicate complete equipment removal. Therefore, it is important that the process of complete equipment removal be reviewed and practiced. These same skills are required of emergency room personnel who must use the same CSI precaution protocols to remove protective athletic equipment following initial radiographic assessment prior to more thorough assessment.

When the decision to remove equipment has been made, the following protocol is suggested for the sports emergency care team.

* If protective helmet removal is necessary:
  - Team member A, maintaining immobilization of the head and neck, transfers stabilization of the head and neck to team member B. This is accomplished by having team member B positioning his or her hands around the athlete's neck such that his or her fingers cradle and support the cervical spine from C7 to the occiput.

  - Team member A then prepares the helmet for removal by cutting the chinstraps and removing the cheek pads. If it is possible to extract the facemask prior to removing the helmet, it becomes easier to tilt the helmet anteriorly without fear of catching the facemask on the athlete's face.

  - Team member A then gently separates the helmet at the ear holes and pulls it over the top of the athlete's head while tilting the helmet forward to clear the occiput.

  - Team member A then uses toweling to pack and fill the 1- to 2-inch gap left between the athlete's head and the ground to prevent hyperextension of the neck.

  - Team member A then retakes control of the head and neck from team member B.

* If shoulder pad removal or both helmet and shoulder pad removal is required:
  - Team member A is positioned above the head of the athlete and is responsible for maintaining stabilization at all times.

  - Team member B cuts through the jersey and chest straps, as well as the jersey sides and any clothing worn under the pads. Next, cut the laces on the front of the pads. When completed at the onset, these steps decrease the amount of time the head must be stabilized off the ground following helmet removal and prior to shoulder pad removal. It also reduces the number of times transfer of stabilization is required.

  - Team member B then cuts the chinstrap of the helmet and pops out the cheek pads.

  - Stabilization is then transferred to team member B.

  - Team member A gently separates the helmet at the ear holes and pulls it over the top of the athlete's head while tilting the helmet forward to clear the occiput.

- After removing the helmet, team member A gently pulls the pads from under the athlete and applies a cervical collar.
- Team member A then resumes stabilization of the head and neck.

SUMMARY OF KEY POINTS

➡ While this chapter emphasizes equipment-intensive sports such as football, lacrosse, and hockey due to the unique challenges that this protective equipment presents during injury management, spinal injuries can result from participation in any sport, and members of the sports emergency care team must always be prepared.

➡ Axial loading is the primary mechanism of injury in CSIs in sports.

➡ Spinal shock affects the spinal cord and neural tissues in 2 stages that can be identified as a primary and secondary phase of injury.

➡ The best method of managing spinal injuries in sports is through prevention.

➡ The initial injury assessment of an athlete with a potential CSI begins with an assessment of the athlete's circulation, airway, and breathing, followed by assessing for severe bleeding, shock, and spinal injury.

➡ Frequent practice with all members of the sports emergency care team is essential.

➡ Acute on-field management can have a significant impact on the extent of secondary injury suffered by athletes with spinal injuries.

➡ Upon determining a mechanism of injury that could involve the cervical spine, the sports emergency care team must immediately immobilize the athlete's head and neck in a neutral position to minimize spinal motion and to provide an optimal position for airway management.

➡ For the athlete with protective football or hockey equipment, the combination of properly fitted shoulder pads and helmet provide adequate immobilization. If equipment does not fit properly, is partially dislodged, or if the facemask cannot be removed in a reasonable amount of time, the equipment may need to be removed.

➡ Every situation involving a potential CSI in an athlete wearing protective equipment is unique, and sports emergency care providers should be trained in removal of protective equipment in the field if the situation requires such action.

➡ The 6-plus-person lift and lift and slide techniques have been shown to produce less head and cervical spine movement when transferring an injured athlete to a rigid support as compared to the log-roll.

➡ Removal of the athlete's facemask as a precautionary measure prior to transport significantly eases the work of EMS should breathing emergency arise during transport.

➡ There are several different fastening systems that are used to secure facemasks to football helmets, and sports emergency care professionals must be prepared to efficiently remove each of these facemask fasteners during care for a critically injured athlete.

➡ The use of a cordless screwdriver should be considered a primary means of facemask removal, as research has demonstrated greater efficiency and less movement of the head and cervical spine using a cordless screwdriver as opposed to other methods.

REVIEW QUESTIONS

1. Under what circumstances should football protective equipment be left in place when managing an athlete with a potential CSI? When should equipment be removed?
2. Explain why lacrosse helmets may need to be removed in the field.

3. Why is the "combined tool" approach the best way to manage facemask removal?
4. Describe contraindications for placing the spine in a neutral position.
5. Describe the advantages and disadvantages of the log-roll and 6-plus-person lift.

REFERENCES

1. Swartz EE, Boden BP, Courson RW et al. National Athletic Trainers' Association position statement: acute management of the cervical spine-injured athlete. *J Athl Train.* 2009;44(3):306-331.
2. Otis JC, Burnstein AH, Torg SJ. Mechanisms and pathomechanics of athletic injuries to the cervical spine. In: Torg JS, ed. *Athletic Injuries to the Head, Neck, and Face.* 2nd ed. St. Louis, MO: Mosby; 1991:438-456.
3. Boden BP, Tacchetti RL, Cantu RC, Knowles SB, Mueller FO. Catastrophic cervical spine injuries in high school and college football players. *Am J Sports Med.* 2006;34:1223-1232.
4. Associated Press. Tackle leaves Idaho State defensive back paralyzed. *Missoulian.* Sept 24, 1996:2C.
5. Bell J. Doctors: Brown got fast, effective care. *USA Today.* Dec 23, 1997:1C.
6. Torg J. *Prevention of cervical spine injuries.* Presentation at: Adam Taliaferro Foundation Medical Workshop; September 19, 2006; Voorhees, NJ.
7. Heck JF, Clarke KS, Peterson TR, Torg JS, Weis MP. National Athletic Trainers' Association position statement: head-down contact and spearing in tackle football. *J Athl Train.* 2004;39;101-111.
8. Otis JC. Biomechanics of spine injury. In: Cantu RC, ed. *Neurologic Athletic Head and Spine Injuries.* Philadelphia, PA: WB Saunders Co; 2000:6-21.
9. Swartz EE, Floyd RT, Cendoma MJ. Cervical spine functional anatomy and the biomechanics of injury due to compressive loading. *J Athl Train.* 2006;40:155-161.
10. Heck J. The incidence of spearing during a high school's 1975 and 1990 football seasons. *J Athl Train.* 1996;31(1):31-36.
11. Cantu RC, Meuller FO. Catastrophic spine injuries in football (1977-1989). *J Spinal Disord.* 1990;3:227-231.
12. Cantu RC, Meuller FO. Catastrophic football injuries: 1977-1998. *Neurosurgery.* 2000;47:673-675; discussion 675-677.
13. Christopher and Dana Reeve Foundation Paralysis Resource Center: Spinal Cord Tutorial 101. http://www.christopherreeve.org/atf/cf/%7B3d83418f-b967-4c18-8ada-adc2e5355071%7D/SCI%20Tutorial%20101.PDF. Accessed September 29, 2012.
14. Buchanan LE, Nawoczenski DA. An overview. In: Buchanan LE, Nawoczenski DA, eds. *Spinal Cord Injury: Concepts and Management Approaches.* Baltimore, MD: Williams & Wilkins; 1987:11-18.
15. Riser TV, Mudiyam R, Waters RL. Orthopedic evaluation of spinal cord injury and management of vertebral fractures. In: Adkins HV, ed. *Spinal Cord Injury.* New York, NY: Churchill Livingstone; 1985:1-36.
16. Wilberger JE. Athletic cervical spinal cord and spine injuries. In: Cantu RC, ed. *Neurologic Athletic Head and Spine Injuries.* Philadelphia, PA: WB Saunders Co; 2000:144-152.
17. Podolsky S, Baraff LJ, Simon RR, Hoffman JR, Larmon B, Ablon W. Efficacy of cervical spine immobilization methods. *J Trauma.* 1983;23:461-465.
18. Waters RL, Apple DF, Meyer PR, Cotler JM, Adkins RH. Emergency and acute management of spinal trauma. In: Stover S, DeLisa JA, Whiteneck GG, eds. *Spinal Cord Injury: Clinical Outcomes from the Model Systems.* Gathersburg, MD: Aspen; 1995:21-25.
19. Go BK, DeVivo MJ, Richards SJ. The epidemiology of spinal cord injury. In: Stover S, DeLisa JA, Whiteneck GG, eds. *Spinal Cord Injury: Clinical Outcomes from the Model Systems.* Gaithersburg, MD: Aspen; 1995:21-25.
20. Polumbo MA, Hulstyn MJ, Fadale PD, O'Brien T, Shall L. The effect of protective football equipment on alignment of the injured cervical spine. *Am J Sp Med.* 1996;24(4):446-452.
21. Vegso JJ, Torg JS. Field evaluation and management of cervical spine injuries. In: Torg JS, ed. *Athletic Injuries to the Head, Neck, and Face.* 2nd ed. St. Louis, MO: Mosby; 1991:426-437.
22. Cantu RC. The cervical spinal stenosis controversy. *Clin Sports Med.* 1998;17(1):121-126.
23. Crosby ET. Airway management in adults after cervical spine trauma. *Anesthesiology.* 2006;104(6):1293-1318.
24. De Lorenzo RA. A review of spinal immobilization techniques. *J Emerg Med.* 1996;14(5):603-613.
25. Gabbott DA, Baskett PJ. Management of the airway and ventilation during resuscitation. *Br J Anaesth.* 1997;79(2):159-171.
26. Lennarson PJ, Smith D, Todd MM, et al. Segmental cervical spine motion during orotracheal intubation of the intact and injured spine with and without external stabilization. *J Neurosurg.* 2000;92(suppl 2):201-206.
27. Gosch HH, Gooding E, Schneider RC. An experimental study of cervical spine and cord injuries. *J Trauma.* 1972;12:570.
28. Phillips BJ. Spinal cord injuries: a suggested approach. *The Internet Journal of Emergency Medicine.* 2004;2(1).DOI: 10.5580/d97.
29. American Red Cross. Injuries. In: American Red Cross, ed. *Standard First Aid.* St. Louis, MO: Mosby; 1993.

30. Feld F. Management of the critically injured football player. *J Athl Train.* 1993;28(3):206-212.

31. Ray R, Lunchies C, Bazuin D, Farrell R. Airway preparation techniques for the cervical spine-injured football player. *J Athl Train.* 1995;30(3):217-221

32. Kleiner DM, Almquist JL, Bailes J, et al. *Prehospital Care of the Spine-Injured Athlete. A Document From the Inter-Association Task Force for Appropriate Care of the Spine-Injured Athlete.* Dallas, TX: Inter-Association Task Force for the Appropriate Care of the Spine-Injured Athlete; 2001.

33. Block JJ, Kleiner DM, Knox KE. Football helmet face mask removal with various tools and straps. *J Athl Train.* 1995;31(suppl 2):11.

34. Kleiner DM. Face mask removal vs face mask retraction. *J Athl Train.* 1995;31(suppl 2):32.

35. Knox KE, Kleiner DM. EMT shears effectiveness for face mask removal. *J Athl Train.* 1995;31(suppl 2):17.

36. Rehberg RS. Rating face mask removal tools. *NATA News.* January 1995:26-27.

37. Swartz EE, Armstrong CW, Rankin JM, Rodgers B. A 3-dimentional analysis of face mask removal tools in inducing helmet movement. *J Athl Train.* 2002;37:178-184.

38. Gale SD, Decoster LC, Swartz EE. The combined tool approach for face mask removal during on-field conditions. *J Athl Train.* 2008;43(1):14-20.

39. Copeland AJ, Decoster LC, Swartz EE, Gattie ER, Gale SD. Combined tool approach is 100% successful for emergency football face mask removal. *Clin J Sport Med.* 2007;17(6):452-457.

40. Decoster LC, Shirley CP, Swartz EE. Football face-mask removal with a cordless screwdriver on helmets used for at least one season of play. *J Athl Train.* 2005;40:169-173.

41. Hanak M, Scott A. Spinal trauma. In: Hanak M, Scott A., eds. *Spinal Cord Injury: An Illustrated Guide for Health Care Professionals.* New York, NY: Springer; 1983:24-33.

42. Waninger KN. Management of the helmeted athlete with suspected cervical spine injury. *Am J Sports Med.* 2004;32:1331-1350.

43. Swartz EE, Norkus SA, Cappaert T, Decoster LC. Football equipment design affects face mask removal efficiency. *Am J Sports Med.* 2005;33:1210-1219.

44. Banerjee R, Palumbo MA, Fadale PD. Catastrophic cervical spine injuries in the collision sport athlete, part 2: principles of emergency care. *Am J Sports Med.* 2004;32:1760-1764.

45. Delbridge TR, Auble TE, Garrison HG, Menegazzi JJ. Discomfort in healthy volunteers immobilized on wooden backboards and vacuum mattress splints. *Prehospital and Disaster Med.* 1993;8(suppl 2):S63.

46. Del Rossi G, Horodyski M, Powers ME. A comparison of spine board transfer techniques and the effect of training on performance. *J Athl Train.* 2003;38:204-208.

47. Del Rossi G, Horodyski MH, Conrad BP, Di Paola CP, Di Paola MJ, Rechtine, GR. The 6-plus-person lift transfer technique compared with other methods of spine boarding. *J Athl Train.* 2008;43(1):6-13.

48. Cendoma MJ. Evaluation of various face mask removal techniques. *NATA News.* April 2006:14-18.

49. Donaldson WF, Lauerman WC, Heil B, Blanc R, Swenson T. Helmet and shoulder pad removal from a player with a suspected cervical spine injury. A cadaveric model. *Spine.* 1998;23(16):1729-1732.

50. Lovell ME, Evans JH. A comparison of spinal board and the vacuum stretcher, spinal stability and interface pressure. *Injury.* 1994;25(3):7-8.

51. Johnson DR, Hauswald M, Stockhoff CY. Comparison of a vacuum splint device to a rigid backboard for spinal immobilization. *Am J Emerg Med.* 1996;14(4):369-372.

52. Prinsen RK, Syrotuik DG, Reid DC. Position of the cervical vertebrae during helmet removal and cervical collar application in football and hockey. *Clin J Sport Med.* 1995;5(3):155-161.

53. Jenkins HL, Valovich TC, Arnold BL, Gansneder BM. Removal tools are faster and produce less force and torque on the helmet than cutting tools during face-mask retraction. *J Athl Train.* 2002;30(3):217-221.

54. Jahre C, Pavlov H, Deck MDF. Computed tomography and magnetic imaging of cervical spine trauma. In: Torg JS, ed. *Athletic Injuries to the Head, Neck, and Face.* 2nd ed. St. Louis, MO: Mosby; 1991:412-425.

55. Pavlov H. Radiographic evaluation of the cervical spine and related structures. In: Torg JS, ed. *Athletic Injuries to the Head, Neck, and Face.* 2nd ed. St. Louis, MO: Mosby; 1991:384-411.

56. Wales LP, Knopp RK, Morishima MS. Recommendations for evaluation of the acutely injured cervical spine: a radiologic algorithm. *Ann Emerg Med.* 1980;9:422-428.

57. Swenson TM, Lauerman WC, Blanc RO, Donaldson WF. Cervical spine alignment in the immobilized football player. Radiographic analysis before and after helmet removal. *Am J Sports Med.* 1997;25(2):226-230.

58. Waninger KN. On-field management of potential cervical spine injury in helmeted football players: leave the helmet on! *Clin J Sports Med.* 1998;8(2):124-129.

59. Metz CM, Kuhn JE, Greenfield ML. Cervical spine alignment in immobilized hockey players: radiographic analysis with and without helmets and shoulder pads. *Clin J Sports Med.* 1998;8(2):92-95.

60. Sherbondy PS, Hertel JN, Sebastianelli WJ. The effect of protective equipment on cervical spine alignment in collegiate lacrosse players. *Am J Sports Med.* 2006;34:1675-1679.

61. LaPrade RF, Schnetzler KA, Broxerman RJ, Wentorf F, Wendland E, Gilbert TJ. Cervical spine alignment in the immobilized ice hockey player. A computed tomographic analysis of the effects of helmet removal. *Am J Sports Med.* 2000;28:800-803.

62. Bronus S. Put me in the game, coach. *J Emerg Med Srvc.* 1993;18(2):26-37.
63. Segan RD, Cassidy C, Bentkowski J. A discussion of the issue of football helmet removal and suspected cervical spine injuries. *J Athl Train.* 1993;28(4):294-305.

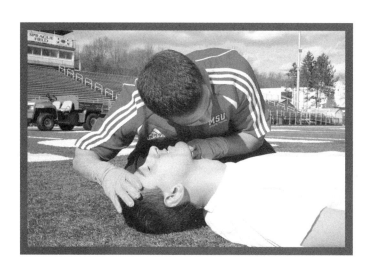

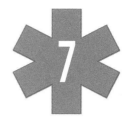

Unconsciousness and Seizures

David A. Middlemas, EdD, ATC

Scenario 1

You are providing medical coverage for a high school ice hockey game. One of your players gets the puck and begins to accelerate toward the goal in an attempt to score. He is checked hard by one of the defensemen from the other team and goes down on the ice. He slides into the boards head first and is lying on the ice motionless. You approach the athlete and begin your primary survey. The athlete does not respond to your attempts to get a response.

What do you do?

Scenario 2

You have graciously agreed to serve on the medical staff for a local triathlon. The participants in this event range in age from their early 20s to mid-60s. You are called to assist a participant who has collapsed at the halfway mark of the running portion of the event. Upon your arrival you find a woman in her late 50s or early 60s lying on the ground with some people around her. She is not responsive, but is breathing and has a pulse.

What do you do?

"Are you all right? Can you hear me?" These are 2 questions for which sports emergency care personnel always hope the answer is "yes." Changes in a person's level of consciousness can range from mild disorientation or confusion to unconsciousness. Changes in level of consciousness indicate impairment of normal brain function or brain injury in almost every instance. Emergencies in the athletic venue resulting in changes in the victim's state of consciousness can occur from injury events or changes in brain function as a result of a medical condition or disease.

Rehberg RS.
Sports Emergency Care: A Team Approach,
Second Edition (pp 95-107).
© 2013 SLACK Incorporated.

This chapter will focus on the causes of unconsciousness and seizure events. We will also learn the strategies and methods of recognizing and caring for victims of emergencies involving changes in level of consciousness and/or seizures.

THE ATHLETE IS DOWN AND DOES NOT RESPOND!

In both of the scenarios at the beginning of the chapter, the athlete has suffered an event that rendered him or her unconscious and unable to provide information that would be essential for providing the correct emergency care. When an athlete is down on the field or court and does not respond, sports emergency care personnel must identify the potential reasons the victim is unconscious in order to determine and carry out a care plan that will stabilize the victim and prevent further injury. Sports emergencies involving loss of consciousness require the emergency care provider to develop skills that allow for collecting the required information from the environment, coaches, officials, other athletes, and bystanders. Loss of consciousness can occur as a result of an injury or a crisis resulting from a medical condition. It is important to know the events leading up to the athlete becoming unconscious because they are essential in determining the course of care for this individual.

The unconscious victim presents a challenge during the process of patient assessment because he or she is not able to provide the sports emergency care team with the verbal feedback normally used to determine the extent of injury or illness. In the best of situations, sports emergency care personnel are in a position to observe the events preceding the athlete's becoming unconscious. They would be able to see any contact or collision that caused the injury or to witness the victim's collapse. Witnessing what happened provides the caregiver with information that directs the course of care, but in reality this is not always possible.

Unfortunately, in the world of youth, scholastic, and collegiate athletics, sports emergency care personnel cannot be present at all events. There are many venues in which multiple practices or contests are held in different locations simultaneously. Help may be summoned and often arrives at the scene of the emergency after the fact. Whether or not the events leading up to the athlete's becoming unconscious were observed by the emergency care provider, he or she must be skilled in evaluating the situation and taking the appropriate actions. Therefore, let's start with assessing the patient and the situation.

ASSESSMENT OF THE ATHLETE WITH LOSS OF CONSCIOUSNESS

Take a moment to look back at the 2 opening scenarios presented at the beginning of the chapter. In the hockey example, you observed the events leading up to the athlete becoming unconscious. In the triathlon example, you did not witness the collapse. In the second situation, information about the events leading up to the incident must be collected without the victim's input or the luxury of witnessing the collapse. Sports emergency care personnel should start by observing the environment in which the athlete became unconscious and the position in which the victim is found to begin piecing together what happened and the possible extent of injury or illness.

As in any other emergency, conducting a primary survey to determine the presence of life-threatening conditions and the stability of the victim is the first order of business. It is a good premise to adopt the mindset to assume the worst and hope for the best. Young athletes who become unconscious during practice or competition are often involved in some sort of contact or collision. Immediate immobilization of the spine and head is always warranted in unobserved athletic emergencies resulting in unconsciousness, even when the cause may not appear to be a result of contact. In so doing, you will always protect the victim from things that could make the condition worse while completing your assessment. Aggravation of a possible spinal fracture could result in temporary or permanent paralysis, deterioration of vital signs, loss of consciousness, or death.

Initial patient assessment should follow the CAB Sx3 format (circulation, airway, breathing, severe bleeding, shock, and spinal injury; discussed in Chapter 3). If the athlete is responsive, has blood circulating through the body, has a stable airway, and is breathing, the athletic trainer can then move on to a secondary survey. If the athlete is not responsive, preparations need to be made to provide basic life support in the event breathing and/or pulse stop.

The assessment of breathing and pulse should usually be done in the position in which the athlete is found. Athletes will often be found lying on their side or face down after a collision or incident that would cause unconsciousness during practice or a game. Evaluating the athlete without moving him or her will allow you to determine the presence of breathing and pulse without potentially aggravating possible head or neck injuries. If the athlete is unconscious leaving him or her prone or side lying, this position will provide the same protection to a patent airway as having the victim in the recovery position by allowing any fluids or vomit to readily drain. Primary assessment of unconscious victims that have not suffered collision or trauma should also be performed in the position in which the victim is found.

When the athlete does not respond or the response is so incoherent or diminished that it is obvious that he or she is in distress, emergency medical services (EMS) should be activated immediately. Because the amount of time it takes for EMS to arrive varies greatly depending on your location, athletic trainers must be prepared to continue to monitor vital signs and provide basic life support in the event breathing and/or pulse stop. Pulse rate and quality, respiration rate and quality, blood pressure, and other vital signs should be assessed and the results recorded at 5-minute intervals while waiting for EMS to arrive.

Athlete Down and Motionless

While approaching:
  Observe the athlete's position
  Observe the surroundings for potential causes or mechanisms of injury

When you reach the athlete's side:
  Check for responsiveness—the athlete does not respond!
  Stabilize the head and neck
  Activate your emergency action plan
  Call 911 or your local emergency number to activate EMS
  Complete primary survey—CAB Sx3

While waiting for EMS to arrive:
  Prevent any motion of the victim's head and neck
  Monitor the victim's vital signs at 5-minute intervals
  Monitor and treat the victim for shock
  Write the results of the assessment on a piece of tape or paper for the EMS
  personnel to take with the athlete (a bystander can help with this, if necessary)

TAKING IT TO A HIGHER LEVEL

Assessment of the athlete's responsiveness involves more than just seeing whether or not he or she responds to you. Evaluating the changes in a person's level of consciousness also involves determining the quality and coherence of that response. The role of the sports emergency care

Table 7-1
GLASGOW COMA SCALE

Total = E + V + M

Eye Opening (4)	Verbal (5)	Motor Response (6)
4 = Spontaneous	5 = Normal conversation	6 = Normal
3 = To voice	4 = Disoriented conversation	5 = Localizes to pain
2 = To pain	3 = Words, incoherent	4 = Withdraws to pain
1 = None	2 = No words, only sounds	3 = Decorticate posture
	1 = None	2 = Decerebrate
		1 = None

personnel in this situation is to assess the athlete for diminished or abnormal brain function by evaluating basic neurological functions such as dizziness, balance, vision, eye movement, memory, and the ability to speak.

A tool commonly used to assess neurological status in serious injury or illness is the Glasgow Coma Scale.[1] This easy-to-administer scale evaluates an individual's response to stimuli, the quality of verbal responses, and ability to move. The scale is broken into 3 components—eye opening response (E), verbal response (V), and motor response (M). The victim is scored in each of the 3 categories, adding the 3 scores to give a total score. Because these 3 types of activities are important indicators of quality of brain function and neurological status, the scores in each of the individual categories and the total Glasgow Coma Score are reported. The administration of the Glasgow Coma Scale and its scoring are summarized in Table 7-1. The scale can be a useful tool in assessing the severity of the condition of an athlete who is unconscious or who is experiencing an altered level of consciousness. Glasgow scores are reported in the format E + V + M = Total Score. Simply reporting the total does not provide the physician with information as to which categories had stronger or weaker performance by the patient. Reporting the score on each section and the total gives insight as to the nature of neurological deficit for the individual patient. Generally speaking, a total Glasgow score between 13 and 15 would indicate mild brain injury, 9 to 12 would indicate moderate brain injury, and a total of 8 or less would indicate significant loss of normal brain function.

Amnesia is the inability to accurately remember information. It is important to determine whether amnesia is present in individuals with head injury or significantly altered brain function by asking the victim questions to which he or she should know the answers. It is also important to remember to ask questions to which the interviewer knows the answer; otherwise it may be impossible to determine whether the athlete is answering appropriately. For example, asking the athlete questions about what he or she ate for breakfast may not be a question to which the interviewer will know the answer. Questions referring to place ("Do you know where you are?"), time ("What is the date?" "Approximately what time is it?"), person ("Can you tell me your name? Do you remember my name?"), and event ("What are you doing here? What team are you playing?") are all appropriate questions to which the interviewer and the athlete should know the answer.

There are 2 types of amnesia for which you should assess the athlete on the field. Retrograde amnesia is the inability to remember events before the time of the injury. Anterograde amnesia (sometimes referred to as *post-traumatic amnesia*) is the inability to remember events after the time of injury. When dealing with victims suffering memory loss, it is important to continue to reassess

Table 7-2	
ASSESSMENT OF MEMORY LOSS	
Retrograde Amnesia	*Anterograde Amnesia*
Ask questions about information or events occurring before the injury.	Ask questions about information or events after the injury.
What is your name? What were you doing before you got hit? Where are you? What day is it? Who am I?	Provide a list of unrelated words to remember: Light Spoon Flower Radio Dog

memory function at frequent intervals. This is done to see if there are any changes that could indicate the injury or condition is worsening with time. Worsening anterograde amnesia could be an indication of intracranial bleeding, which is an emergency. Table 7-2 gives examples of the types of questions one might ask to assess memory loss.

It is also important to perform a physical examination that is focused on evaluating the status of brain function. In addition to the things discussed previously, assessing the victim for headache, vision, pupillary response, eye movement, facial muscles, tongue motion, and ability to speak clearly provides feedback on brain function. Because these activities are controlled directly by the brain through cranial nerves, any abnormalities are very likely indications of injury or damage to the brain. Refer to Chapter 8 for additional information on assessing cranial nerve function.

Serious or critical injuries or medical emergencies affecting the brain can result in significant damage to the portions of the brain controlling motor function. Although these situations rarely occur in the athletic venue, it is important that the sports emergency care team member recognize the signs of these emergencies. When serious brain damage occurs, the victim may present in one of two abnormal positions or postures indicating significant damage to the brain. Decorticate posturing is identified by flexion of the fingers, wrists, and elbows with the forearms on the chest. The legs are extended and rotated slightly inward. Decorticate posturing indicates damage along the pathway controlling messages from the cortex of the brain to the spinal cord. Patient position occurs because the mechanisms that inhibit flexion of the upper extremities and extension of the lower extremities have been damaged. Decerebrate posturing presents with both the upper and lower extremities in extended positions. The arms will be at the patient's sides, and the neck will be arched into extension. Decerebrate posture in the unconscious patient indicates possible damage to the brainstem, which is more serious than that indicated by the decorticate posture. It is possible for a patient to go from decorticate to decerebrate over time as the patient's brain condition worsens. Both positions are presented in Figure 7-1.

The information from the patient assessment that you have recorded should be given to the paramedic or emergency medical technician (EMT) as part of the process of patient transfer. When a collision or other contact is part of the mechanism of injury or there is reason to suspect possible cervical injury, the athlete's head and spine must be immobilized while waiting for the ambulance. The methods and procedures for these situations are covered in Chapter 6.

Figure 7-1. (A) Decerebrate posturing. (B) Decorticate posturing.

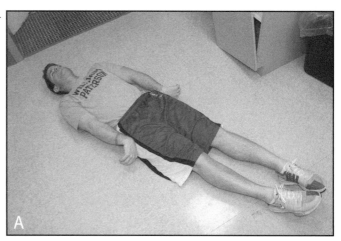

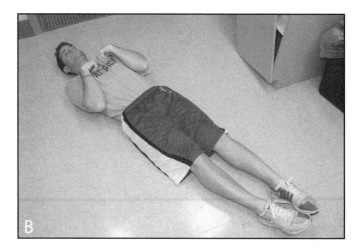

UNDERSTANDING LOSS OF CONSCIOUSNESS

An individual's level of consciousness can range from completely aware, responsive, and functional to unconscious and unresponsive—and pretty much anywhere in between. In this section, we will explain some of the common causes of unconsciousness that may be seen in the sports emergency care environment. Some of these are related to injury and some are not. Having a better understanding of the common causes of unconsciousness and types of conditions you may encounter will help you to decide what actions to take.

SYNCOPE

Sometimes an individual may pass out without any immediately obvious reason. Syncope occurs when someone becomes unconscious and recovers quickly without assistance. Common names for syncope include *fainting, passing out, collapsing,* or *blackout.* These episodes are usually accompanied by loss of voluntary muscle tone, hence, the victim stumbles or falls to the floor if standing or slumps forward in a chair if sitting.

Victims of syncope may have changes in vital signs similar to someone in shock. In addition to becoming unresponsive, the patient may present with pale skin that may be cool to the touch, rapid weak pulse, increase in breathing rate, and drop in blood pressure. For example, an individual having a syncopal episode may have pale skin, a weak pulse at the rate of 110 beats per minute, irregular breathing at the rate of 24 breaths per minute, and a blood pressure of 90/60 mm Hg. All of these symptoms are consistent with conditions in which blood flow to the brain is diminished.

By its very definition, when someone has a syncopal episode (passes out), the condition is often temporary, and the victim usually recovers on his or her own without medical assistance. It is possible that he or she may only have a partial loss of consciousness, becoming disoriented, confused, and lightheaded, temporarily losing awareness of surroundings. More benign causes of syncopal episodes include upsetting emotional events, psychogenic shock, response to illness (ie, cold or flu), or orthostatic hypotension. Syncope can also be caused by more serious conditions that cause diminished blood flow to the brain, including dehydration and cardiogenic shock.

Syncope is a common cause for emergency room visits. Syncope should be considered as a potential diagnosis in any situation where there is an unexplained fall or unexplained brief loss of consciousness, especially if the individual becomes alert and aware shortly after the incident. The return of awareness after collapse is also consistent with the return of blood flow to the brain when the patient becomes horizontal. Recovery is usually spontaneous in many cases. Emergency care for the condition involves protecting the victim from injury during the collapse and assessment for significant injury or illness. It is common for individuals to refuse EMS or medical treatment after recovering from a syncopal episode. Reasons for refusing medical care may include embarrassment, the person feeling as though he or she has returned to normal, or the possibility that this has happened before in response to emotionally traumatic events. Regardless, sports emergency care personnel should be thorough in their assessment, taking the time to rule out any serious underlying cause for the episode. Although most syncopal episodes are benign, their occurrence may be indicative of an underlying significant cardiovascular problem.

STUPOR

Stupor is defined as a decreased state of mental activity or awareness that can be associated with drowsiness or diminished response. One possible description of stupor is that it is short of unconsciousness and the patient can be awakened or will respond to stimuli. It is possible that someone who is stuporous will respond to the rescuer but will then return to his or her state of disorientation or semiconsciousness. The response may be incoherent or appear disoriented. As always, the need for emergency care directly relates to the stability of the patient's vital signs, the amount of disorientation, and the difficulty in arousing the patient. When an individual is difficult to arouse, provides incoherent responses, and/or returns to the semiconscious state after being aroused, EMS should be activated for care and transportation to an emergency room.

Stupor can occur as a result of head injury or secondary to shock. It can also be a symptom of drug or alcohol abuse, advanced heat illness, insulin shock, or hyperglycemia. It is important to determine the underlying cause of stupor in active individuals who become semiconscious or drowsy, which may also require emergency care and/or psychological intervention.

COMA

Coma is defined as a deep state of unconsciousness during which the patient does not react or respond to stimuli in the environment. Individuals who are comatose do not respond to verbal, visual, tactile, or painful stimuli. It is not unusual for someone in a coma to have a Glasgow score of E = 1, V = 1, M = 3, or a total of 5 or less. Someone who becomes comatose has suffered serious loss of brain function. Coma can often happen as a result of serious head injury or after consuming large amounts of alcohol or drugs. Coma can also occur after severe diabetic reaction or hemorrhage in the brain. Although not seen frequently in the athletic venue, the possibility of an athlete suffering deep unconsciousness after a head injury is real. In sports such as soccer, ice hockey, and rugby, in which high-force collisions occur between athletes' heads, or in high-speed events such as equestrian, motocross, or racing, athletes have the real possibility of significant head injury from collisions or falls. Extreme sports such as freestyle skateboarding and snowboarding, BMX events, and half pipe skate, bike, and snow sports have gained popularity with recreational and club participants in recent years. These activities all involve aerial stunts from which participants, even when wearing a helmet, can suffer head trauma resulting in unconsciousness. Athletic trainers and other medical personnel must be prepared to provide basic life support in the event of unconsciousness due to injury.

HEAD TRAUMA

In many athletic activities, the participants are exposed to contact and collisions leading to the possibility of head injury during the normal course of play. Sports like football, ice hockey, motor sports, lacrosse, baseball, and softball require that players wear protective helmets while participating. On the other hand, helmets are not required in many other activities in which collisions and falls occur regularly, including soccer, rugby, wrestling, gymnastics, rodeo, and recreational skiing and snowboarding. Incidents involving head injuries and unconsciousness have occurred in all of these sports.

When a victim is unconscious immediately after a fall or collision, the sports emergency care team member must assume that there is significant head injury and the high possibility of spinal injury. Immediate on-the-field spinal immobilization, assessment of vital signs, and preparation for the possibility of providing basic life support are paramount. EMS must be called immediately, and the athlete should be only removed from the playing area on a spineboard by ambulance.

Unconsciousness does not always happen immediately when an athlete suffers a head injury. There are times when the injury in the brain that results from a head injury is the result of bleeding within the skull. If the bleeding continues long enough to place enough pressure on the brain tissue within the skull, the victim's neurological status will begin to worsen. It is often the speed at which the neurological signs and symptoms change that provides the best indicator of the severity of the bleeding. (Details on intracranial injuries are presented in Chapter 8.)

MEDICAL AND SUBSTANCE-RELATED CAUSES OF UNCONSCIOUSNESS

There will be times when an athlete may present with changes in the signs and symptoms normally related to brain function that cannot be attributed to an injury event. Changes in mental function, including unconsciousness, can be can be caused by any one of many medical conditions. The sports emergency care team must be prepared for the possibility of caring for an unconscious victim when dealing with individuals from all stages of the life span. At times, the cause of the unconsciousness, such as a heart attack or fainting, may be easily recognized. Often the cause of a victim's loss of consciousness may not be obvious to the rescuer. Regardless, the role of the first responder is to provide basic life support, call EMS, and pass on the information collected about the situation to the ambulance crew for the emergency room physician's use in making an appropriate diagnosis.

Unfortunately, the world of sports is not immune to the negative effects of substance abuse that may lead to unconsciousness. The athletic trainer or other sports emergency care provider needs to be aware of the signs and symptoms that indicate the potential presence of alcohol or drugs in the victim's system. Key factors in determining the urgency of the situation include the quality of the patient's breathing, pulse, and neurological status. Observing and recording whether these signs and symptoms are stable or changing and the length of time the symptoms have been present provides the emergency room physician with vital information. Regardless of its cause, loss of consciousness is a medical emergency and EMS should be activated. The athlete should never be allowed to return to activity until cleared by a physician.

Some Things to Look for in Unconscious Victims With Undetermined Cause

Irregular breathing
Unusually enlarged or extra small pupils
Unusually slow or rapid pulse
Strange smells on victim's breath
Vomiting
Reddish face and heavy sweating
High or low body temperature
Hallucinations

You are a high school athletic trainer. Today's responsibilities include providing medical coverage for a basketball game. In the third quarter, one of the players on the visiting team stops playing, looks confused, and says something to one of his teammates. Suddenly his entire body becomes rigid, and he collapses to the floor. His teammate catches him on the way down. When you approach him, he starts to have full body convulsions.
What is happening? What do you do?

SEIZURES

Changes in a person's level of consciousness may be due to the occurrence of sudden, uncontrolled, abnormal electrical activity in the brain. This condition may present itself in different ways. Depending on where in the brain the abnormal activity takes place, the victim can have a blank stare, minor twitches, convulsions, and/or unconsciousness. Seizures can be caused by a number of problems, including epilepsy, head injury, fever, poisoning, and insulin shock (hypoglycemia). The causes of seizures may not be determined in as many as 50% of the individuals having one.[2]

The athlete is said to have a generalized seizure when abnormal electrical activity takes place throughout the entire brain. Because the entire brain is involved, the patient is likely to become unresponsive and unaware of surroundings, become unconscious, and collapse. The most common type of generalized seizure is the tonic-clonic, or grand mal, seizure. The tonic phase involves stiffening of the muscles of the body, at which point the victim will collapse. There will be muscle spasms and convulsions of the limbs after the tonic phase; this is called the *clonic* phase. The seizure will end after a couple of minutes. The person will be tired, potentially irritable for a short time, and is said to be postictal.

Efforts should not be made to restrain someone having convulsions because it is not possible to stop the seizure and injury to the victim or rescuer can occur. The primary focus in providing emergency care for an athlete having a seizure is to protect him or her from injury and to monitor vital signs and condition until he or she has regained consciousness and awareness (Figure 7-2). Although it may appear that the victim is not breathing during a seizure, there is sufficient air exchange. After the seizure ends, the athletic trainer should be in a position to provide support and assistance as the patient reorients to the environment and deals with any embarrassment.

Figure 7-2. Protecting the seizure patient.

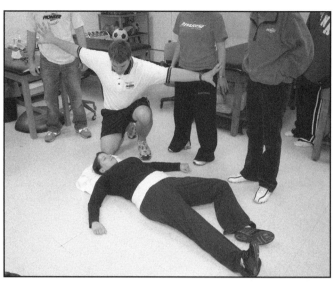

A partial seizure happens when only part of the brain is affected by the abnormal electrical activity. In this case, spasm will be limited to the area controlled by the affected part of the brain. In the case of a partial seizure, the victim will most likely not lose consciousness and should recover fairly quickly on his or her own.

When the athlete has a partial seizure that generalizes into a grand mal seizure, it will usually be preceded by an aura, which is a period of altered sensation before the onset of the seizure. The individual may describe flashing lights, a feeling of warmth, or unusual sights, smells, or tastes before the seizure begins. The aura serves as a warning to individuals with a seizure disorder that a seizure is imminent, providing time to sit down or get to a location to minimize injury from the seizure.

When an individual has a seizure disorder such as epilepsy, he or she is usually aware of the signs of oncoming seizure and the sequence of events that take place during a seizure. In such cases, management of the situation during the seizure is the primary concern of the caregiver, and EMS may not be indicated. For such individuals, the primary causes of seizure are usually forgetting to take seizure medication, physical or emotional stress, or underlying illness. In the vast majority of situations, the athlete will recover spontaneously without significant incident in a matter of a few minutes.[3]

After the seizure, the individual is likely to experience extreme fatigue, memory loss, confusion, fear, embarrassment, muscle soreness, bruising, and headache. These reactions are normal for someone who has just had a seizure event. The term *postictal* refers to the period of time after a seizure when the person is experiencing these types of symptoms. The postictal period usually lasts approximately 5 to 30 minutes. In most cases the victim will want to sleep.[3]

Not all seizures involve violent convulsions or muscle contractions. Some individuals who have a seizure disorder may experience seizures in which the major element of the event is the change in their level of consciousness. Called *absence seizures*, or *petit mal seizures*, their common identifying factor is a sudden impairment of consciousness that will affect the victim's activities. The victim may appear to suddenly "space out," having a blank stare, slowed or stopped speech, or stopping an activity or motion midstream. This type of seizure usually lasts less than 30 seconds and occurs more commonly in children between 5 and 15 years of age.

Seizures become an emergency situation when they last longer than 5 minutes, when they repeat without the person regaining consciousness in between, if the victim is injured during the seizure, or if the person does not return to normal consciousness and alertness afterward. The condition in which a seizure continues or repeats over a period of at least 30 minutes is sometimes called *status epilepticus*. It indicates ongoing abnormal seizure activity in the brain and requires emergency medical intervention.

When a seizure takes place after head injury or as a result of a medical emergency, EMS should be activated immediately, and the sports emergency care provider must be prepared to provide support for breathing and pulse. Brain damage from head trauma, poisoning, insulin shock, or other medical emergency can be significant and life threatening. Any information the sports emergency care provider can provide to the physician will be important in determining the nature and extent of brain injury and the course of care.

Seizure Types: How They Present and What to Do		
	Presentation	*Emergency Care*
Tonic-clonic seizure	*May experience an aura* *May tell you he or she feels strange or different* *Muscles stiffen and victim collapses* *Muscle spasms and convulsions* *Postseizure symptoms*	*When the athlete tells you he or she feels the seizure coming on, tell him or her you are there to help* *Clear the area of objects on which the victim can become injured* *Have the athlete sit or lie down* *Protect the victim's head from injury during the convulsions* *Call EMS* *Provide reassurance and care as needed after the seizure has ended*
Absence seizure	*Sudden change in level of consciousness* *Possible "blank stare"* *Suddenly stops what he or she is doing: "motion suspended mid-stream"* *May not collapse or fall*	*Stay with victim and protect him or her in case he or she falls* *Victim will usually recover quickly* *Athlete is done participating for the day*

OTHER POINTS TO CONSIDER

Concerns sometimes arise regarding the participation of individuals with conditions such as epilepsy or other seizure disorders in sports. Anyone with an underlying medical condition that can result in altered states of consciousness or brain function should consult his or her physician before attempting new, demanding activities. In general, individuals whose epilepsy or seizure disorder is not controlled should refrain from sports or activities that could increase the chances of a seizure occurring. A seizure disorder is considered under control when the athlete is taking the appropriate medication as ordered by a physician and has been seizure-free for a period of time determined by the doctor.

Certain activities that could significantly increase the possibility of a seizure, such as boxing, should be avoided. Activities in which serious injury could result if an individual had a seizure during the activity, such as rock climbing or sky diving, may also be contraindicated for some individuals. On the other hand, many contact sports, like lacrosse, hockey, and possibly football, may be allowed with physician consent. In these cases, it is essential that the athlete has the proper protective equipment and that it fits properly. The sports emergency care team must work together to ensure a safe playing situation for the athlete concerned. Epilepsy and other neurological disorders are not necessarily grounds for disqualification from sports or physical activity.

Summary of Key Points

➡ When an athlete is down on the field or court and does not respond, sports emergency care personnel must identify the potential reasons the victim is unconscious in order to determine and carry out an emergency care plan that will stabilize the victim and prevent further injury.

➡ Initial patient assessment should follow the CAB Sx3.

➡ When the athlete does not respond, or the response is so incoherent or diminished that it is obvious that he or she is in distress, EMS should be activated immediately.

➡ Evaluating the changes in a person's level of consciousness involves determining the quality and coherence of that response.

➡ Serious or critical injuries or medical emergencies affecting the brain can result in significant damage to the portions of the brain controlling motor function, and victims may present in decorticate or decerebrate posturing, depending on the area of the brain injured.

➡ Syncope, also known as fainting, passing out, collapsing, or blackout, occurs when someone becomes unconscious and recovers quickly without assistance.

➡ Stupor, a decreased state of mental activity or awareness that can be associated with drowsiness or diminished response, can occur as a result of head injury or secondary to shock.

➡ Coma is defined as a deep state of unconsciousness during which the patient does not react or respond to stimuli in the environment. Sports emergency care personnel must be prepared to provide basic life support in the event of unconsciousness due to injury.

➡ When a victim is unconscious immediately after a fall or collision, the sports emergency care team member must assume that there is significant head injury and the high possibility of spinal injury.

➡ Unconsciousness does not always happen immediately when an athlete suffers a head injury.

➡ The world of sports is not immune to the negative effects of substance abuse that may lead to unconsciousness.

➡ Changes in a person's level of consciousness may be due to the occurrence of sudden, uncontrolled, abnormal electrical activity in the brain, which may present as a seizure.

➡ Anyone with an underlying medical condition that can result in altered states of consciousness or brain function should consult his or her physician before attempting new, demanding activities.

Review Questions

1. When approaching the down athlete, what should the sports emergency care provider be observing?

2. What is the Glasgow Coma Scale? Describe how the scale is used.

3. Describe "syncope," "stupor," and "coma."

4. What are the signs and symptoms that might indicate a substance-related cause of unconsciousness?

5. Explain proper care for seizures.

REFERENCES

1. Teasdale G, Jennett B. Assessment of coma and impaired consciousness: a practical scale. *Lancet.* 1974;2(7872):81-84.
2. National Institute of Neurological Disorders and Stroke. *Seizures and epilepsy: Hope through research.* http://www.ninds.nih.gov/disorders/epilepsy/detail_epilepsy.htm. Accessed October 1, 2012.
3. The Center for Epilepsy and Seizure Education. *The ICE (International classification of epilepsies).* http://www.epilepsy.cc/index.php?option=com_content&view=article&id=123&Itemid=131. Accessed October 1, 2012.

BIBLIOGRAPHY

American Red Cross. *Emergency Medical Response.* Yardley, PA: Staywell Publishing; 2011.

Booher JM, Thibodeau GA. *Athletic Injury Assessment.* 4th ed. New York, NY: McGraw Hill; 2000.

Ebell MH. Syncope: initial evaluation and prognosis. *Am Fam Physician.* 2006;74(8):1367.

Guskiewicz KM, Bruce SL, Cantu RC, et al. National Athletic Trainers' Association position abatement: management of sport-related concussion. *J Athl Train.* 2004;39(3):280-297.

Harmon KG. Assessment and management of concussion in sports. *Am Fam Physician.* 1999;60(3)887-892, 894.

Luke A, Micheli L. Sports injuries: emergency assessment and field-side care. *Pediatr Rev.* 1999;20:291-300.

McCrory P, Meeuwisse W, Johnston K, et al. Consensus statement on concussion in sport: the 3rd International Conference on Concussion in Sport held in Zurich, November 2008. *Br J Sports Med.* 2009;43(suppl 1):i76-i90.

Meyer C. Using the Glasgow Coma Scale: for accurate results, experience counts. *Am J Nurs.* 1991;91(7):14

National Registry of Emergency Medical Technicians, Inc. Advanced level practical examination: patient assessment—trauma. https://www.nremt.org/nremt/downloads/Pediatric_Intraosseous_Infusion.pdf. Accessed September 29, 2012.

O'Connor FG, Levine BD, Childress MA, Asplundh CA, Oriscello RG. Practical management: a systematic approach to the evaluation of exercise-related syncope in athletes. *Clin J Sport Med.* 2009;19(5):429-434.

Pollak AN, ed. *Emergency Care and Transportation of the Sick and Injured.* 9th ed. Boston, MA: Jones and Bartlett Publishers; 2005.

Prentice WE. *Arnheim's Principles of Athletic Training.* 12th ed. New York, NY: McGraw Hill; 2006.

Spitz MC, Towbin B, Honigman B, Shantz D. Emergency seizure care in adults with known epilepsy. *J Epilepsy.* 1996;9(3):159-164.

Valente LR. Seizures and epilepsy. *Clinician Reviews.* 2000;10(3):79.

Warren WL, Bailes JE. On the field evaluation of athletic head injuries. *Clin Sports Med.* 1998;17(1):13-26.

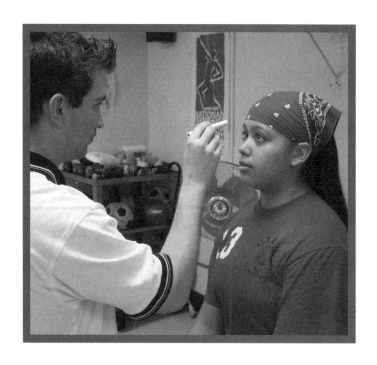

Management of
Traumatic Brain Injury

Casey Christy, MA, ATC, CSCS

While covering a football game, your starting quarterback reports to you on the sideline. He says he has a slight headache and feels "out of it." The coach thinks he "looks fine," that he "just got his bell rung," and expects him to return for the next offensive series.
What do you do?

The awareness and management of traumatic brain injuries has changed dramatically in recent years. Concussions have received considerable attention in the media, creating more awareness of brain injury risks and the long-term effects of repeated concussions. Many states have enacted concussion laws that outline both concussion management and return to play guidelines, in addition to mandating concussion education for athletes, parents, coaches, physicians, and athletic trainers. It is important for sports emergency care personnel to remain current with the latest head injury management guidelines. It is equally important to educate others, including athletes, coaches, parents, physicians, and school staff members about concussion recognition and management. This will help ensure optimal safety and recovery for the brain-injured individual.

It is estimated that 1.6 to 3.8 million sports- and recreation-related concussions occur each year in the United States.[1] However, this number is likely higher since many concussions go unreported. One study found only 47% of high school football players actually reported their concussions.[2] Postseason questionnaires have revealed 15% to 25% of high school football players claimed to have concussion symptoms during the season, many of whom did not report their symptoms to anyone at the time of their injury.[3]

For the purposes of this chapter, traumatic brain injuries are divided into 2 main categories—concussions and intracranial bleeding injuries—the latter of which are vascular emergencies including epidural hematoma, subdural hematoma, and cerebral contusion. An intracranial bleeding injury represents a structural vascular injury that differs from a concussion. In fact, by

Rehberg RS.
Sports Emergency Care: A Team Approach,
Second Edition (pp 109-128).
© 2013 SLACK Incorporated.

definition, the diagnosis of concussion implies that a more severe injury, such as a brain contusion or bleed, is not present.[4]

Although it was initially thought that a concussion produced only a temporary disturbance of brain function due to neuronal, chemical, or neuroelectrical changes without gross structural damage, it is now known that structural damage with loss of brain cells can occur with some concussions.[5] Axonal stretch injury and swelling, in particular, are 2 factors contributing to brain dysfunction following a concussive injury.[4]

CLINICALLY RELEVANT ANATOMY

The brain is divided into the following 4 sections: the brainstem, cerebellum, diencephalon, and cerebrum.

The brainstem consists of the medulla oblongata, pons, and midbrain. It functions as a 2-way conduction path. Sensory nerves carry impulses up the spinal cord, through the brainstem to other parts of the brain. Motor nerves carry impulses down from higher parts of the brain through the brainstem to the spinal cord. The brainstem also houses the "vital center," which controls heartbeat, respirations, and blood vessel diameter. Twelve pairs of cranial nerves are attached to the undersurface of the brain, extending from the brainstem. These nerve fibers communicate with the head and neck and with structures in the thoracic and abdominal cavities.[6] Extending through the brainstem is an important network of nerves called the *reticular activating system*, which regulates an individual's level of consciousness. Since the brainstem is fixed relative to the more movable cerebrum above and spinal cord below, it may sustain damage when the cerebrum moves or rotates as a result of head impact.[7]

The cerebellum is the second largest part of the brain and lies under the occipital lobe of the cerebrum. It functions to produce smooth, coordinated body movements and helps to maintain posture and equilibrium.

The diencephalon is located between the brainstem below and the cerebrum above, and it consists of the hypothalamus and thalamus. The hypothalamus, as its name suggests, is located below the thalamus and is vital to many body functions. The role of the hypothalamus is quite varied, affecting every cell in the body. It makes hormones that are released into the blood, maintains body temperature, helps regulate water balance and sleep cycles, and even controls appetite. The hypothalamus is also involved with the vital center functions and controls emotions such as pleasure, fear, anger, and pain. The thalamus relays information from the sensory organs of the body to the cerebral cortex and associates emotions with these senses. It also plays a role in the arousal or "alerting mechanism."[6]

The cerebrum is the largest part of the brain and is the main area of focus when discussing traumatic brain injuries such as concussions and intracranial bleeding injuries. The cerebrum is divided into 4 lobes, named for the bones located over them: frontal, parietal, temporal, and occipital. The frontal lobes control conscious thought, concentration, planning, problem solving, speech, and muscle action. The parietal lobes help interpret sensory information and aid in understanding speech and in choosing words to express thoughts and feelings. The temporal lobes house the auditory areas, while important visual functions occur in the occipital lobes. The cerebral cortex is a thin layer of gray matter (2 to 5 mm thick) that makes up the outermost part of the cerebrum and contains 75% of the neuron cell bodies within the nervous system.[8]

The brain is surrounded by a fluid-filled membrane called the *meninges*, which is continuous with the spinal cord. The meninges consist of 3 layers—the outer dura mater, the middle arachnoid mater, and the inner pia mater. The dura mater is dense, fibrous, inelastic tissue that encloses the brain. A layer of fat containing vital arteries lies over the dura mater.[6,8,9] The middle meningeal artery, the largest branch that supplies the dura mater, is of particular significance. A skull fracture may tear this artery, leading to an epidural hematoma, which is discussed later in this chapter.[7,10] The arachnoid mater is very delicate tissue lining the inner dura mater. Veins are located in the subdural space, between the dura mater and arachnoid. Cerebrospinal fluid fills the subarachnoid spaces between the arachnoid mater and pia mater and within the brain's ventricles, 4 interconnected cavities located deep inside the brain.[6,8,9] The brain is "suspended" in cerebrospinal fluid, and this fluid helps to protect the brain by acting as a cushion.

INJURY MECHANISMS

Head injuries commonly result from a blow or jolt to the head or from the head striking an object such as the ground or another individual. Research indicates the most common injury mechanism is contact with another player, with head-to-head contact being the most frequent mechanism specifically.[11] A blow to the body can also jolt the head and cause a traumatic brain injury. These mechanisms commonly result in an acceleration-deceleration motion to the head, with or without a rotational component, resulting in tissue damage.

The terms *diffuse* and *focal* are used to describe the nature of different types of brain injuries. Diffuse brain injuries are characterized by a widespread disruption of neurological function as commonly seen with a concussion. Focal brain injuries are life-threatening intracranial bleeding injuries.

Two basic types of brain injury mechanisms exist: coup and contrecoup. A coup injury results from trauma to a nonmoving head, such as when one is struck by a kicked or batted ball. Maximal brain injury occurs directly beneath the point of impact. A contrecoup injury occurs when a moving head strikes a nonmovable object, such as a gym floor or soccer goal post.[12] Because the brain floats freely within cerebrospinal fluid, it moves at a rate that is different from that of the skull in response to a collision or force to the head.[13] As a result, the brain may "bounce" or "twist" within the skull, similar to yolk "bouncing" inside an eggshell. A contrecoup injury causes this type of brain-shifting within the skull, producing maximal brain damage on the side opposite of the impact.

Regardless of the specific mechanism, cells and cell membranes are stretched or torn with either coup or contrecoup injuries. There is no evidence indicating which type of injury is worse or that symptoms present any differently.[12,14] Damaged tissue leads to the abnormal movement of potassium, calcium, glutamate, and other substances in and out of injured brain cells, disrupting normal brain function.[14]

After a traumatic brain injury, brain cells need an increased amount of glucose as a fuel to repair themselves. However, at the same time, cerebral blood flow decreases as a result of the injury, impairing glucose levels. This "metabolic mismatch" of increased energy needs and decreased energy stores places the brain at risk for catastrophic damage should a second trauma occur before the initial injury resolves.[15-17]

CONCUSSION

A *concussion* is defined as a complex pathophysiological process involving the brain, induced by traumatic biomechanical forces.[18] Simply stated, a concussion is a brain injury that results in a temporary disruption of neurological function. One does not need to lose consciousness to suffer a concussion. In fact, less than 10% of sports-related concussions actually involve loss of consciousness.[12] This is an important point when educating athletes, coaches, and parents. In a study of youth coaches, 42% believed that a concussion only occurs when an athlete loses consciousness.[19]

SIGNS AND SYMPTOMS

According to the Third International Conference on Concussion in Sport,[18] the suspected diagnosis of concussion can include one or more of the following general components:

Table 8-1
CONCUSSION SIGNS AND SYMPTOMS

Signs Observed by Others	Symptoms Reported by the Athlete
Appears dazed	Headache
Is confused about what to do	Nausea
Forgets plays	Fatigue
Is unsure of game, score, or opponent	Balance problems or dizziness
Moves clumsily	Double or fuzzy vision
Answers questions slowly	Feeling sluggish or slowed down
Loses consciousness	Feeling foggy or groggy
Cannot recall events prior to the hit	Concentration or memory problems
Cannot recall events after the hit	Light or noise sensitivity
"Vacant stare"	Ringing in the ears
	Sleeplessness, excess sleep, or fatigue

---

* Somatic symptoms (ie, headache, dizziness, or tinnitus)
* Cognitive symptoms (ie, "feeling in a fog" or "feeling slowed down")
* Emotional symptoms (ie, sadness or nervousness)
* Physical signs (ie, amnesia or loss of consciousness)
* Behavioral changes (ie, irritability, mood swings, or personality changes)
* Cognitive impairment (ie, slowed reaction time or sleep disturbances)

If one or more of these general components is present, a concussion should be suspected. The athlete must be immediately removed from play, and the appropriate management strategy should be instituted.[18] The possible signs and symptoms of concussion are numerous and may also include disorientation, confusion, nausea, vomiting, light or noise sensitivity, fatigue, difficulty concentrating, pupil dilation, or blurred vision.[12] Table 8-1 provides a summary of the common signs and symptoms of concussion.[14]

It is important for sports emergency care personnel to understand that even one sign or symptom, even if brief, resulting from a direct or indirect blow to the head, is indicative of a possible concussion. Research indicates concussed high school football players whose symptoms "cleared" within 15 minutes showed increased symptoms and lower memory scores 36 hours postinjury on neurocognitive testing compared to baseline. Furthermore, neurocognitive scores did not return to baseline until 6 days postinjury.[20] Emergency care personnel must remember the true effects of a concussion may not be apparent immediately following the injury, signs and symptoms may manifest or worsen at a later time, and some athletes may not report any concussion symptoms because of a strong desire to play or their competitive nature.

While concussion signs and symptoms can be quite varied, research has identified what is most commonly seen in the athletic population. For example, in one study the top 3 signs and symptoms among nearly 400 concussed collegiate athletes were headache (40%), dizziness (15%), and confusion (9%). Loss of consciousness and amnesia occurred in only 4% and 6% of the cases, respectively.[21] Headache is by far the most commonly reported symptom following concussion, occurring in up to 86% to 93% of concussed athletes in other studies.[11,17]

INTRACRANIAL BLEEDING INJURIES

Although less common, intracranial bleeding (also known as *cerebral hematoma*) can occur with some head injuries. These pathologies include epidural hematoma, subdural hematoma, and cerebral contusion. The skull fits tightly around the brain, similar to a well-fitted football helmet, leaving little room to accommodate intracranial bleeding or swelling. Therefore, any bleeding or swelling that may occur can increase intracranial pressure, causing permanent neurological injury or death.[22]

In general, loss of consciousness, cranial nerve deficits, mental status deterioration, and worsening symptoms raise the concern for intracranial bleeding. Additional red flags include unequal or unreactive pupils, disorientation, seizure, a gradual increase in blood pressure, or a decrease in respiration or pulse rate. Signs or symptoms presenting after an initial lucid (asymptomatic) period may also indicate intracranial bleeding.[9,12] The possibility of intracranial bleeding underscores the importance of a thorough evaluation (including serial re-evaluations), frequent postinjury monitoring, and providing clear instructions to caregivers about serious warning signs that may require immediate medical attention. An athlete with a head injury should not be left alone following the injury in case the condition worsens. The following section summarizes the characteristics of the most common types of intracranial bleeding injuries.

EPIDURAL HEMATOMA

Head trauma can cause tearing of the meningeal arteries, which are embedded in bony grooves in the skull. Most individuals with an epidural hematoma have a skull fracture that lacerates the meningeal blood vessels.[23] Arterial blood pressure causes blood accumulation and a hematoma to rapidly occur between the dura and skull, usually within minutes to hours after the impact. The athlete may lose consciousness after the hit, but may then demonstrate a lucid interval with no signs or symptoms for a period of time after regaining consciousness. Symptoms slowly begin to develop such as headache, dizziness, nausea, pupil dilation (usually on the same side of the injury), altered consciousness, or drowsiness, as the hematoma enlarges and compresses the brain. Declining consciousness, decreasing pulse or respirations, or convulsions may follow. An epidural hematoma is a medical emergency and a computed tomography (CT) scan is needed to make the diagnosis.[9]

SUBDURAL HEMATOMA

A subdural hematoma occurs when blood vessels between the dura mater and brain are stretched or torn and low-pressure, venous bleeding occurs in the subdural space.[9] Subdural hematomas are classified into 2 different types—acute and chronic. Acute subdural hematomas are more common and present symptoms within 48 to 72 hours, while chronic hematomas may not cause symptoms until 30 days after the trauma.[24] Clinically, an athlete with an acute subdural hematoma may present awake and alert with no focal neurological deficits. However, an athlete with a sizeable acute subdural hematoma will typically have a significant neurological deficit and altered consciousness that may progress to coma. Skull fracture is less commonly associated with subdural hematoma than epidural hematoma. A chronic subdural hematoma is defined as a hematoma present 3 weeks or more after an injury. In this case, the initial hemorrhage may be small, however, bleeding or oozing of blood may continue, leading to dangerous intracranial pressure. Clinical symptoms can include personality change, neurological deficits, or simply a progressive or severe headache. Like an epidural hematoma, a subdural hematoma is a medical emergency and the diagnosis is confirmed by a CT scan.[23,25]

CEREBRAL CONTUSION

Also known as *intracerebral hemorrhage*, a cerebral contusion results in a zone of brain damage consisting of life-threatening brain bleeding, cerebral infarction, necrosis, and edema. Considered one of the most common traumatic brain lesions seen on radiographic evaluation, this injury may evolve over hours and days after the injury. The clinical course of individuals with a cerebral contusion varies greatly, which may include normal function initially, progressing to neurological deterioration including coma.[23]

THE HEAD INJURY EVALUATION PROCESS

Sports emergency care personnel will typically encounter an individual with a head injury in 1 of 3 possible scenarios: an injured athlete down on the field, an athlete who comes off to the sideline and notifies the medical or coaching staff of the injury, or the athlete who presents during or after an athletic event in the athletic training office. Regardless of the injury scenario, sports emergency personnel must be aware that each can present with a life-threatening emergency.

EVALUATING THE DOWN ATHLETE

The injury evaluation process of the head-injured athlete who is down on the field begins with a primary survey of consciousness level, respiration, and cardiac status. Checking the athlete's circulation, airway, and breathing is the critical first step in the evaluation process. During this process, always assume a spinal cord injury until proven otherwise. If the athlete is unconscious, not breathing, or does not have a pulse, emergency hospital transport procedures are to be initiated immediately. The emergency responder administers defibrillation, rescue breathing, and/or cardiopulmonary resuscitation (CPR) as indicated. An athlete who is unconscious, or is regaining consciousness but is still disoriented or confused, should be managed as if a cervical spine injury is present. Vital signs should be monitored every 1 to 2 minutes. Talking to a semiconscious athlete is encouraged to bring about full consciousness.[22] The emergency responder then performs a secondary survey to determine the presence of other injuries, such as fractures, dislocations, and bleeding.

Several red flags indicate immediate head and spine immobilization and transport to the nearest hospital by ambulance[12]:

* Loss of consciousness
* Deterioration of neurological function
* Decreasing level of consciousness
* Decrease or irregularity in respirations
* Decrease or irregularity in pulse
* Unequal, dilated, or unreactive pupils
* Any signs or symptoms of associated injuries, spine or skull fracture, or bleeding
* Mental status changes such as lethargy, difficulty maintaining arousal, confusion, or agitation
* Seizure activity
* Lucid interval
* Any apprehension on the part of the athlete or emergency personnel regarding moving to the sideline for further evaluation

If the athlete is fully conscious and alert, and shows no red flags indicative of emergency immobilization and transport, assessment of the athlete may continue on the sideline.

SIDELINE AND OFFICE EVALUATION

The sideline and office head injury evaluation process are similar. They apply to situations in which it was determined that a down athlete may safely be removed to the sideline for a more thorough evaluation, or when an athlete presents to the athletic training facility during or after an athletic event to report a head injury.

The Sport Concussion Assessment Tool 2 (SCAT2)[18] is a head injury evaluation method based on a point system that sports emergency care personnel can utilize to evaluate a concussion for either situation and is described in detail later in this chapter (Figure 8-1). Regardless of whether this specific tool is utilized, it is important for sports emergency care personnel to understand that a complete head injury evaluation consists of carefully assessing 8 essential components: history and observation, orientation and memory, level of consciousness, signs and symptoms, cognitive function, cranial nerve function, balance, and coordination. Since signs and symptoms may not appear immediately, can worsen over time, or present after a lucid interval, serial evaluations are critical. The injured athlete should be re-evaluated frequently right after the injury, as well as the days and weeks that follow as indicated. It is recommended that sports emergency care personnel create a head injury evaluation form that consists of assessment methods for each component to ensure consistent and thorough examinations or utilize the provided SCAT2 tool. The following components serve as the foundation for a complete head injury evaluation.

History and Observation

Details on what happened and how it happened should be obtained from the athlete and any witnesses. This includes the nature and location of the head impact and uncovering any history of prior head injuries. The athlete's ability to interact normally with teammates, coaches, and the emergency responders must be monitored and can provide a subtle clue to the presence of a concussion or worsening symptoms.

Orientation and Memory

Research indicates simple orientation of person, place, and time are not reliable measures for evaluating orientation and memory in the athletic setting.[26,27] That being said, basic questions such as asking the day of the week, the current month and year, the venue location, and the time of day (within 1 hour) should be utilized to gain an overall assessment of orientation and memory. However, emergency personnel must be aware of the limited use and reliability of these questions. The modified Maddocks questions involve more specific inquiries that include asking the athlete to identify the current opponent, who scored last in the current game, and the outcome from the last game played.[18] The inability to recall information or events that took place prior to the head injury is called *retrograde amnesia*. Examples include the game score, the opponent, or the last play that was called.[18] The inability to recall information or events that took place after the head injury is called *anterograde amnesia*. Examples include failure to recall coming off the field or failure to recall a discussion that took place on the sideline after the injury occurred.

Level of Consciousness

Evaluating and re-evaluating whether the athlete is fully conscious and alert or lethargic is critical in identifying a worsening condition. In addition, sports emergency care personnel must also consider the possibility of a lucid interval.

Signs and Symptoms

A graded symptom checklist is recommended to ensure a consistent, thorough, and quantified exam and can be used for serial evaluations. An extensive checklist of signs and symptoms that should be evaluated and re-evaluated are outlined in Figures 8-1[18] and 8-2.[12]

NAME: _____

SPORT: _____

DATE/TIME OF INJURY: _____

DATE/TIME OF ASSESSMENT: _____

AGE: _____GENDER: M   F

GRADE _____ SCHOOL _____

EXAMINER: _____

The SCAT 2 Symptom Evaluation

How do you feel? You should score yourself on the following symptoms, based on how you feel now.

	None		Moderate			Severe	
Headache	0	1	2	3	4	5	6
"Pressure in head"	0	1	2	3	4	5	6
Neck Pain	0	1	2	3	4	5	6
Nausea or vomiting	0	1	2	3	4	5	6
Dizziness	0	1	2	3	4	5	6
Blurred Vision	0	1	2	3	4	5	6
Balance problems	0	1	2	3	4	5	6
Sensitivity to light	0	1	2	3	4	5	6
Sensitivity to noise	0	1	2	3	4	5	6
Feeling slowed down	0	1	2	3	4	5	6
Feeling like "in a fog"	0	1	2	3	4	5	6
"Don't feel right"	0	1	2	3	4	5	6
Difficulty concentrating	0	1	2	3	4	5	6
Difficulty remembering	0	1	2	3	4	5	6
Fatigue or low energy	0	1	2	3	4	5	6
Confusion	0	1	2	3	4	5	6
Drowsiness	0	1	2	3	4	5	6
Trouble falling asleep	0	1	2	3	4	5	6
More emotional than usual	0	1	2	3	4	5	6
Irritability	0	1	2	3	4	5	6
Sadness	0	1	2	3	4	5	6
Nervous or Anxious	0	1	2	3	4	5	6

Total number of symptoms (Maximum possible 22) _____

Symptom SCORE

22 minus positive symptoms: _____ of 22

Symptom Severity Score
(Sum of all scores. Max possible 22x6=132)   _____

Do the symptoms get worse with physical activity ☐ y   ☐ n

Do the symptoms get worse with mental activity ☐ y   ☐ n

Overall rating
If you know the athlete well prior to injury, how different is the athlete acting compared to his/her usual self? Please check one response
☐No different   ☐ very different   ☐ unsure

PHYSICAL SIGNS SCORE

Was there loss of consciousness/unresponsiveness? Y   N
If yes, how many minutes: _____

Was there a balance problem/unsteadiness?   Y   N

Physical signs score (1 pt. for each negative) _____ of 2

GLASGOW COMA SCALE (GCS)

Best eye response (E)

No eye opening _____	1
Eyes opening in response to pain _____	2
Eyes opening to speech _____	3
Eyes opening spontaneously _____	4

Best verbal response (V)

No verbal response _____	1
Incomprehensible sounds _____	2
Inappropriate words _____	3
Confused _____	4
Oriented _____	5

Best motor response (M)

No motor response _____	1
Extension to pain _____	2
Abnormal flexion to pain _____	3
Flexion/withdrawal to pain _____	4
Localizes to pain _____	5
Obeys commands _____	6

Glasgow Coma score (E +V + M) _____ of 15
GCS should be recorded for all athletes in case of subsequent deterioration.

Sideline Assessment – Maddocks Score
Modified Maddocks questions (1 pt. for each correct)

At what venue are we at today?	0	1
Which half is it now?	0	1
Who scored last?	0	1
What team did you play last?	0	1
Did you win your last game?	0	1

Maddocks score: _____ of 5

Maddocks score is validated for sideline diagnosis of concussion only and is not included in the summary score for serial testing.

Coordination Exam
Upper Limb Coordination – Finger-to-nose task:

Which arm was tested: right   left

Scoring: 5 correct repetitions in < 4 sec. = 1

Coordination score: _____ of 1
Must fully touch nose and fully extend elbow after touching nose.

Figure 8-1A. SCAT2. (Reprinted with permission from McCrory P, Meeuwisse W, Johnston K, et al. Consensus statement on concussion in sport: the Third International Conference on Concussion in Sport held in Zurich, November 2008. *J Athl Train.* 2009;44[4]:434-448.)

Cognitive Assessment
Standardized Assessment of Concussion (SAC)

Orientation (1 pt. for each correct)

What month is it?	0	1
What is today's date?	0	1
What day of the week is it?	0	1
What year is it?	0	1
What time is it right now? (within 1 hr.)	0	1

Orientation score _____ of 5

Immediate Memory (1 pt. for each correct)

List	Trial 1	Trial 2	Trial 3	Alternative Words		
Elbow	Y N	Y N	Y N	candle	baby	finger
Apple	Y N	Y N	Y N	paper	monkey	penny
Carpet	Y N	Y N	Y N	sugar	perfume	blanket
Saddle	Y N	Y N	Y N	table	sunset	lemon
Bubble	Y N	Y N	Y N	wagon	iron	insect

(Circle all words used. The athlete should repeat words in order. Complete all 3 trials regardless of score on trail 1 & 2. Do not inform the athlete that delayed recall will be tested. Total score equals sum across all 3 trials).

Immediate memory score _____ of 15

Concentration
Digits Backwards (1 pt. possible for each string length)

			Alternativedigitlist		
4-9-3	Y	N	6-2-9	5-2-6	4-1-5
3-8-1-4	Y	N	3-2-7-9	1-7-9-5	4-9-6-8
6-2-9-7-1	Y	N	1-5-2-8-6	3-8-5-2-7	6-1-8-4-3
7-1-8-4-6-2	Y	N	5-3-9-1-4-8	8-3-1-9-6-4	7-2-4-8-5-6

Months in Reverse Order (1 pt. for entire sequence correct)

Dec-Nov-Oct-Sept-Aug-Jul-Jun-May-Apr-Mar-Feb-Jan   Y   N

Concentration score _____ of 5

Scoring data from the SCAT2 or SAC should not be used as a stand alone method to diagnose concussion, measure recovery, or make return to

Balance Examination
Modified BESS Test

Non-dominant foot:	Right	Left

Double-leg Stance (20 seconds)   _____ of 10

Single-leg Stance (20 seconds)   _____ of 10

Tandem Stance (20 seconds)   _____ of 10
(Non-dominant foot in back)
Trials are scored by counting all errors or deviations from the proper stance during the three 20 second intervals.
Types of errors include:
Hands off iliac crest
Opening eyes
Step, stumble or fall
Moving hip into >30 degrees abduction
Remaining out of testing position >5 seconds

Balance exam score (30-total errors) _____ of 30

Cognitive Assessment
Standardized Assessment of Concussion (SAC)
Delayed Recall
Ask athlete to recall the list of words read earlier in any order.

Elbow	candle	baby	finger
Apple	paper	monkey	penny
Carpet	sugar	perfume	blanket
Saddle	table	sunset	lemon
Bubble	wagon	iron	insect

Overall Score

Test Domain	Score
Symptom score	_____ of 22
Physical signs score	_____ of 2
Glasgow coma score (E +V+M)	_____ of 15
Coordination score	
_____ of 1	
Balance score	_____ of 30
Subtotal	**_____ of 70**
Orientation score (SAC)	_____ of 5
Immediate memory score (SAC)	_____ of 15
Concentration score (SAC)	_____ of 5
Delayed recall score (SAC)	_____ of 5
SAC subtotal	**_____ of 30**
SCAT2 total	**_____ of 100**
Maddocks total	**_____ of 5**

Figure 8-1B. SCAT2. (Reprinted with permission from McCrory P, Meeuwisse W, Johnston K, et al. Consensus statement on concussion in sport: the Third International Conference on Concussion in Sport held in Zurich, November 2008. *J Athl Train.* 2009;44[4]:434-448.)

Graded Symptom Checklist (GSC)					
Symptom	**Time of Injury**	**2-3 hours post-injury**	**24 hours post-injury**	**48 hours post-injury**	**72 hours post-injury**
Blurred vision					
Dizziness					
Drowsiness					
Excess sleep					
Easily distracted					
Fatigue					
Feel "in a fog"					
Feel "slowed down"					
Headache					
Inappropriate emotions					
Irritability					
Loss of consciousness					
Loss of orientation					
Memory problems					
Nausea					
Nervousness					
Personality change					
Poor balance/ coordination					
Poor concentration					
Ringing in ears					
Sadness					
Seeing stars					
Sensitivity to light					
Sensitivity to noise					
Sleep disturbance					
Vacant stare/ glassy eyed					
Vomiting					

NOTE: The GSC should be used not only for the initial evaluation but for each subsequent follow-up assessment until all signs and symptoms have cleared at rest and during physical exertion. The ATC has completed the column for the initial signs and symptoms, we ask the parent/ guardian to assist in the follow-up grading of symptom severity on a scale 0-6, where 0= not present, 1=mild, 3=moderate, and 6=most severe.

Figure 8-2. Sample graded symptom checklist.

Cognitive Testing

Several techniques can be used to evaluate cognitive function and concentration. For example, 5 words can be provided for the athlete to immediately repeat back to the examiner. The athlete can be asked to state the same 5 words 10 minutes later (without the examiner repeating the words) to evaluate delayed recall and the presence of anterograde amnesia. Additional testing can involve stating the months in reverse order beginning with the current month or the 100-7 test. For the 100-7 test, the athlete is first asked to subtract 7 from 100. If the correct answer of 93 is provided, the athlete is asked to then subtract 7 from 93. This process is continued and the examiner notes if the athlete is able to correctly identify the answer sequence (93, 86, 79, 72, etc). Asking the athlete to repeat back a series of single digits in reverse order is another cognitive evaluation method and is described in Figure 8-1.

Cranial Nerve Function

The cranial nerves can be quickly tested as follows: sense of smell (I), visual acuity (II), eye tracking and pupil reactivity (III, IV, VI), biting down (V), facial expressions (VII), hearing and balance (VIII), swallowing (IX, X), neck strength (XI), and tongue protrusion (XII).[9,28] A complete list of cranial nerves and methods to assess each nerve is provided in Table 8-2.

Table 8-2
CRANIAL NERVE ASSESSMENT

Cranial Nerve	Function	Test
I. Olfactory nerve	Smell	Ask athlete to identify familiar odors
II. Optic nerve	Visual acuity	Ask athlete to read scoreboard, eye chart, etc
III. Oculomotor nerve	Pupillary reaction	Use penlight to determine if pupils are equal and reactive to light
IV. Trochlear nerve	Eye movements	Using a penlight, ask athlete to track the light medially, laterally, inferiorly, and superiorly
V. Trigeminal nerve	Facial sensation	Ask athlete if light facial touch is perceived normally, ask athlete to bite down
VI. Abducens nerve	Lateral eye movement	Using a penlight, ask athlete to track the light in a medial and lateral direction
VII. Facial nerve	Facial expression	Ask athlete to smile, wrinkle forehead
VIII. Acoustic nerve	Hearing, balance	Snap next to each ear to check hearing, conduct balance tests such as tandem stance, or Balance Error Scoring System
IX. Glossopharyngeal nerve	Swallowing, voice	Ask athlete to swallow, speak
X. Vagus nerve	Swallowing, gag reflex	Ask athlete to swallow; using a tongue depressor, check gag reflex
XI. Spinal nerve	Neck strength	Check isometric strength of neck muscles, shoulder shrug
XII. Hypoglossal nerve	Tongue movement and strength	Ask athlete to stick out his or her tongue and move medially and laterally

Balance Testing

The tandem stance test is a simple way to quickly assess postural stability as part of the overall head injury evaluation and to specifically evaluate the acoustic nerve. The athlete stands with the dominant foot directly in front of the nondominant foot in a heel-to-toe stance. With the hands on the hips and the eyes closed for 20 seconds, the athlete attempts to maintain balance without any errors. The evaluator counts the number of errors during the 20-second period. Any of the following body movements is considered an error: one or both hands are lifted off the hips; a step, stumble, or fall; lifting of the forefoot or heel; or remaining out of the testing position for more than 5 seconds.[18] The tandem stance test is included in the SCAT2 evaluation tool (see Figure 8-1). It can be used as an isolated test or incorporated into the Balance Error Scoring System (BESS) discussed in the Return to Play section of this chapter.

Coordination Testing

The finger-to-nose test can be utilized to evaluate coordination and is also included in the SCAT2 evaluation tool (see Figure 8-1). With the shoulder flexed to 90 degrees, the athlete attempts to touch his or her index finger to the tip of his or her own nose and then touch the examiner's fingertip 5 consecutive times (fully extending the elbow), as accurately and as quickly as possible in less than 4 seconds.[18]

PHYSICIAN REFERRAL

Once the initial sideline or office evaluation is completed and a head injury is identified, sports emergency care personnel must determine if an urgent, same-day, or nonurgent physician evaluation is appropriate. All concussions should be evaluated by a physician who has experience dealing with head injuries; however, it is important to determine if the athlete can be safely monitored for the time being, or if he or she must see a physician more urgently. Immobilization and transport by ambulance to the nearest hospital for an urgent physician evaluation is indicated if any of the previously mentioned red flags are present. If none of these red flags are present, the athlete can be monitored closely with serial evaluations and advised to see a physician promptly for follow-up evaluation. Serial assessments should be given every 5 minutes on the sideline until the athlete's condition improves, looking for any red flags that indicate an urgent physician evaluation or signs and symptoms that warrant a same-day physician evaluation. This is perhaps one of the most critical measures the sports emergency care provider should take when dealing with any type of head injury. If any of the following occur, a minimum of a same-day physician evaluation is indicated[12]:

* Amnesia
* Increase in blood pressure
* Cranial nerve deficits
* Vomiting
* Motor, sensory, or balance deficits subsequent to the initial on-field assessment
* Postconcussion symptoms that worsen or do not improve over time
* Additional postconcussion symptoms as compared to the initial evaluation
* Athlete is still symptomatic at the end of the game
* Postconcussion symptoms that begin to interfere with the athlete's daily activities including sleep disturbances or cognitive difficulties

HOME CARE

If it has been determined that a same-day physician evaluation is not necessary, the athlete should be provided with a copy of the initial graded symptom checklist and instructed to complete the checklist again with a caregiver 2 to 3 hours after the injury. Any worsening or additional symptoms warrant an immediate physician evaluation. Caregivers, such as family and friends, must be advised about the importance of close monitoring and the warning signs that indicate an urgent physician evaluation. Verbal instructions and an information sheet (Figure 8-3) should be provided. The athlete should report daily to the athletic trainer for re-evaluation and completion of the graded symptom checklist at 24-hour intervals until all signs and symptoms resolve.

There is still some debate about the necessity of nighttime wake-ups following a concussion. Wake-ups disrupt the athlete's normal sleep pattern, which can lead to increased symptoms due to sleep deprivation. However, the athlete should be awakened at night periodically to check for a decreased level of consciousness and persistent or worsening symptoms if any of the following occur: the athlete experienced any loss of consciousness, had a period of amnesia, or still has significant symptoms at bed time.

Concussion Injury Information

Head Injuries and Concussions

Any head, face or jaw injury can result in a concussion and has the potential to be dangerous. A concussion is a brain injury that results in a temporary disruption of neurological function. **One does not need to lose consciousness to suffer a concussion.** In fact, less than 10% of sports-related concussions actually involve loss of consciousness. A concussion often results from a blow or jolt to the head or body, or from the head striking an object such as the ground or another athlete. Because the brain floats freely within cerebrospinal fluid, it moves at a rate that is different from that of the skull in response to a collision or force to the head. As a result, the brain may "bounce" or "twist" within the skull, similar to yolk "bouncing" inside an eggshell. Although less common, bleeding in the brain can occur with some head injuries. **Loss of consciousness, mental status deterioration and worsening symptoms raise the concern for a bleeding injury.**

What are the signs and symptoms of a concussion?

Signs Observed by Others

- Appears dazed
- Is confused about what to do
- Forgets plays
- Is unsure of game, score or opponent
- Moves clumsily
- Answers questions slowly
- Loses consciousness (rare)
- Shows behavior or personality changes
- Can't recall events prior to the hit
- Can't recall events after the hit
- Clear fluid or bleeding coming from the ears or nose indicates a possible skull fracture

Symptoms Reported by Athlete

- Headache
- Nausea
- Fatigue
- Balance problems or dizziness
- Double or fuzzy vision
- Feeling sluggish or "slowed down"
- Feeling foggy or groggy
- Concentration or memory problems
- Confusion
- Light or noise sensitivity
- Ringing in the ears
- Sleeplessness or excess sleep

Second Impact Syndrome

Second Impact Syndrome is a dangerous condition that can occur if an athlete returns to sports before full recovery. If you receive a second blow to the head (even a relatively minor one) before the symptoms of the initial concussion have cleared, the consequences can be deadly.

A second blow to the head after a concussion can cause the brain to lose its ability to regulate blood flow properly. Engorgement of the blood vessels occurs which places excessive pressure on the brain. This pressure can result in rapid respiratory failure, coma and even death.

Prevention

Do not return to sports after a concussion until your symptoms have completely resolved and you have been cleared by your physician or athletic trainer.

For more information

about concussions, visit the athletic trainers website...

Observe the athlete: Check your son or daughter frequently for any signs or symptoms after any direct or indirect head trauma. Consult a physician immediately if there is any question of a concussion. Note that a severe or worsening headache, particularly when accompanied by vomiting or rapidly declining mental status may signal a life-threatening brain-bleeding injury.

Important Phone Numbers:
Athletic Trainers: (xxx) xxx-xxxx   School Physician (xxx) xxx-xxxx

Figure 8-3. Sample home instruction information sheet.

Concussed athletes should avoid aspirin or nonsteroidal anti-inflammatories since these medications thin the blood and may potentially increase the risk of intracranial bleeding. It is generally acceptable for the athlete to take acetaminophen for a concussion-related headache; however, sports emergency care personnel should advise the athlete to check with a physician before taking any medication.[12]

The athlete should be advised to rest from both physical and cognitive activities, the latter of which includes schoolwork, playing video games, computer use, texting, extended TV viewing, and using other electronic devices.

ACADEMIC ACCOMMODATIONS

Temporary academic accommodations are sometimes necessary during concussion recovery due to concentration difficulties and other cognitive deficits. This may include reduced school work, home instruction, increased time for tests, or perhaps no tests for a period of time, at the discretion of the treating physician. The athletic trainer can provide general written information about academic accommodations at the time of injury so this can be discussed during the physician evaluation (Figure 8-4).[29]

THE ASYMPTOMATIC ATHLETE

If the athlete presents with absolutely no signs or symptoms following head trauma, he or she must still undergo a complete head injury evaluation and serial re-evaluations every few minutes as previously described. If the athlete continues to remain free of any concussion signs or symptoms, the sports emergency care provider must exertionally test the athlete on the sideline to ensure he or she is completely symptom-free both at rest and with exertion before returning to play. Suggested exertional testing includes pushups, situps, sprints, and other noncontact functional activities. Athletic trainers must take into consideration the strong desire to play and lack of forthright symptom reporting with some athletes and the possibility of delayed symptoms or a lucid interval when making return to play decisions for the individual who claims to have no symptoms after head trauma. The athlete should be monitored closely if returned to play and re-evaluated after the game. A head injury information sheet should also be provided as a precaution.

Any athlete with a suspected concussion or who presents with any concussion signs or symptoms should not return to play the same day of injury, and should follow the return to play procedures (outlined later in the Return to Play section of this chapter) at the direction of a physician.

CATASTROPHIC INJURIES: SECOND IMPACT SYNDROME AND INTRACRANIAL BLEEDING

With a 50% fatality rate, second impact syndrome (SIS) is a rare but potentially fatal injury that occurs when an athlete receives a second head injury before complete recovery from a previous concussion can take place. The brain loses its ability to regulate blood flow, leading to blood vessel engorgement, cerebral edema, and intracranial pressure. This can cause rapid respiratory failure, coma, permanent neurological injury, and possibly death. Brainstem failure may occur in 2 to 5 minutes. The second blow may be minor, but can cause SIS if symptoms are still present from the previous concussion at the time of the second impact.[22,30]

Dear Physician,

Some concussed athletes may need academic accommodations when recovering from their head injury due to cognitive impairment or other concussion symptoms.

According to the Zurich International Concussion Consensus Statement[1], "the cornerstone of concussion management is physical and <u>cognitive rest</u> until symptoms resolve and then a graded program of exertion prior to medical clearance and return to play. "

The following are examples of temporary academic accommodations that may help with reducing cognitive load, thereby minimizing post-concussion symptoms and allowing the student to better participate in the academic process during the injury period:

- Tests: extra time to complete tests, testing in a quiet environment, reduced length of tests or eliminating tests

- Workload reduction: decreased class work, homework, projects, etc.

- Tutoring

- Reduced note-taking: pre printed class notes, outlines ahead of time, etc.

- Physical Education limitations or restrictions

- Attendance Restrictions: full or half days as tolerated, no school until _____ then half/full days as tolerated, homebound instruction

Should you find any of these or other academic accommodations necessary, please provide a written note to the student and instruct the student to present the note to the guidance department. Thank you.

[1] McCrory et al. Consensus Statement on Concussion in Sport: The 3rd International Conference on Concussion in Sport. *Journal of Athletic Training.* 2009; 44(4):434-448.

Figure 8-4. Sample academic accommodations letter.

In a study of high school and college football players, researchers evaluated the records of 94 severe head injuries that occurred over a 13-year period, the majority of which were subdural hematomas. Half of these injuries resulted in permanent neurological injury, and 8 of the athletes died as result of their head injury. Of the 94 injuries 92 were high school athletes, indicating younger athletes may be more vulnerable to a severe head injury than the older athlete. The authors discovered nearly 60% of the catastrophically injured athletes had a prior head injury (most were in the same season) and about 40% were playing with neurological symptoms at the time of the catastrophic event.[31]

Adolescent athletes appear more likely to suffer from SIS and other severe head injuries than college-aged or other adult athletes. Nearly all of the cases of SIS have occurred to athletes younger than 18 years old (KM Guskiewicz, personal communication, 2010). Several theories have been proposed as to why younger athletes are more vulnerable than adult athletes. First, the brain is not fully developed at a younger age. Second, blood vessels in the brain tear more easily in the younger athlete. Third, the skull is thinner in the younger athlete, providing less brain protection.[32] The risk of SIS and intracranial bleeding underscore the critical importance of making certain the athlete is asymptomatic and completely recovered before returning to play.

CHRONIC TRAUMATIC ENCEPHALOPATHY

Chronic traumatic encephalopathy (CTE) is a condition associated with repetitive brain trauma that has been identified in athletes. CTE may involve gradual and progressive neurological deterioration, memory disturbances, dementia, behavioral and personality changes, parkinsonism, and speech and gait abnormalities. Atrophy of the cerebral hemispheres and abnormal protein deposits in the brain are associated with this disorder as a result of repeated concussions.[33] The long-term consequences of repeated concussions and the effects of CTE and other postconcussion disorders reinforce the importance of appropriate mild traumatic brain injury management.

RETURN TO PLAY

The combination of a thorough clinical exam, use of a symptom checklist, and neurocognitive testing is recommended when making return to play decisions.[34] In addition, athletes should be medically cleared and complete a gradual, stepwise, asymptomatic exercise program before returning to play after a concussion. At no time should an athlete still having any postconcussion signs or symptoms be permitted to return to play.

A gradual exercise program is a critical part of the return to play protocol, and may begin once the athlete is symptom-free for an appropriate period of time and has been cleared by a physician to begin exercising. The required asymptomatic period is dependent upon the latest published concussion guidelines and may also be based on institutional or state policies, and possibly state law. Individualized variations of the asymptomatic period may occur based on the severity or duration of the concussion signs or symptoms, any prior concussion history, and the proximity to the current concussion. Additional conditions that may modify concussion management and return to play include prolonged loss of consciousness, age, sport, style of play, and medication use. The presence of migraines, depression, learning disability, attention deficit hyperactivity disorder, sleep disorder, or other mental health issues may also affect return to play.

Table 8-3 outlines the exercise progression based on recommendations made by the Third International Conference on Concussion in Sport held in Zurich, Switzerland.[18] Each step should take 24 hours. If any postconcussion symptoms occur in the stepwise program, the athlete should drop back to the previous asymptomatic level and try to progress again after a further 24-hour period of rest has passed.[18]

Neurocognitive testing is a tool commonly used in making return-to-play decisions; however, such testing should not be the sole basis of determining when an athlete can return to activity.[12] Paper-and-pencil and computer-based programs are available in which pre-injury baseline scores are compared to postinjury scores to monitor and determine recovery. Some concussed athletes fail their postinjury neurocognitive testing compared to baseline when claiming to be asymptomatic.[34] Therefore, objective data provided by such testing measures are valuable adjuncts to the return to play protocol, particularly if the athlete is not forthright with self-reported symptoms.

Table 8-3
GRADUAL RETURN TO PLAY PROTOCOL

Rehabilitation Stage	Functional Exercise	Goals
1. No activity	Complete cognitive and physical rest	Recovery
2. Light aerobic exercise	Walking, stationary cycling, skating	Increase heart rate
3. Sport-specific exercise	Running or skating drills, no head impact	Add movement
4. Noncontact training drills	Progress to more complex training drills (ie, passing drills in football, soccer, or hockey), may begin weight training	Exercise, coordination, and cognitive load
5. Full-contact practice	Participation in normal training activities with medical clearance	Restore athlete's confidence, coaching staff assesses athlete's functional skills
6. Return to play	Normal game play	

The Balance Error Scoring System (BESS) is another evaluation tool to gauge concussion recovery and is best used when compared to a baseline score. The athlete uses 3 stances (double-leg with feet together, single leg, and tandem) on both a firm and foam surface with eyes closed for 20 seconds. The examiner counts the number of errors (see Balance Testing section earlier in this chapter) for each trial to evaluate postural stability.[12]

Although concussion recovery rates can be highly variable, most concussed athletes recover within 3 weeks.[35] Prolonged post-traumatic headache (60 hours or longer), symptoms of fatigue, tiredness, "fogginess," or the presence of 3 symptoms or more initially after the injury are associated with longer recovery and return to play times after a concussion. With regard to predicting a quicker recovery, post-traumatic headache lasting less than 24 hours is associated with shorter recovery time.[36] Research indicates adolescent athletes have longer recovery rates compared to adult athletes.[18] For example, high school football players take longer to recover from concussion compared to professional football players, particularly with regard to memory and reaction time.[32] The combination of increased severe head injury risk, SIS, and slower recovery rates among adolescents indicates younger athletes must be treated more conservatively.

Sports emergency care personnel must document all aspects of concussion management, including the return to play activity progression and any other evaluation methods utilized. Figure 8-5 provides a sample form that can be utilized to record the athlete's exercise progression following a concussion.

Concussion Recovery and Graded Exercise Program Log				
Name:_____				
Injury Date:_____				
First Asymptomatic Date:_____				
Neurocog. Test WNL:_____				
Cleared fo Full Activity Date:_____				

Date	Activity	Signs/Symptoms?	ATC Comments	AT Initials
	Stationary Bike 10 mins			
	Running 15 mins			
	Non-contact drills			
	Non-contact practice			
	Full-contact practice			

Figure 8-5. Sample form to document stepwise activity progression.

SUMMARY OF KEY POINTS

➡ It is estimated that 1.6 to 3.8 million sports- and recreation-related concussions occur each year in the United States. However, this number is likely higher since many concussions go unreported.

➡ Diffuse brain injuries are characterized by a widespread disruption of neurological function as commonly seen with a concussion. Focal brain injuries are life-threatening intracranial bleeding injuries.

➡ Athletes who have suffered a concussion may present with one or more of a number of symptoms. Less than 10% of sports-related concussions actually involve loss of consciousness.

➡ Although less common, intracranial bleeding (also known as cerebral hematoma) can occur with some head injuries. These pathologies include epidural hematoma, subdural hematoma, and cerebral contusion.

➡ The injury evaluation process of the head-injured athlete who is down on the field begins with a primary survey of consciousness level, respiration, and cardiac status. Checking the athlete's circulation, airway, and breathing is the critical first step in the evaluation process.

➡ The SCAT2 is a head injury evaluation method based on a point system that sports emergency care personnel can utilize to evaluate a concussion.

➡ All concussions should be evaluated by a physician who has experience managing head injuries.

➡ Serial assessments should be given every 5 minutes on the sideline until the athlete's condition improves, looking for any red flags that indicate an urgent physician evaluation or signs and symptoms that warrant a same-day physician evaluation.

➡ If it has been determined that a same-day physician evaluation is not necessary, the athlete should be provided with a copy of the initial graded symptom checklist and instructed to complete the checklist again with a caregiver 2 to 3 hours after the injury. Any worsening or additional symptoms warrant an immediate physician evaluation.

➡ Temporary academic accommodations are sometimes necessary during concussion recovery due to concentration difficulties and other cognitive deficits.

➡ If the athlete presents with absolutely no signs or symptoms following head trauma, he or she must still undergo a complete head injury evaluation and serial re-evaluations every few minutes.

➡ Any athlete with a suspected concussion or who presents with any concussion signs or symptoms should not return to play the same day of injury, and should follow the return to play procedures outlined in this chapter at the direction of a physician.

➡ SIS is a rare but potentially fatal injury that occurs when an athlete receives a second concussion before symptoms of a first concussion have resolved.

➡ CTE is a condition associated with repetitive brain trauma that has been identified in athletes. The long-term consequences of repeated concussions and the effects of CTE and other postconcussion disorders reinforce the importance of appropriate mild traumatic brain injury management.

➡ The combination of a thorough clinical exam, use of a symptom checklist, and neurocognitive testing is recommended when making return to play decisions. In addition, athletes should be medically cleared and complete a gradual, stepwise, asymptomatic exercise program before returning to play after a concussion. At no time should an athlete still having any postconcussion signs or symptoms be permitted to return to play.

REVIEW QUESTIONS

1. What is the difference between a "diffuse" brain injury and a "focal" brain injury?
2. Define concussion.
3. Name the components of concussion symptoms, and give an example of each.
4. What is difference between epidural and subdural hematoma?
5. Describe the proper emergency care for an athlete suspected of having a concussion.

REFERENCES

1. Langlios JA, Rutland-Brown W, Wald M. The epidemiology and impact of traumatic brain injury: a brief overview. *J Head Trauma Rehabil*. 2006;21(5):375-378.
2. McCrea M, Hammeke T, Olsen G, Leo P, Guskiewicz K. Unreported concussion in high school football players: implications for prevention. *Clin J Sport Med*. 2004;14(1):13-17.
3. Gerberich SG, Priest JD, Boen JR, Straub CP, Maxwell RE. Concussion incidences and severity in secondary school varsity players. *Am J Public Health*. 1983;73(12):1370-1375.
4. Grady MF. Concussion in the adolescent athlete. *Curr Prob Pediatr Adolesc Health Care*. 2010;40(7):154-169.
5. Cantu RC. Posttraumatic retrograde and anterograde amnesia: pathophysiology and implications in grading and safe return to play. *J Athl Train*. 2001;36(3):244-248.
6. Thibodeau GA, Patton KT. The nervous system. In: *Structure and Function of the Body*. 13th ed. St. Louis, MO: Mosby Elsevier; 2008.
7. Booher JM, Thibodeau GA. Head and face injuries. In: *Athletic Injury Assessment*. 2nd ed. St. Louis, MO: Times Mirror/Mosby College Publishing; 1989.
8. Shier D, Butler J, Lewis R. Nervous system II: divisions of the nervous system. In: *Hole's Human Anatomy and Physiology*. 12th ed. New York, NY: McGraw-Hill; 2010.
9. Prentice W. The head, face, eyes, ears, nose, and throat. In: *Arnheim's Principles of Athletic Training: A Competency-Based Approach*. 14th ed. New York, NY: McGraw-Hill; 2011.
10. Gray H. The blood-vascular system. In: Pick TP, Howden R, eds. *Gray's Anatomy*. New York, NY: Bounty Books; 1977.
11. Meehan WP, d'Hemecourt P, Comstock RD. High school concussions in the 2008-2009 academic year: mechanism, symptoms and management. *Am J Sports Med*. 2010;38(12):2405-2409.
12. Guskiewicz KM, Bruce SL, Cantu RC, et al. National Athletic Trainers' Association position statement: management of sports-related concussion. *J Athl Train*. 2004;39(3):280-297.
13. Viano DC, Casson IR, Pellman EJ, Zhang L, King AI, Yang KH. Concussion in professional football: brain responses by finite element analysis: part 9. *Neurosurgery*. 2005;57(5):891-916.
14. National Federation of State High School Associations. A parent's guide to concussion in sports. April 2010. www.nfhs.org/WorkArea/DownloadAsset.aspx?id=4243. Accessed October 1, 2012.

15. Thompson HJ, Lifshitz J, Marklund N, et al. Lateral fluid percussion brain injury: a 15 year review and evaluation. *J Neurotrauma*. 2005;22(1):42-75.

16. Bergschneider M, Hovda DA, Shalmon E, et al. Cerebral hyperglycolysis following severe traumatic brain injury in humans: a positron emission tomography study. *J Neurosurgery*. 1997;86(2):241-251.

17. Sabini RC, Reddy CC. Concussion management and treatment considerations in the adolescent population. *Phys Sportsmed*. 2010;38(1):139-146.

18. McCrory P, Meeuwisse W, Johnston K, et al. Consensus statement on concussion in sport: the Third International Conference on Concussion in Sport held in Zurich, November 2008. *J Athl Train*. 2009;44(4):434-448.

19. Valovich Mcleod TC, Schwartz C, Bay RC. Sport-related concussion misunderstandings among youth coaches. *Clin J Sports Med*. 2007;17(2):140-142.

20. Lovell MR, Collins MW, Iverson GL, Johnston KM, Bradley JP. Grade 1 or "ding" concussions in high school athletes. *Am J Sportsmed*. 2004;32(1):47-54.

21. Gessel LM, Fields SK, Collins CL, Dick RW, Comstock RD. Concussions among United States high school and collegiate athletes. *J Athl Train*. 2007;42(4):495-503.

22. Guskiewicz KM, McCrea M. Head injuries. In: Starkey C, Johnson G, eds. *Athletic Training and Sports Medicine*. Sudbury, MA: Jones and Bartlett Publishers; 2006:557-578.

23. Bailes JE, Hudson V. Classification of sport-related head trauma: a spectrum of mild to severe injury. *J Athl Train*. 2001;36(3):236-243.

24. White RJ. Subarachnoid hemorrhage: the lethal intracranial explosion. *Emerg Med Clin North Am*. 1994;12(2):74.

25. Robinson RG. Chronic subdural hematoma: surgical management in 133 patients. *J Neurosurgery*. 1984;61(2):263-268.

26. Maddocks DL, Dicker GD, Saling MM. The assessment of orientation following concussion in athletes. *Clin J Sports Med*. 1995;5(1):32-35.

27. McCrea M, Kelly JP, Kluge J, Ackley B, Randolph C. Standardized assessment of concussion in football players. *Neurology*. 1997;48(3):586-588.

28. Oliaro S, Anderson S, Hooker D. Management of cerebral concussion in sports: the athletic trainer's perspective. *J Athl Train*. 2001;36(3):257-262.

29. McGrath N. Supporting the student-athlete's return to the classroom after a sport-related concussion. *J Athl Train*. 2010;45(5):492-498.

30. Cantu RC. Second impact syndrome: a risk in any contact sport. *Phys Sportsmed*. 1995;20(12):27-34.

31. Boden BP, Tacchetti RL, Cantu RC, Knowles, SB, Mueller FO. Catastrophic head injuries in high school and college football players. *Am J Sports Med*. 2007;35(7):1075-1081.

32. Pellman EJ, Lovell MR, Viano DC, Casson IR. Concussion in professional football: recovery of NFL and high school athletes assessed by computerized neuropsychological testing—part 12. *Neurosurgery*. 2006;58(2):263-274.

33. McKee AC, Cantu RC, Nowinski CJ, et al. Chronic traumatic encephalopathy in athletes; progressive tauopathy after head injury. *J Neuropathol Exp Neurol*. 2009;68(7):709-735.

34. Broglio SP, Macciocchi SN, Ferrara MS. Neurocognitive performance of concussed athletes when symptom free. *J Athl Train*. 2007;42(4):504-508.

35. Collins M, Lovell, MR, Iverson GL, Maroon IT. Examining concussion rates and return to play in high school football players wearing newer helmet technology: a three-year prospective cohort study. *Neurosurgery*. 2006;58(2):275-286.

36. Makdissi M, Darby D, Maruff P, Ugoni A, Brukner P, McCrory PR. Natural history of concussion in sport: markers of severity and implications for management. *Am J Sports Med*. 2010;38(3):464-471.

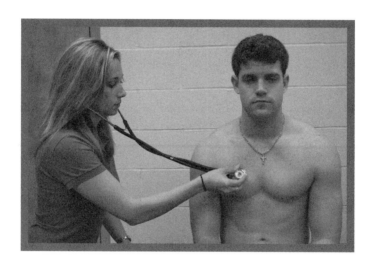

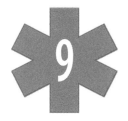

Injuries to the Thoracic Region

Michael A. Prybicien, MA, ATC, CSCS, CES, PES

> *Shortly before the end of the lacrosse game, one of your players reports to you complaining of a sudden stabbing pain in his right pectoral and lateral axillary regions. He tells you he feels out of breath, and his respiratory rate and heart rate are elevated. You listen to his breathing with a stethoscope and notice decreased lung sounds on his right side. He has no history of respiratory problems, but you noticed he took a hard hit a few minutes earlier in the game. He becomes pale and his skin is cool and clammy. Upon placing him in the recovery position, he complains that the pain in his chest increases.*
> *What would you do?*

Acute thoracic injuries can be among the most serious in sports because they can impose a threat of long-term disability, and in the most severe cases even death. They have the potential to be catastrophic in nature because they can affect the spinal cord, nerves around the spinal cord (which are responsible for motor and sensory activity), and even the heart, lungs, and various other organs. Fortunately, thoracic injuries are usually nonemergency acute conditions such as sprains, strains, and contusions.

REVIEW OF CLINICALLY RELEVANT ANATOMY

The thorax (Figure 9-1) is a bone cavity that is formed by 12 pairs of ribs that join posteriorly with the thoracic spine and anteriorly with the sternum. The intercostal neurovascular bundle runs along the inferior surface of each rib. The inner side of the thoracic cavity and the lung itself are lined with a thin layer of tissue called the *pleura*. The space between the 2 pleural layers is normally only a potential space. However, this space may be occupied by air, forming a pneumothorax, or blood, forming a hemothorax. This potential space can hold 3 L of fluid on each side in an adult.

Rehberg RS.
Sports Emergency Care: A Team Approach,
Second Edition (pp 131-140).
© 2013 SLACK Incorporated.

Figure 9-1. Anterior view of the thorax. (Illustration by Joelle Rehberg, DO.)

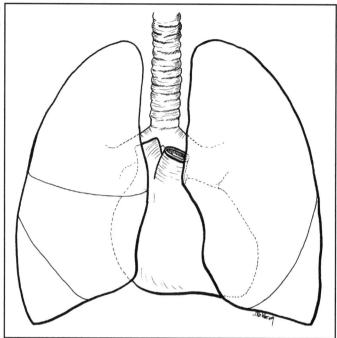

One lung occupies each thorax cavity. The mediastinum is between the chest cavity and contains the heart, aorta, superior and inferior vena cava, trachea, major bronchi, and esophagus. The spinal cord is protected by the vertebral column. The diaphragm separates the thoracic organs from the abdominal cavity. The upper abdominal organs, including the spleen, liver, kidneys, pancreas, and stomach, are protected by the lower rib cage. Any patient with a penetrating thoracic wound (ie, javelin) at the level of the nipples or lower should be assumed to have an abdominal injury as well as a thoracic injury. Similarly, blunt deceleration injuries such as direct blows from a helmet or other body parts can often injure both the thoracic and abdominal structures.

The thoracic spine consists of 12 vertical columns (vertebrae) connected by "facet joints." A disc with a lining and a center filled with a gelatinous substance lies between each of these vertebrae. These discs act as shock absorbers and provide the spinal column with its flexibility. When an athlete runs and jumps, these discs absorb the impact as well as prevent the vertebrae from grinding against one another.

Four muscle groups—the abdominals, the extensors, and 2 sets of paraspinal muscles—control the thoracic spinal column. Within the spinal cord is a massive trunk of nerves that runs down the length of the spinal column from the brain to the sacrum. Smaller nerves branch out from the main trunk at each vertebra. These nerves travel to the arms, torso, and the legs. The brain can send out electrical impulses through these nerves to the various tissues to make them function. The brain can also receive feedback from the tissues through these nerves.

EVALUATION AND ASSESSMENT

When evaluating an athlete with a possible thoracic injury, sports emergency care providers should always assume the worst because it is extremely important that potential life-threatening injuries are not overlooked. During the initial evaluation, search first for the most serious injuries. As with any athletic injury, the mechanism of injury is extremely important in caring for the most severe thoracic injuries. Thoracic injuries may be the result of blunt or penetrating trauma. Blunt trauma, which can occur in most contact sports, can result in a force being distributed over a large area, and visceral injuries occur from deceleration, shearing forces, compression, or bursting. Penetrating injuries, which are less common, can occur from objects that are inadvertently on the field or court surface or objects that are airborne such as a javelin. The distribution of forces is typically over a much smaller area in penetrating injuries.

Often, thoracic injury causes tissue hypoxia. Tissue hypoxia may result from the following:

* Inadequate oxygen delivery to the tissues secondary to airway obstruction

* Hypovolemia from blood loss

* Asymmetrical lung expansion

* Changes in pleural pressures from tension pneumothorax

* Pump failure from severe myocardial injury

The major symptoms of chest injury include shortness of breath, chest pain, and respiratory distress. Signs indicative of chest injury include shock, hemoptysis, cyanosis, chest wall contusion, flail chest, open wounds, distended neck veins, tracheal deviation, or subcutaneous emphysema. Check the lungs for the presence, quality, and equality of breath sounds. Life-threatening, sports-related thoracic injuries should be identified immediately. Some sports-related thoracic injuries will be detected during the primary survey while others may not be detected until a more detailed examination is conducted.

The following injuries are detected during the initial assessment:	*The following injuries are more likely to be detected during the detailed examination:*
Airway obstruction	*Traumatic aorta rupture*
Tension/traumatic pneumothorax	*Tracheal or bronchial tree injury*
Spontaneous pneumothorax	*Myocardial contusion*
Massive hemothorax	*Diaphragmatic tear*
Flail chest	*Esophageal injury*
Cardiac tamponade	*Pulmonary contusion*
	Sternal fractures/contusion
	Rib fractures/contusions
	Costochondral separation/dislocation
	Thoracic spine fracture
	Thoracic muscle strains

AIRWAY OBSTRUCTION

Airway obstruction recognition is vital. Airway management is a challenge that must be met in the care of the life-threatening sports injury. Refer to Chapter 4 for additional information on management of airway and breathing emergencies. Finally, always assume a spinal injury in the unconscious down athlete when securing the airway.

TENSION PNEUMOTHORAX

A tension pneumothorax (sometimes known as *traumatic pneumothorax*) can occur when a one-way valve is created from either blunt or penetrating trauma. Air can enter but cannot leave the pleural space. This causes an increase in the intrathoracic pressure, which will collapse the

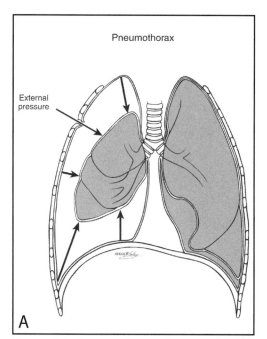
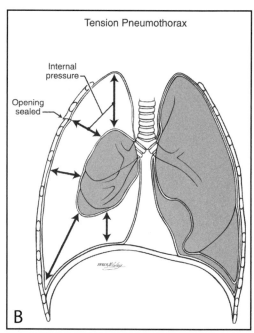

Figure 9-2. Pneumothorax. (Reprinted with permission from O'Connor DP, Fincher AL. *Clinical Pathology for Athletic Trainers: Recognizing Systemic Disease.* 2nd ed. Thorofare, NJ: SLACK Incorporated; 2008.)

lung and increase pressure on the mediastinum. This pressure will eventually collapse the superior and inferior vena cava, resulting in a loss of venous return to the heart. A shift of the trachea and mediastinum away from the side of the tension pneumothorax will also compromise ventilation of the other lung, although this is a late phenomenon.

Clinical signs of a tension pneumothorax (Figure 9-2) include apprehension, agitation, cyanosis, diminished breath sounds and hyperresonance to percussion on the affected side, cold and clammy skin, distended neck veins, and hypotension. Tracheal deviation, or a shifting of the trachea toward the side of the functioning lung, is usually a late sign (if at all), and its absence does not rule out a tension pneumothorax.

Spontaneous Pneumothorax

When a pneumothorax occurs in the absence of any traumatic injury or disease, it is called a *spontaneous pneumothorax.* This type of pneumothorax is rare in athletes, but can be fatal if not appropriately detected and managed. Diagnosis depends on a thorough understanding of possible presenting signs and symptoms such as chest pain, dyspnea, and diminished breath sounds.

Regardless of whether a pneumothorax occurs spontaneously or from trauma, early and accurate diagnosis is essential. The classic complaint of an athlete with a pneumothorax is chest pain. The pain can be vague but is usually localized to the side of the affected lung and can radiate to the shoulder, neck, and/or back. Often pain can be associated with dyspnea on exertion and/or a dry cough. Other classic findings of pneumothorax include tachypnea, tachycardia, hyperresonance to percussion of the affected chest area, diminished breath sounds, and fremitus on the side of the affected lung.

Although the factors that cause or contribute to a spontaneous pneumothorax are not clearly understood, it has been suggested that a family history and a tall, thin body build can be associated factors.

Table 9-1
MANAGEMENT OF SPONTANEOUS AND TENSION PNEUMOTHORAX AND HEMOTHORAX

- Establish an open airway
- Activate EMS if not on the scene
- Treat for shock
- Provide supplemental oxygen (avoid positive pressure ventilation)
- Place in a position of comfort, or if lying, with affected side down (this occasionally helps)
- Monitor oxygen saturation with pulse oximeter
- Rapid transport to hospital

Sports-related spontaneous pneumothorax has been documented in weight lifting, football, and jogging. Most cases of spontaneous pneumothorax, however, are not related to exertion or activity.

Clinical signs of a spontaneous pneumothorax include apprehension, agitation, sharp unilateral chest pain, a history of vigorous coughing, and decreased lung sounds unilaterally.

This patient must be transported rapidly to the hospital (Table 9-1) so chest decompression can be performed. A chest tube will also be necessary upon arrival to the hospital.

MASSIVE HEMOTHORAX

A hemothorax (Figure 9-3) occurs when blood enters the pleural space. A massive hemothorax occurs as a result of at least 1500 cc blood loss into the thoracic cavity. Each thoracic cavity may contain up to 3000 cc of blood. A massive hemothorax is more commonly caused by a penetrating trauma, but it can also occur from a blunt trauma. Either mechanism of injury may disrupt a major pulmonary or systemic vessel. As blood accumulates within the pleural space, the lung on the affected side is compressed. If enough blood accumulates, the mediastinum will be shifted away from the hemothorax. The inferior and superior vena cava and the contralateral lung are compressed. Thus, the blood loss is complicated by hypoxemia.

Clinical signs and symptoms of massive hemothorax are produced by both hypovolemia and respiratory compromise. The patient may be hypotensive from blood loss and compression of the heart or great veins. Anxiety, apprehension, and confusion are the results of hypovolemia and hypoxemia. Signs and symptoms of hypovolemic shock may be apparent followed by difficulty breathing. The neck veins are usually flat, breath sounds are decreased or absent on the side of the injury, and chest percussion is dull.

FLAIL CHEST

Flail chest (Figure 9-4) is defined as a fracture of 2 or more adjacent ribs in at least 2 places. These injuries typically occur in contact sports like football, hockey, wrestling, and lacrosse. In rare cases, they may occur from a severe torsion mechanism in a noncontact sport. The result is a segment of the chest wall that is not in continuity with the thorax. A lateral flail chest or anterior flail chest (sternal separation) may result. With posterior rib fractures, the heavy

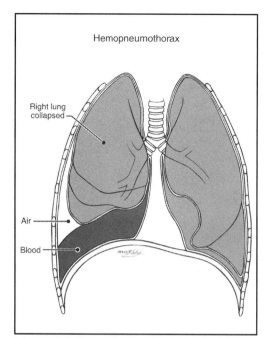

Figure 9-3. Hemothorax. (Reprinted with permission from O'Connor DP, Fincher AL. *Clinical Pathology for Athletic Trainers: Recognizing Systemic Disease.* 2nd ed. Thorofare, NJ: SLACK Incorporated; 2008.)

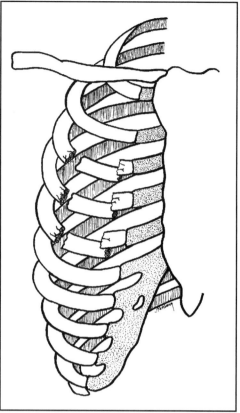

Figure 9-4. Flail chest. (Illustration by Joelle Rehberg, DO.)

musculature usually prevents the occurrence of a flail segment. The flail segment moves with paradoxical motion relative to the rest of the chest wall. The force necessary to produce injury also bruises the underlying lung tissue, and the pulmonary contusion can also contribute to hypoxia. The patient is at risk for the development of the other conditions already discussed in this chapter (a hemothorax or pneumothorax). With a large flail segment, the patient may be in marked respiratory distress. Pain from the chest wall injury exacerbates the already impaired respiration from paradoxical motion and the underlying lung contusion. Palpation of the chest may reveal crepitus in addition to the abnormal respiratory movement.

Management of flail chest includes stabilizing the flail segment with manual pressure or a bulky dressing or pillow secured to the chest. Treat for pneumothorax or hemothorax if signs and symptoms are present.

Tracheal or Bronchial Tree Injury

Injuries to the trachea or bronchial tree are rare in sports because they are usually the result of a penetrating or blunt trauma. The signs and symptoms must be recognized because it can be a fatal condition. Penetrating upper airway injuries can be associated with major vascular injuries and extensive tissue destruction. Signs and symptoms include shortness of breath, mediastinal shift, subcutaneous emphysema, and hemoptysis. Mechanism of injury and history are vital, and the clinical findings may be subtle. In this blunt injury, either the trachea or mainstream bronchus will be ruptured. The signs that may be present can include subcutaneous emphysema of the chest, face, or neck or even associated pneumothorax or hemothorax.

Management of tracheal or bronchial tree injury includes maintaining an open airway, activating emergency medical services ([EMS] if not already on scene), administering high-flow supplemental oxygen, and transporting the athlete to the hospital immediately.

DIAPHRAGMATIC TEARS

Tears in the diaphragm may result from a severe blow to the abdomen and can occur in a large variety of sporting events. A sudden increase in intra-abdominal pressure, such as a kick, punch, or elbow to the abdomen, may tear the diaphragm and allow herniation of the abdominal organs into the thoracic cavity. This occurs more commonly on the left side than the right side because the liver protects the right diaphragm. The blunt trauma may produce large radial tears in the diaphragm. Penetrating trauma may also produce holes in the diaphragm, but those tend to be small.

This injury may be difficult to diagnose, even in the hospital. The clinical signs may include marked respiratory distress, diminished breath sounds, and infrequent bowel sounds, which may be heard when the chest is auscultated. The abdomen may present with a sucked-in appearance if a large quantity of abdominal contents is in the chest.

Management for diaphragmatic tears includes treating for shock, assisting with breathing, supplemental oxygen, and immediate transfer to a medical facility.

ESOPHAGEAL INJURY

Injury to the esophagus is usually produced by a penetrating trauma, and it is rare in sports. However, sports emergency care personnel must be able to recognize this injury because it can be fatal if unrecognized. Signs and symptoms of esophageal injury include stridor, hoarseness, dysphagia, subcutaneous emphysema, and oropharyngeal/nasopharyngeal bleeding. Management of associated trauma is extremely important as well. Treat for shock, provide supplemental oxygen, and package the patient as soon as possible and transport to a hospital because operative repair will be required for this injury.

PULMONARY CONTUSION

A pulmonary contusion is a common injury that occurs from blunt trauma. Bruising of the lung results from passage of a shock wave through the tissue. Injuries involving high velocity rather than slow crushing are more likely to cause pulmonary contusion. Contusion of the lung may produce marked hypoxemia.

Pulmonary contusions are rarely diagnosed on physical examination. The mechanism of injury may suggest blunt chest trauma, and thus there may be obvious signs of chest wall trauma such as bruising, rib fractures, or flail chest. These suggest the presence of an underlying pulmonary contusion. Crackles may be heard on auscultation but are rarely heard in the emergency room and are nonspecific. Patients with pulmonary contusions should be referred to a physician for further evaluation.

STERNAL FRACTURE/CONTUSION

Sternal fractures result from a high-impact blunt trauma to the chest. While it is more common in automobile accidents than in sports, it can still occur in sports. Sports emergency care personnel must be aware of this injury because it can result in an injury to the underlying cardiac muscle.

Clinical signs and symptoms of this injury may be point tenderness over the sternum that will worsen with deep inspiration or forceful expiration. Signs of shock may indicate an injury to the underlying tissue. In the field, it is difficult sometimes to differentiate between the sternal contusion and fracture, and an X-ray will help make the differential diagnosis.

RIB FRACTURES/CONTUSIONS

Rib contusions are common in sports. These injuries occur more frequently in collision sports like football, hockey, lacrosse, and wrestling but can also occur in other sports. A direct blow to the rib cage can contuse intercostal muscles or fracture them if the blow is severe enough.

Because the intercostal muscles are essential to breathing, the athlete may experience sharp pain with expiration, inspiration, coughing, laughing, or sneezing. There will be point tenderness over the rib cage and pain with compression of the rib cage.

Rib fractures are especially common in collision sports. Fractures can be caused by direct and indirect trauma. Ribs 5 through 9 are the most commonly fractured.

The direct-blow rib fracture causes the most serious damage because the external force fractures and displaces the ribs inward. Such a mechanism may completely displace the bone and cause fragmentation. The fragments may cut, tear, or perforate the tissue of the pleurae (hemothorax) or they may collapse one lung (pneumothorax). Contrary to the direct injury, the indirect fracture usually causes the rib to fracture outward, producing an oblique or transverse fracture. Stress fractures can also occur. Repetitive movements like throwing or rowing or repetitive coughing or sneezing can result in a rib stress fracture.

Rib fractures are either easily detectable due to a deformity or difficult to detect. An athlete should always be examined thoroughly for any underlying conditions that may occur. The athlete should be stabilized and immediately transported to a medical facility if there is a possibility of an unstable fracture.

COSTOCHONDRAL SEPARATION/DISLOCATION

Costochondral separations occur from a direct blow to the anterolateral aspect of the thorax or indirectly from a sudden twist or fall on a ball that compresses the rib cage.

The costochondral injury displays many signs that are similar to the rib fracture, with the exception of the location of the pain. The pain location of this injury will be localized in the junction of the rib cartilage and rib. The athlete will complain of sharp pain with sudden movement of the trunk and difficulty breathing deeply. There is point tenderness.

Management of costochondral separations and dislocations includes ice and referral to a physician for follow-up.

THORACIC SPINE FRACTURE

Thoracic spinal fractures can occur whenever forces exceed the strength and stability of the spinal column. Thoracic spine fractures are uncommon in sports but need to be recognized because spinal cord injuries represent the second most serious long-term morbidities resulting from thoracic trauma, with traumatic aortic rupture being the first.[1]

Fractures most commonly occur in the lower thoracic vertebrae and are less common in the upper and mid-thoracic vertebrae. The ribs and the orientation of the facets stabilize the upper thoracic spine (T1–T10). However, at the T12–L1 junction, increased range of motion allows combinations of acute hyperflexion and rotation. The mechanisms of thoracolumbar spine trauma are hyperflexion, vertical compression, hyperextension, and shearing injury.

Hyperflexion injury includes flexion with compression, lateral flexion, flexion-rotation, and flexion-distraction injuries. These mechanisms can occur in collision sports and some non-contact sports. A vertical compression mechanism results in burst injuries of the vertebral body. Hyperextension injuries result in posterior spinal compression fractures, while shearing injury can cause subluxation or dislocation of the spinal column.

Management of Thoracic Spine Injury/Trauma

Maintain spinal immobilization
Establish an open airway
Activate EMS
Treat for shock
Administer high concentration oxygen
Monitor oxygen saturation with a pulse oximeter
Transport the athlete rapidly to a hospital
Notify medical direction

The athlete may experience pain or point tenderness in the thoracic region or paralysis below the chest or waist with a thoracic spine injury. The lower extremities may be cool.

CONCLUSION

Most thoracic injuries, although rare in sports, can be life threatening in nature. It is important to recognize these life-threatening conditions because it is vital that the athlete receives prompt intervention, EMS activation, and transport to the nearest hospital. It is extremely important that most of the injuries in this chapter are recognized by the sports emergency care team and treated properly in the field because it may help save the athlete's life.

SUMMARY OF KEY POINTS

➡ Acute thoracic injuries can be among the most serious in sports because they can impose a threat of long-term disability, and in the most severe cases even death.

➡ A tension pneumothorax can occur when a one-way valve is created from either blunt or penetrating trauma. A spontaneous pneumothorax is a rare condition found occasionally in athletes and occurs in the absence of trauma or disease.

➡ A hemothorax occurs when blood enters the pleural space.

➡ Flail chest is defined as a fracture of 2 or more adjacent ribs in at least 2 places, and typically occurs in contact sports like football, hockey, wrestling, and lacrosse.

➡ Penetrating upper airway injuries to the trachea or bronchial tree can be associated with major vascular injuries and extensive tissue destruction.

➡ Tears in the diaphragm may result from a severe blow to the abdomen, causing a sudden increase in intra-abdominal pressure.

➡ Esophageal injuries are produced by penetrating trauma and are rare in sports.

➡ A pulmonary contusion is a common injury that occurs from blunt trauma and may produce marked hypoxemia.

➡ Sternal fractures result from a high-impact blunt trauma to the chest.

➡ Rib contusions and fractures are common in sports. These injuries occur more frequently in collision sports like football, hockey, lacrosse, and wrestling and cause sharp pain with expiration, inspiration, coughing, laughing, or sneezing. Rib fractures are either easily detectable due to a deformity or difficult to detect.

➡ Costochondral injury displays many signs that are similar to the rib fracture, with the exception of the location of the pain. The pain location of this injury will be localized in the junction of the rib cartilage and rib.

➡ Thoracic spine fractures are uncommon in sports but need to be recognized because spinal cord injuries represent the second most serious long-term morbidities resulting from thoracic trauma, with traumatic aortic rupture being the first.

REVIEW QUESTIONS

1. Define tension pneumothorax, spontaneous pneumothorax, and hemothorax.
2. What is the proper care for flail chest?
3. What are the signs and symptoms of a pulmonary contusion?
4. What is the most common mechanism of injury for a thoracic spinal fracture?
5. What is the most important concern in managing a tracheal or bronchial tree injury?

REFERENCES

1.   Nadalo LA, Chew FS. Thoracic spinal trauma imaging. http://emedicine.medscape.com/article/397896-overview. Accessed September 30, 2012.

BIBLIOGRAPHY

Anderson MK. *Foundations of Athletic Training: Prevention, Assessment and Management.* 4th ed. Baltimore, MD; Lippincott Williams and Wilkins; 2009.

Campbell JE. *BTLS: Basic Trauma Life Support for the EMT-B and the First Responder.* Upper Saddle River, NJ: Pearson Prentice Hall; 2004.

Ciocca M. Pneumothorax in a weight lifter: the importance of vigilance. *Phys Sportsmed.* 2000;28(4):97-103.

Curtin SM, Tucker AM, Gens DR. Pneumothorax in sports: issues in recognition and follow-up care. *Phys Sportsmed.* 2000;28(8):23-32.

Copass MK, Gonzales L, Eisenberg MS, Soper RG. *EMT Manual.* 3rd ed. Philadelphia, PA: WB Saunders Co; 1998.

Micheli LJ. *The Sports Medicine Bible.* New York, NY: Harper Perennial; 1995.

Prentice W. *Arnheim's Principles of Athletic Training: A Competency-Based Approach.* 14th ed. New York, NY: McGraw-Hill; 2011.

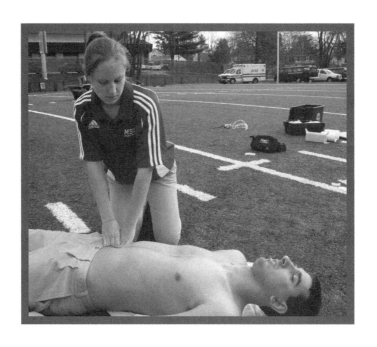

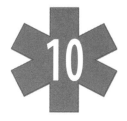

Abdominal and Pelvic Injuries

David A. Middlemas, EdD, ATC

> *As a member of the medical team for the local martial arts competition, you have the responsibility to provide on-the-mat medical care for the athletes during the fighting competitions. During a bout, one of the athletes is kicked in the upper abdomen. He goes to his knees, takes a couple of moments to gather himself, and then continues the bout. A few minutes later, he collapses and is complaining of abdominal pain. You approach the athlete to begin your assessment.*
> *What is wrong? How bad is it? What do you do?*

Emergencies involving the abdominal and pelvic regions are not uncommon in sports. Athletes and others participating in exercise are subject to pain and discomfort resulting from injuries or illness involving the internal organs of the abdomen. The sports emergency care team members providing emergency care for individuals participating in sports need to be aware of the potential causes of abdominal problems in athletes, their signs and symptoms, and their role in recognizing the nature and extent of injury so the athlete can be referred for appropriate medical care.

Many sports and physical activities involve intentional and unintentional collisions with other athletes, impact with sports implements, and high-velocity movement and twisting. The ability of the sports emergency care team member to recognize and interpret the effects of events in exercise and sports on the internal organs of the abdomen is essential to determining the extent of injury and the need for immediate action. This chapter will provide the reader with an overview of the anatomy of the abdominopelvic region, assessment of abdominal injuries, and medical conditions and guidelines for immediate care.

Rehberg RS.
Sports Emergency Care: A Team Approach,
Second Edition (pp 143-159).
© 2013 SLACK Incorporated.

Figure 10-1. The abdominopelvic cavity. (Illustration by Joelle Rehberg, DO.)

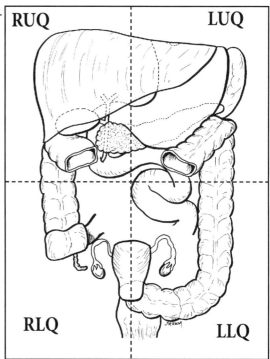

REVIEW OF CLINICALLY RELEVANT ANATOMY

The abdominal cavity is defined as the area below the thoracic cavity that contains many of the body's internal organs. It is separated from the thorax by the diaphragm and lined with a membrane called *peritoneum*. The lower portion of the abdominal cavity surrounded by the pelvis, vertebra, and sacrum is called the *pelvic region* (Figure 10-1).

The location of the organs in the abdomen and pelvis is usually described by dividing the abdomen into 4 quadrants. The abdominal quadrants are defined by drawing a vertical and horizontal line through the navel. The quadrants and the structures located within them are shown in Figure 10-1. The quadrants are called the left upper quadrant (LUQ), right upper quadrant (RUQ), left lower quadrant (LLQ), and right lower quadrant (RLQ). The quality of communication between medical professionals and the accuracy of injury records is improved when everyone involved in the care of the injured athlete uses the same terminology.

The liver, gallbladder, spleen, pancreas, and the digestive organs (stomach, small intestine, and large intestine) are contained in the abdominal cavity. The urinary bladder and female reproductive organs are in the pelvic region, with male genitalia being external. It is important to note that the kidneys are not within the abdomen. They are located outside the peritoneum behind the abdominal cavity, covered by the muscles of the back and protected by the lower ribs.

To assist in understanding the nature of emergencies in the abdominopelvic region and their implications, it is important to understand the basic structure and functions of the organs in this region. It is helpful to divide the organs into 2 categories—hollow organs and solid organs (Table 10-1).

Hollow organs either allow materials to pass through them, as in the stomach and intestines, or serve as "holding tanks" for materials until they are needed or expelled from the body, as in the gallbladder or urinary bladder. As a rule, hollow organs tend to be injured less in sports and

Table 10-1
CATEGORIES OF ORGANS OF THE ABDOMINAL AND PELVIC CAVITIES

Solid Organs	*Hollow Organs*	*Reproduction*
Liver	Stomach	Female: ovaries, uterus, and vagina
Spleen	Small intestine	Male: scrotum, testes, and penis
Pancreas	Large intestine	
Kidney	Gallbladder	
	Urinary bladder	

physical activity because they are at significantly less risk when they are empty. The best way to prevent injuries to the hollow organs is to have them as empty as possible when participating in sports or exercise. Such things as not eating immediately before competition and urinating before a game or practice significantly reduce the risk of injury to digestive organs and the urinary bladder.

Solid organs do not have cavities inside them to hold or store fluids. They tend to have significant blood supplies that are necessary to complete their functions. The solid organs include the liver, spleen, pancreas, kidneys, ovaries, and testes. The very fact that these organs will not easily compress when suffering a collision, combined with their ample blood supply, place them at a higher risk of bruising or tearing with potentially life-threatening bleeding.

The liver, primarily located in the RUQ, is the largest solid organ of the body. It has many functions, including making bile, converting glucose to glycogen for storage, producing urea, and storing multiple substances for the body. As a result of these critical functions, it has a very rich blood supply. Injuries to the liver can result in serious bruising or significant bleeding into the abdominal cavity.

The spleen is located in the LUQ of the abdomen. Its job is to filter blood and to store red blood cells and platelets. It has a plentiful blood supply and is at risk for injury from blows to the upper abdomen. It is also important to note that the spleen swells in individuals who have had mononucleosis, thus increasing the risk of injury from contact or collision.

Although the kidneys are located outside the abdominal cavity, their function of producing urine is critical to the body. The kidneys, which are on the back of the body, are somewhat protected by the ribs. The process of filtering waste products from the blood produces urine. It then flows through the ureters to the urinary bladder, which is located in the lower abdominal cavity. Because the kidneys are the primary filters that remove waste from the bloodstream, they have a very rich blood supply. Although the lower ribs cover the kidneys, blows to the kidneys can cause significant injuries.

The majority of reproductive organs in women are within the abdominal cavity. The ovaries, uterus, fallopian tubes, and vagina are internal, placing them at significantly less risk for injury than the male's external reproductive anatomy. The male reproductive anatomy is more likely to be injured from a direct blow or collision due to the fact that it is external. The penis, which has a rich blood supply, and the testes, which are solid, have little protection.

AVOIDING INJURY

Preventing abdominal injuries in athletes is very important and requires the efforts of many individuals. The sports emergency care team member, coach, official, parents, and even the athlete can be essential to preventing or reducing the occurrence of abdominal trauma in sports. By working together, everyone can ensure that athletes have the proper equipment, learn and use correct sports technique, and that rules are appropriately taught and enforced.

Protective equipment for the abdominal region includes such items as baseball and softball chest protectors and extensions for shoulder pads in sports such as football and ice hockey. In order to get the best protection possible, the coach and sports emergency care team member must work together to ensure that protective equipment is in good repair, meets required standards, and fits the athlete properly. The athlete is a critical link in helping to keep his or her equipment safe. Reporting damaged or ill-fitting equipment allows for immediate repair or adjustment of any problems before an injury occurs.

Proper technique in those sports where contact and collision are part of the game is essential to reducing injury. Coaches and officials can work together to reduce the occurrence of injury by teaching proper methods of contact and collision and to appropriately penalize those who abuse the rules.

Finally, there are times where the best method for preventing a potentially devastating situation is to disqualify an individual from participation in certain activities where the potential for injury is unacceptable for that person. Examples of situations in which a physician might disqualify an athlete from participation in collision or contact sports may include absence of a paired organ, such as a kidney or eye, or a medical condition that could place the athlete in danger. It may be appropriate in these situations to substitute an activity with lower risk of injury for the involved athlete.

EVALUATION AND RECOGNITION OF ABDOMINAL INJURIES

Many of the emergencies encountered in the athletic venue can be assessed by directly visualizing and touching the injured tissue. However, evaluation of injuries and medical conditions in the abdominal region requires the practitioner to apply knowledge and skills that will allow him or her to recognize emergencies without the ability to directly access the affected organ or tissue. This section will help the caregiver to understand the use of vital signs to recognize illnesses and injuries requiring indirect methods of evaluation.

We begin our discussion with an explanation of the concept of "indirect methods of evaluation." Unlike such things as open wounds or bruising, injuries to internal organs and structures require the caregiver to evaluate the status of an affected body part by looking at "something else." Usually that "something else" is one or more of the vital signs. The caveat here is that a victim who has been participating in exercise or sports will likely have vital signs that are different from those of a resting patient immediately before the injury occurs. These differences, which may be interpreted as abnormal for the average person, are the norm or baseline for determining the extent of injury in someone who was physically active at the time he or she was hurt. It is important for the emergency caregiver to be familiar with these differences as he or she begins the assessment (Table 10-2). A summary of the differences is presented in Chapter 3.

In athletic situations, injuries to the abdomen usually involve a collision with another athlete, running into an object such as a wall or fence, or being struck by an athletic implement like a bat or stick. These impacts often occur in the course of play, and the injured athlete may or may not appear to be injured immediately after the incident. The primary concern in these situations is that of internal bleeding from damaged internal organs, especially those with ample blood supply, like the liver, spleen, and kidneys. Injuries to these structures have the potential to be life threatening and may require surgery. It is important for the sports emergency care team member to collect information quickly and efficiently in situations in which abdominal trauma may be present. Decisions relating to the possible extent of injury and immediate course of care will depend on the caregiver's ability to assess the situation and get the athlete to appropriate medical care in a timely fashion.

Table 10-2
EXAMPLES OF CHANGES IN DIAGNOSTIC SIGNS AND WHAT THEY MAY INDICATE

Diagnostic Sign	Change	Possible Cause
Blood pressure	Below normal	Internal bleeding
Pulse	Weak, rapid	Shock Internal bleeding
Respirations	Rapid	Internal injury Internal bleeding Pain
Skin color	Pale Bruising	Shock Internal bleeding Evidence of direct blow
Abdominal palpation	Rigidity Guarding	Internal bleeding Pain Injury to internal organ

In the ideal situation, abdominal injury assessment begins with observation of the events leading up to the injury and the mechanism of injury. For example, a running back in football who is struck in the middle of the back with another player's helmet may have a kidney injury, or a lacrosse player who gets the butt of another player's stick thrust into the LUQ of the abdomen might have ruptured the spleen. In order to gain the most information from observing the events leading up to an injury, the caregiver must have an understanding of the anatomy of the injured body region and the possible injuries that can result from the event causing the injury.

It is not unusual for the sports emergency care team member to be called to the location of an injury after it has occurred. The disadvantage in these situations is that he or she was not able to witness the mechanism of injury. Information about how the injury occurred must be gathered by observing the injured athlete and surroundings as one approaches and by asking questions of the athlete, coaches, officials, and other players to determine how the accident happened and the extent of possible injuries. It is usually best to take the history using a structured interview format such as the SAMPLE history (signs/symptoms, allergies, medications, past medical history, last oral intake, events leading to injury illness; see Chapter 3 for more details).

Like any emergency situation, the first concern of the caregiver is to assess the injured athlete for the presence of severe or potentially devastating injuries or conditions. When life-threatening problems such as absence of breathing or pulse or severe bleeding are present, the sports emergency care team member should take the appropriate actions to immediately deal with the problem. When the injured athlete is determined to be in no immediate danger, a more thorough examination, or secondary survey, that can focus on the potential abdominal injury should take place.

Understanding what caused the injury is particularly helpful when dealing with internal injuries because the sports emergency care team member must make decisions about injured organs that cannot be directly seen or touched. The care provider should ask the patient where and how the blow to the abdomen took place and what the patient felt immediately at the time of injury. Questions about the nature and intensity of any pain, lightheadedness or dizziness, nausea, and

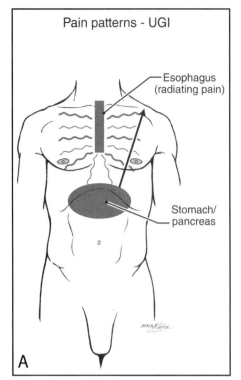
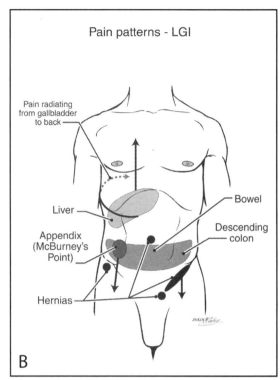

Figure 10-2. Referred pain patterns. (Reprinted with permission from O'Connor DP, Fincher AL. *Clinical Pathology for Athletic Trainers: Recognizing Systemic Disease.* 2nd ed. Thorofare, NJ: SLACK Incorporated; 2008.)

any other abnormal feelings or sensations at the time of injury and afterward will help the rescuer get an overall understanding of the possibility of internal injury to the athlete.

After determining the mechanism of injury, one of the first concerns in assessing abdominal injuries is the location and nature of the patient's pain. Generally, the injured athlete will have pain at the location of the injury. For example, if a hockey player has an injury to the liver after being checked into the boards, one would expect pain in the RUQ of the abdomen; if the spleen is ruptured after being hit in the abdomen with a lacrosse stick, one would expect pain in the LUQ of the abdomen and so on. Victims of internal organ injuries may have pain or soreness at places away from the injured structure in addition to pain at the location of the injury. This phenomenon is called *referred pain*. Referred pain is a condition in which pain from an injury or illness in one part of the body presents in another location of the body. One example is Kehr's sign, which is a referred pain pattern for an injury to the spleen in which the patient will have pain or soreness in the left shoulder. Some referred pain patterns are presented in Figure 10-2.

Questions about lightheadedness, nausea, and changes in sensations around the abdomen provide information about whether or not there might be internal bleeding from injured structures in the abdomen. Because any bleeding from abdominal injuries cannot be directly observed, the caregiver must look for signs and symptoms that indicate the presence of secondary conditions caused by the internal bleeding. A secondary condition is one that occurs as a result of an injury or illness existing in the body. The most significant secondary condition when it comes to suspecting the possibility of internal bleeding is shock, of which lightheadedness, dizziness, and nausea are symptoms.

Remember that a comprehensive patient history will collect information from the athlete, the other players in the area, officials, and coaches about the causes of the injury and the patient's condition. The answers to questions about what happened, the presence and nature of any pain, and other feelings or sensations help the caregiver understand the potential severity of the injury and set the basis for the hands-on portion of the patient assessment.

THE PHYSICAL EXAMINATION

The sports emergency care team member will conduct a physical assessment after collecting information about the nature and cause of the injury to verify what was learned in the history and to pinpoint the specific structures that may have been injured. The physical examination should assess appropriate vital signs and include palpation of the abdomen.

A primary concern of the sports emergency care team member when caring for patients with potential internal bleeding from injuries to solid internal organs, like the liver and spleen, is the onset of shock. The sports emergency care team member should be prepared to assess the rate and quality of the athlete's pulse and respirations. It is also important to assess the victim's blood pressure. As with any other bleeding injury, changes in vital signs provide information about the patient's current status and the stability of his or her condition. Vital sign assessment should focus on changes that indicate the possibility of internal bleeding, such as a weak rapid pulse, changes in rate and quality of breathing, drop in blood pressure, pale skin, and sweating. Patients with significant blood loss may also present with changes in their level of consciousness consistent with those of patients in shock.

Injuries to hollow organs present the additional problem of leakage of their contents into the abdominal cavity. The presence of such things as urine or bowel contents in the abdominal cavity creates the additional dangers of significant infection in the abdominal region and inflammation and irritation of the lining of the cavity. This is called *peritonitis*. The sports emergency care team member may find elevated body temperature, elevated skin temperature, and severe abdominal pain. These conditions may require surgery and/or the administration of antibiotics by the physician, and—if not treated promptly—may be life threatening.

Palpation of the abdomen (Figure 10-3) can be very helpful in determining the nature and extent of injuries to the region. Abdominal assessment should include the ability to recognize guarding, abdominal rigidity, and rebound tenderness. Guarding occurs when the athlete tightens the muscles of the abdominal wall when the sport emergency care team member applies pressure to the abdomen at a point where the athlete has pain. Guarding can be an indication of acute abdominal pain and/or inflammation to internal organs and serves as an attempt to protect the area from additional aggravation. Abdominal rigidity presents as contraction of the muscular walls of the abdomen so that the abdomen feels firm or hard to the touch of the evaluator. It can indicate swelling in the abdomen, possibly related to bleeding, abdominal pain, or patient apprehension about being touched. Pain upon quickly releasing the abdominal wall after slow pressure is called *rebound tenderness*. It is an indicator of pain in the abdominal lining and happens in response to the rapid stretching of the irritated tissue after pressure. It is a sign commonly found in individuals with acute appendicitis.

When you assess someone for abdominal injury, remember to complete the following:
Take a thorough history.
Determine the events leading up to the injury and what actually happened.
Take and record the patient's vital signs.
Take them again frequently to look for any changes that may indicate a change in the patient's status.
Palpate the abdomen. Note any rigidity or guarding.

Figure 10-3. Palpation of the abdomen.

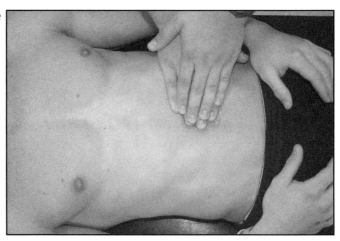

ABDOMINAL AND PELVIC INJURIES

Direct blows to the abdomen can result in injuries ranging from surface contusions and muscle bruises to significant internal organ damage. This section will present some common abdominal injuries, their common causes, and how they usually present.

Blows to the anterior surface of the abdomen tend to cause injuries to the organs and structures in the abdominal cavity where the impact took place. Because solid organs such as the liver and spleen are located in the upper 2 quadrants of the abdomen, internal bleeding is of particular concern when the athlete is struck at that location. Staying with the classification of internal injuries into those involving either solid or hollow organs, let us first look at how injuries to some of the solid organs might present themselves.

SOLID ORGAN INJURIES

The spleen is located under the stomach in the LUQ of the abdomen. Contusions or rupture of the spleen can occur as a result of a direct blow to the LUQ. Athletic activities that might result in injury to the spleen include such things as tackling in football, collisions or checking in ice hockey, or being struck in the abdomen with a sports implement such as a stick or bat. The victim will have pain in the LUQ. In addition, spleen injuries may present with Kehr's sign. If the spleen is ruptured, there will be internal bleeding, which may be delayed by the organ's ability to splint itself. When this happens, internal bleeding, and hence the signs and symptoms of shock, begin sometime after the injury takes place. Patient evaluation will often reveal tenderness in the LUQ, possibly rebound tenderness, nausea, and signs and symptoms of shock. Athletes in contact and collision sports with medical conditions such as mononucleosis are at increased risk of spleen injury due to enlargement of the organ. Physician clearance should be obtained before these athletes return to their sports activities.

The liver is the largest solid organ in the body. It occupies the majority of the RUQ and is susceptible to contusion or laceration from direct blows to the abdomen. Like the spleen, it is highly vascularized and injuries have the potential to bleed into the abdomen relatively quickly. Victims of a lacerated liver may have pain on deep palpation, rebound tenderness, and nausea and can develop signs and symptoms of shock fairly quickly. Referred pain may present in the center of the chest and under the left arm.

Blows to the back can cause injury to the kidneys. Contusions or lacerations to the kidneys can result in internal bleeding. Often an injury to the kidney will present with localized pain over the "flank" that may be intense and burning. Palpation of the back in the area of the kidneys can elicit tenderness. The victim of a kidney contusion or laceration might also have a burning sensation while urinating, blood in his or her urine (hematuria), loss of the ability to urinate, and/or referred pain in the lower abdominal region.

HOLLOW ORGAN INJURIES

Injuries to hollow organs like the urinary bladder, stomach, and intestines can usually be prevented by having them as empty as possible before activities with the potential for collisions or contact. Although some bleeding can occur with injuries to these organs, the main concern is the spilling of contents into the abdominal cavity, causing inflammation, infection, and peritonitis. Generally speaking, these victims will present with abdominal pain, tenderness on palpation, abdominal guarding, and signs and symptoms of inflammation and infection, including fever and soreness. There may also be nausea and vomiting.

An injury to the urinary bladder can occur from a direct blow to the midline in the pelvic region. Spilling of urine into the abdominal cavity can cause severe pain and inflammation in the lower abdomen.

Open wounds in the abdominal cavity or those involving penetrating objects present the possibility of internal bleeding and infection. Open abdominal injuries can occur from sports implements such as the javelin or a ski pole or collisions with equipment such as metal fence posts.

Injuries to the genitalia can occur in sports in which there is the possibility of being struck in the groin area by a ball or sports implement or in a collision with another athlete. Because the majority of female reproductive organs are internal, genital injuries in female athletes are not very common in sports. Direct blows to the genital area can cause contusions or lacerations, which the sports emergency care team member can care for using ice or appropriate bandaging. The sports emergency care team member should take care to protect the privacy or modesty of the victim at all times by moving to a private area or covering the athlete with a blanket or other available item. Males, on the other hand, have a higher risk of genital injury because the anatomy is outside the abdominal cavity. Injuries to male genitalia include contusions to the scrotum, testes, and penis; testicular torsion; and laceration or entrapment of anatomy in clothing or equipment. Athletes participating in activities in which there is a risk of injury to the external genitalia should be required to wear a cup protector.

Blows to the groin area can result in painful injuries to the external anatomy in males. It is not uncommon for contusions and lacerations to happen as a result of being hit by another athlete, a ball, or sports implement. Lacerations to the penis are of concern because of the rich blood supply in the area, and thus they have the potential to bleed freely. Lacerations to the scrotum can be superficial or deep enough to expose and damage the testicle. Superficial wounds that are bleeding can be treated the same as any other laceration, taking care to preserve the victim's dignity. Deeper lacerations involving the penis or scrotum should be considered emergent and the athlete transported by ambulance to the emergency room.

Closed injuries to the male genitals can be very serious. A direct blow to the groin can result in deep contusion or fracture of a testicle or tearing of a blood vessel in the scrotum. In either case the situation is an emergency. Disruption of blood supply to the testicle can possibly result in loss of the organ if not cared for by a physician immediately and properly. These sorts of injuries present with significant pain in the scrotal area accompanied by significant swelling in the scrotum and require immediate transportation to the emergency room.

Testicular torsion is a medical emergency that can result in loss of blood supply and possibly result in loss of the testicle. In this condition the testicle can rotate in the scrotum. When this happens, the blood supply can be cut off. The patient complains of sudden pain and swelling on one side of the scrotum or in one of the testes. Testicular torsion is often the result of a predisposing situation in which the testicle is not adequately attached to the inside of the scrotum.

This condition is seen most frequently in boys but has been seen in adults. The condition must be addressed promptly with surgery to restore the blood supply.

EMERGENCY CARE OF ABDOMINAL AND PELVIC INJURIES

When suspecting abdominal injury, it is important to continue monitoring the patient's vital signs for changes that would indicate the possibility of internal bleeding. The sports emergency care team member should evaluate the injured athlete's pulse, respirations, skin color and temperature, and—when possible—blood pressure. Weak rapid pulse; rapid shallow breathing; pale, cool, and clammy skin; and decreased blood pressure are all indicators of internal bleeding that will send the patient into shock. The injured athlete may also complain of nausea and dizziness and may vomit.

> *Once an abdominal injury is suspected, the following steps should be taken:*
> *Activate the emergency action plan.*
> *Place the victim in a comfortable position. The recovery position will assist in maintaining a patent airway in the event the patient is nauseated or vomits.*
> *Treat for shock.*
> *If the victim does not have a spinal or head injury, elevate the feet and legs.*
> *Maintain the athlete's body temperature by using a blanket, jacket, or some other covering when necessary.*

It is important that the victim's vital signs be assessed for changes at regular intervals while waiting for the ambulance and during transportation to the hospital. Do not give the injured athlete anything to eat or drink because internal injuries may require surgery. Because the sports emergency care team member is not able to control internal bleeding directly, it is important to be prepared to provide basic life support in the event the patient's condition should worsen significantly.

There are times when an athlete may suffer an abdominal injury with an impaled object. One example of this would be an individual struck in the abdomen with a javelin. As with all injuries involving impaled objects, it is important to leave the object in place, pad it, and bandage it where it is. The caregiver must continue to be aware that the visible injury is complicated by the possibility that the javelin (or other object) is also penetrating an internal organ and that moving it could result in significant internal bleeding.

An additional consideration with an impaled sports implement like a javelin is that it may not fit into the back of the ambulance. In rare cases, the sports emergency care team may need to summon rescue personnel for assistance in cutting the impaled object to a length that will allow the victim to be safely transported with it bandaged in place. Professional rescue personnel will have access to specialized equipment such as the Jaws of Life (Hurst, Shelby, NC), which can cut the post or implement with as little movement as possible.

COMMON MEDICAL EMERGENCIES
IN THE ABDOMEN AND PELVIS

There will be times when athletes will have abdominal pain or discomfort that is not a result of an injury or collision. Although the sports emergency care team member cannot directly treat

Table 10-3

SUGGESTED OUTLINE FOR STRUCTURED INTERVIEW FOR ABDOMINAL INJURIES OR CONDITIONS

Abdominal Injury		*Illness*
What happened? (Were you hit? Was there a collision?)		Describe the problem.
Where were you hit?		Have you eaten anything you do not usually eat?
What did you feel at the time of injury?		Please list the symptoms.
Have you had this problem before? Are you nauseous? Have you vomited? Does it hurt?		
O	Onset	When did the problem begin? What caused it?
P	Provokes/ palliates	What makes it better? What makes it worse?
Q	Quality	Describe your pain (ie, is the pain sharp, dull, achy, burning?).
R	Region/radiates	Where does it hurt? Does the pain move or spread?
S	Severity	Rate your pain on a scale from 1 to 10.
T	Timing of the pain	Has it been constant? Does it come and go? How long has the pain been there?

the cause of the problem, assessment and recognition of medical conditions in the abdomen can prevent significant problems. Timely awareness of potentially serious illness will allow the athlete to be referred to a physician for rapid diagnosis and treatment.

The patient is said to have an acute abdomen when he or she suddenly develops abdominal pain. Conditions that can lead to abdominal pain or discomfort can be relatively minor or they can be severe. A physician will be able to determine if the pain can be alleviated through medication and conservative treatment or whether the patient requires more invasive care, such as surgery.

EVALUATING AND RECOGNIZING MEDICAL CONDITIONS IN THE ABDOMEN

The sports emergency care team member should observe the patient for signs indicating the location and intensity of pain. Facial expression, sweating, and posture provide information about the severity of the pain. The athlete may be lying on his or her side with knees drawn up to try to alleviate the pain. It is also important to take a history focusing on the abdomen in order to identify the possible causes of the pain.

The primary focus in taking a history for a person complaining of abdominal pain is the location, nature, and intensity of the pain (Table 10-3). The sports emergency care team member can easily remember what to ask the patient by using OPQRST described in Chapter 3. This mnemonic serves as a reminder to ask about the onset (the start of the problem), provocation and palliation (what makes it feel better or worse), quality (sharp, dull, ache, burning), region (where

Figure 10-4. Assessing bowel sounds.

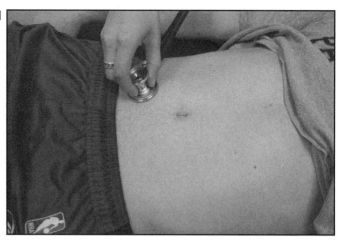

it hurts), severity (how much it hurts), and the timing of the pain. Information about nausea and vomiting, diarrhea, constipation, and fever often provides additional information that identifies the cause of the problem.

The patient's answers from the history will guide the sports emergency care team member in performing a physical exam concentrating on the abdomen. Take the patient's vital signs. The steps in the assessment process should be explained to the patient to reduce stress and apprehension. The 4 quadrants of the abdomen should be palpated. Begin away from the suspected location of the pain and work toward it. Gently press on the regions of the abdomen, feeling for rigidity and/or guarding. Ask the patient if he or she can relax the abdomen. When the location of the pain is identified, check for rebound tenderness. Note the results of the assessment and record the information so it can be communicated to the physician.

The sports emergency care team member can also quickly check to see if the patient's bowel sounds are present (Figure 10-4). The absence of normal bowel sounds can indicate the possibility of such problems as bowel obstruction or significant abdominal injury or illness. Place the head of the stethoscope on the anterior abdomen. Listen to all 4 quadrants of the abdomen. Normal bowel sounds include a combination of squeaking and gurgling sounds, indicating that intestinal contents are being moved through the digestive system. If the sounds are diminished or absent, the information should be recorded in the patient notes and communicated to the physician.

REDUCING THE LIKELIHOOD OF ABDOMINAL PAIN

Many of the nontraumatic causes of abdominal pain, such as acute appendicitis, gall- or kidney stones, and kidney or bladder infections, result from medical conditions or emergencies that cannot be predicted by the patient. There are no effective prevention strategies that target these sorts of conditions. Basic common sense lifestyle choices, such as a well-balanced diet, adequate hydration, and close attention to bodily changes, can help reduce the chances of medically related problems.

EMERGENCY CARE OF THE ACUTE ABDOMEN

The need for emergency transportation and treatment for an individual with abdominal pain would be dictated by the onset and severity of the pain, the possible underlying cause, and the stability of the patient's vital signs. Individuals with moderate to severe abdominal pain accompanied by vital sign changes such as altered pulse or blood pressure, fever, chills, nausea, vomiting, and/or signs of shock should be made as comfortable as possible and monitored while awaiting transportation to a hospital. The location and nature of the pain may provide the sports emergency care team member with clues as to its possible cause, but definitive diagnosis and treatment by a physician are essential for these patients. Under these circumstances, the patient should be given nothing to eat or drink while waiting for the ambulance because it may aggravate the condition or make it more difficult in the event surgery is required.

In many cases, teenagers and adults with relatively minor episodes of abdominal pain or discomfort may have had it before. Such conditions as indigestion, irritable bowel syndrome, or menstrual cramps may be significant enough to affect an athlete's ability to exercise or compete, but they do not usually require emergency transportation and treatment. Athletes who do not have a history of abdominal discomfort should stop their activity, be made comfortable, and be referred to their physician for diagnosis and appropriate treatment. Those who have recurrent or chronic episodes of minor abdominal conditions may have already been advised by their health care provider on how to care for discomfort or minor pain when it occurs. In these situations it is appropriate to assist the athlete in following the instructions he or she has been given by the doctor.

The most effective method of determining the patient's knowledge regarding the abdominal discomfort or pain is by taking a comprehensive history related to the abdominal discomfort. Asking the athlete about when the pain started, the severity of the pain, and factors that worsen or lessen the pain can verify whether or not the episode is a recurrence of an existing problem or something new. Listening carefully to the patient's answers to questions can help the sports emergency care team member to identify whether or not the athlete is familiar with the problem. In any situation in which the athlete has had to stop participation due to abdominal pain or discomfort, it is appropriate to make sure a qualified medical professional has assessed him or her before returning to play. In situations in which the athlete is a minor, it is imperative that the parent or guardian be advised of the situation. In many cases, reviewing the options for follow-up with a physician provides the parent and athlete with information they need and a degree of comfort.

OTHER MEDICAL CONDITIONS OF THE ABDOMEN AND PELVIS

The information in this section presents the signs and symptoms for common medical conditions of the abdomen. This information can help the sports emergency care team member in deciding the potential severity of the problem and the type of assistance that is needed.

Some causes of abdominal discomfort or pain are relatively minor and may resolve with little medical treatment. Other illnesses or conditions causing abdominal pain can be significant and may be life threatening if not diagnosed by a physician and treated properly. The role of the sports emergency care team member is to recognize signs and symptoms in the athlete that indicate potential abdominal illness and facilitate getting the patient to the appropriate medical professional in a timely fashion. Signs and symptoms of medical conditions in the abdomen are presented to provide background information for the sports emergency care team that helps them recognize the athlete's need for medical care.

Problems with the organs of the digestive system often give the patient abdominal pain. The pain can be burning, sharp, dull, or intense.

Dyspepsia is a term that describes pain in the upper abdomen that may come and go but is usually present the majority of the time. Common causes of dyspepsia are gastroesophageal reflux disease (GERD) and stomach ulcers. GERD is a condition in which acid from the stomach splashes out of the upper valve onto the walls of the esophagus. The patient will complain of burning pain in the mid-upper abdomen and/or heartburn. The pain may be constant but is sometimes relieved when the patient eats or takes an antacid. Occasional heartburn may not be a significant problem, but recurrent burning pain in the upper abdomen may be a sign of GERD, which has the potential to cause long-term damage to the esophagus. Stomach ulcers are wounds in the lining of

Figure 10-5. Palpation of McBurney's point.

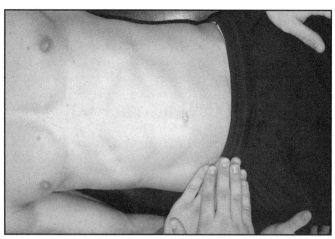

the stomach. They may be caused by stress, a virus, or dietary concerns. Ulcers also present with abdominal pain, burping, nausea, and/or heartburn. The potential for significant bleeding exists if ulcers go untreated because they are open wounds in the stomach lining. A physician should evaluate persistent upper abdominal pain and burning in order to provide proper treatment.

Generalized abdominal pain can result from a number of conditions in the intestinal tract. Intestinal gas can cause significant pain in the abdomen that might be strong enough to cause an athlete to double over. Often "gas pains" are accompanied with increased bowel sounds, or "gurgling," and will resolve themselves.

Irritable bowel syndrome is a term used to describe conditions that cause abdominal pain, diarrhea, and significant discomfort in the abdominal region. The term includes conditions like Crohn's disease and ulcerative colitis. Abdominal pain can also be caused by pockets or folds in the walls of the intestines, called *diverticula*, that become infected or inflamed, causing pain, nausea, vomiting, fever, and changes in bowel habits. This condition is called *diverticulitis*. A physician should properly diagnose and treat an athlete with frequent instances of abdominal pain that persist for a prolonged period of time.

Infection and inflammation of the appendix can cause significant abdominal pain, nausea, vomiting, diarrhea, and fever. Acute appendicitis is often identified by pain in the RLQ of the abdomen, referred pain to the area of the navel, and rebound tenderness at the location of the appendix, called McBurney's point (Figure 10-5). Failure to recognize the signs and symptoms of appendicitis can allow the problem to progress as the infected appendix continues to swell and fill with pus. If left untreated, the appendix will eventually rupture, spreading the infection's contents into the abdomen. When this happens, the patient has a potentially life-threatening condition that causes inflammation to the peritoneal lining and serious infection to the abdominal cavity.

There are medical conditions that do not present as emergencies, but the members of the sports emergency care team may be the first to whom the athlete reports the onset of symptoms relating to the illness. Listening to the pattern of symptoms and performing an initial assessment to determine the potential severity of the condition can be essential to preventing the progression of a condition to a serious problem.

An athlete with discomfort or pain in the RUQ with referred pain to the right shoulder may be suffering from an inflamed gallbladder (cholecystitis) or gallstones. The pain can be aggravated by fatty foods as bile is essential to their digestion. The individual may also have nausea and vomiting, depending on the severity of the condition.

An individual with unexplained abdominal pain, joint ache, fever, loss of appetite, nausea or vomiting, and fatigue may have contracted hepatitis. Hepatitis is a disease that affects the liver and is most often caused by a virus. There are 5 types of hepatitis. Hepatitis type A is the most common in the United States, but cases of type B and C are not uncommon. Hepatitis is contagious and is spread through such routes as unsanitary conditions, blood, feces, and sexual contact. The cause of the symptoms and the proper course of care must be determined by the physician after proper diagnostic testing.

Medical conditions of the urinary tract involve the kidneys, ureters, and bladder. Infections in the urinary tract can present with pain in the lower abdominal region and pubic area. Athletes with kidney infections can have low back soreness or pain, fever, and difficulty urinating. Infections in the urinary bladder, ureters, and/or urethra can cause pain or burning during urination.

The development of kidney stones can cause pain in the flank region of the back that radiates to the genital area. The pain can become severe and even disabling. Abnormal urinary habits and painful urination often occur in patients with kidney stones. Physician intervention is necessary to resolve the problem using one or more of many available treatment methods.

Abdominal pain may present in the female athlete as part of her normal menstrual cycle. Pain in the lower middle portion of the abdominopelvic region may occur in the middle of the menstrual cycle, which is associated with release of the egg from the ovary, or may occur with cramping during the menstrual period. The severity of the pain and cramping varies with the individual. When assessing a female athlete with lower abdominal pain, she is usually able to provide information relating to her normal pattern of pain and cramping during the menstrual cycle.

Sometimes abdominal pain in girls or women is due to medical conditions requiring the attention of their general physician or gynecologist. Patients who develop ovarian cysts can have severe pain in the abdominal or pelvic region and may also present with vaginal bleeding, nausea, and fever. Athletes who suddenly develop these symptoms should be treated as a medical emergency.

Ectopic pregnancy occurs when the fertilized egg implants in the wall of the fallopian tube outside the uterus. Women with a possible ectopic pregnancy can become dizzy and faint, develop low blood pressure, and have vaginal bleeding. It is important to tactfully ask female patients whether they may be pregnant during the history portion of the examination to rule out the possibility of gynecological causes for abdominal pain or symptoms.

We would be remiss in not providing a short discussion of the possibility of sexually transmitted diseases (STD) in the athletic population. The likelihood that sexually active individuals will be seeking advice and treatment from sports emergency care professionals they trust supports the need to recognize the signs of a potential STD. When the athlete communicates the onset of lesions, sores, or unusual skin problems on the genitals; unusual discharges from the penis or vagina; or pain during urination or intercourse, he or she may be communicating the presence of symptoms of STD. The sports emergency care team member should maintain the confidence and dignity of the athlete while strongly encouraging or requiring him or her to seek appropriate medical care for the condition. Since STDs are contagious, strongly encouraging medical follow-up and care provides appropriate care for the athlete and anyone with whom he or she has intimate contact.

Conclusion

The role of the sports emergency care team member or other emergency responder in dealing with emergencies in the abdomen and pelvic regions is to identify the potential causes of the athlete's problem and select the appropriate course of immediate care and referral for medical treatment. In order to be able to provide the best on-site care for the athlete, one should possess the ability to assess victims of both abdominal trauma and those whose abdominal pain may be due to medical conditions. The sports emergency care team member's ability to recognize the signs of significant abdominal injury or illness provides the basis for sound decision making and access to prompt emergency care.

The potential effects of internal bleeding or infection due to such conditions such as a ruptured appendix can be minimized by rapid identification of the problem's cause through effective assessment and immediate access to medical care. Daily contact between the athlete and the sports emergency care team member or other emergency care provider can play the most important role in early recognition of significant abdominal injury or illness by providing the athlete with a trusted professional to whom he or she can go immediately when discomfort, pain, or injury occur.

SUMMARY OF KEY POINTS

➡ Evaluation of injuries and medical conditions in the abdominal region requires the practitioner to apply knowledge and skills that will allow him or her to recognize emergencies without the ability to directly access the affected organ or tissue.

➡ Proper protective equipment and proper technique are essential in reducing injury.

➡ Victims of internal organ injuries may have pain or soreness at places away from the injured structure in addition to pain at the location of the injury. This phenomenon is called referred pain.

➡ Shock is a primary concern of the sports emergency care team member when caring for patients with potential internal bleeding from injuries to solid internal organs, such as the liver and spleen.

➡ Abdominal assessment should include the ability to recognize guarding, abdominal rigidity, and rebound tenderness.

➡ Direct blows to the abdomen can result in injuries ranging from surface contusions and muscle bruises to significant internal organ damage. This section will present some of the common abdominal injuries, their common causes, and how they usually present.

➡ Blows to the anterior surface of the abdomen tend to cause injuries to the organs and structures in the abdominal cavity where the impact took place.

➡ Injuries to hollow organs like the urinary bladder, stomach, and intestines can usually be prevented by having them as empty as possible before activities with the potential for collisions or contact.

➡ Injuries to the genitalia can occur in sports in which there is the possibility of being struck in the groin area by a ball or sports implement or in a collision with another athlete.

➡ When suspecting abdominal injury, it is important to continue monitoring the patient's vital signs for changes that would indicate the possibility of internal bleeding.

➡ The victim's vital signs should be assessed for changes at regular intervals while waiting for the ambulance and during transportation to the hospital.

➡ As with all injuries involving impaled objects, it is important to leave the object in place, pad it, and bandage it where it is.

➡ The sports emergency care team member can easily remember what to ask the patient by using the OPQRST acronym.

➡ The need for emergency transportation and treatment for an individual with abdominal pain is dictated by the onset and severity of the pain, the possible underlying cause, and the stability of the patient's vital signs.

➡ The most effective method of determining the patient's knowledge regarding the abdominal discomfort or pain is by taking a comprehensive history related to the abdominal discomfort.

➡ Generalized abdominal pain can result from a number of conditions in the intestinal tract.

➡ Some abdominal pain in girls or women is due to medical conditions requiring the attention of their general physician or gynecologist.

REVIEW QUESTIONS

1. What conditions might cause abdominal rigidity and guarding?
2. A severe blow to the RUQ of the abdomen might produce what kind of injury?
3. Why is a splenic rupture considered a medical emergency?
4. Describe proper care for a patient with an acute abdomen.
5. What are some causes of severe abdominal pain specific to women?

BIBLIOGRAPHY

American Red Cross. *Emergency Response.* Yardley, PA: Staywell Publishing; 2001.

American Urological Association. Testicular torsion. http://www.urologyhealth.org/urology/index.cfm?article=34. Accessed October 1, 2012.

Booher JM, Thibodeau GA. *Athletic Injury Assessment.* 4th ed. New York, NY: McGraw Hill; 2000.

Cuppett M, Walsh K. *General Medical Conditions in the Athlete.* St. Louis, MO: Mosby; 2005.

Finch R, Banting SW. Commentary: modern management of splenic injury. *ANZ J Surg.* 2004;74(7):513.

Klepac SR, Samett EJ. Spleen trauma imaging. http://emedicine.medscape.com/article/373694-overview. Accessed September 30, 2012.

Kluger Y, Paul DB, Raves JJ, et al. Delayed rupture of the spleen—myths, facts, and their importance: case reports and literature review. *J Trauma.* 1994;36(4):568-571.

Limmer D, O'Keefe M, Dickinson EV, Grant H, Murray B, Bergeron JD. *Emergency Care.* 10th ed. New York, NY: Prentice Hall; 2005.

Penetrating abdominal trauma: guidelines for evaluation. Trauma.org. http://www.trauma.org/index.php/main/article/414/. Accessed October 1, 2012.

Pollak AN, ed. *Emergency Care and Transportation of the Sick and Injured.* 9th ed. Boston, MA: Jones and Bartlett Publishers; 2005.

Prentice WE. *Arnheim's Principles of Athletic Training: A Competency-Based Approach.* 12th ed. New York, NY: McGraw-Hill; 2006.

Tamparo CD, Lewis MA. *Diseases of the Human Body.* 3rd ed. Philadelphia, PA: FA Davis; 2000.

Wright JA. Seven abdominal assessment signs every emergency nurse should know. *J Emerg Nurs.* 1997;23(5):446-450.

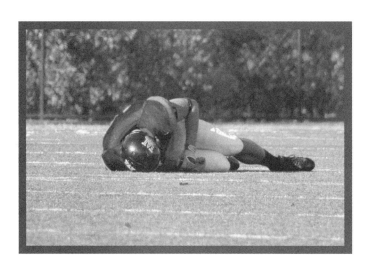

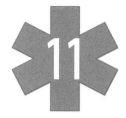

Fractures and Soft Tissue Injuries

Michael A. Prybicien, MA, ATC, CSCS, CES, PES and Louis Rizio, MD

> *A 15-year-old volleyball player is participating in drills during practice. When a teammate spiked the ball over the net, she dove to dig it, and landed on an outstretched arm. You arrive to evaluate the athlete, who is complaining of severe pain in the shoulder. She is guarding the arm by holding it against her side. You note an obvious deformity at the acromioclavicular joint. The area was point tender, but no crepitus was noted. What would you do?*

Fractures, dislocations, and soft tissue injuries are among the most common injuries sustained in sports. This chapter aims to provide a straightforward approach to understanding injuries to bone and soft tissue and the initial evaluation and management of such injuries. Proper initial evaluation and management are critical to ensure the athlete receives the proper medical attention, gets transferred to the hospital for further evaluation when appropriate, and most importantly is protected from further harm.

REVIEW OF CLINICALLY RELEVANT ANATOMY

BONE

This chapter will focus on bones of the extremities. Information on spinal anatomy can be found in Chapter 6. The bones of the arms and legs are long bones, each composed of an epiphyseal, metaphyseal, and diaphyseal segment (Figure 11-1). The epiphyseal segment is the portion of the bone that forms one side of a joint and is typically covered with articular cartilage. The

Rehberg RS.
*Sports Emergency Care: A Team Approach,
Second Edition* (pp 161-178).
© 2013 SLACK Incorporated.

Figure 11-1. Bone. (Illustration by Joelle Rehberg, DO.)

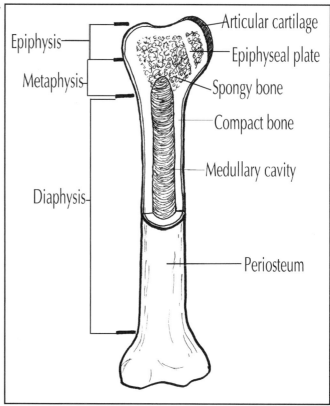

metaphyseal segment is adjacent to the epiphyseal segment. The epiphyseal and metaphyseal segments fuse together once the individual reaches skeletal maturity. In childhood, bone growth occurs at the growth plate, which is between the epiphyseal, metaphyseal, and diaphyseal segments. The diaphyscal segment is the shaft of the long bone and is very strong.

Diaphyseal bone is composed of cortical bone, which is very strong and supports the body's weight. Metaphyseal bone tends to be wider and less tubular in appearance and is the portion of the long bone that forms one end of a joint. This metaphyseal bone is composed of cancellous bone and is not as strong as cortical bone.

JOINTS

The joints of the extremities are called synovial joints. The joint is formed by the proximal end of one bone and the distal end of another bone and is held together by a capsule and ligaments. The ends of each bone are covered with articular cartilage, which provides a low friction surface for motion and also a cushion for shock absorption. The connection of the 2 bones in this type of arrangement allows for motion of the joint; the ligaments and capsule provide stability (Figure 11-2). The capsule of the joint can be divided into a fibrous (outer) layer and synovial membrane (inner) layer. The ligaments that hold the joint stable are often thickenings of the fibrous layer made of dense collagen. The synovial layer makes synovial fluid that bathes and nourishes the cartilage surfaces of the bones forming the joint.

SOFT TISSUE

Soft tissue is a broad term that can be used to describe many tissues in the musculoskeletal system. While the skin can be considered soft tissue and will be covered in the wound management

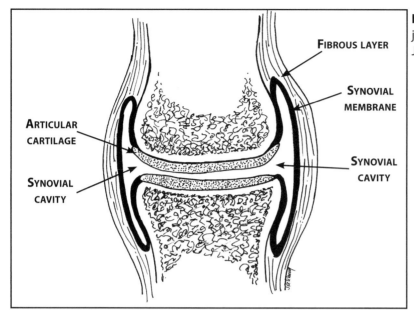

Figure 11-2. Synovial joint. (Illustration by Joelle Rehberg, DO.)

FIBROUS LAYER

SYNOVIAL MEMBRANE

SYNOVIAL CAVITY

ARTICULAR CARTILAGE

SYNOVIAL CAVITY

section of this chapter, for the purposes of this section soft tissue refers to ligaments, tendons, and muscle. All of these structures are composed predominantly of collagen, but the type of collagen varies between the tissues. These soft tissues are critical for the normal functioning and action of joints. These structures allow for motion and stability of the joints they cross.

Ligaments usually attach on either side of the joint and connect one bone to another. Their major function is to provide stability to the joint it crosses. Injury to a ligament is termed a *sprain*. It is a good idea to keep terminology accurate, especially when communicating with other members of the health care system; this avoids confusion and will hopefully convey the message most effectively.

Tendons are the connection between bone and muscle. It is the tendon attachment to bone that allows a muscle to move a joint. Muscle tissue shortens (contracts) under voluntary control to produce movement. Injury to the tendon or muscle is termed a *strain*. Tearing of a tendon can lead to inability to move an extremity or joint, especially if completely torn.

FRACTURES

"Is it broken or just fractured?" There is no distinction between breaks and fractures; they are one in the same. The disruption of the bone's continuity is what defines this injury. Fracture can occur from a direct blow or a rotational (twisting) injury without contact.

EVALUATION

The typical signs of a fracture are pain, swelling, and tenderness over the area. Movement of the extremity will aggravate the athlete's symptoms, and he or she cannot often bear weight on the lower extremity or move the upper extremity due to discomfort. Loss of function of the extremity is usually apparent.

Initial assessment of an injured and potentially fractured extremity includes a careful inspection of the limb, especially the skin. The clothing should be removed around the injured limb for complete inspection. Any wounds over the painful area should be considered indicative of an open

Figure 11-3. Immobilization of wrist and forearm injuries using a SAM splint.

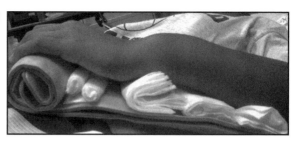

(compound) fracture. Deformity may be present, indicating severe malalignment or displacement of the fractured ends (Figure 11-3). Tenderness over the bone is usually present and sometimes motion can be felt between the fractured ends; this is highly suspicious of a fracture.

A careful assessment of vascular supply and nerve function distal to the injury is vital. Sensory function is assessed grossly by determining the athlete's ability to feel the examiner's touch. This should be done on all surfaces of the limb circumferentially. In addition, an assessment of muscle function below the injury level is performed to determine motor nerve function. For example, ability to move all the toes or fingers up and down can give a gross estimate of nerve function. Any loss of sensation or movement below the injury needs to be documented prior to any splinting or immobilization.

Vascular status or circulation is evaluated as well. Pulses should be felt below the level of the injury. In addition, a cold, very white (pallor), or blue extremity signals severe injury to the blood supply of the extremity. Capillary refill is not a reliable method of determining adequacy of the blood supply to the limb. All pulses felt or not felt need to be documented prior to transfer or immobilization.

INITIAL TREATMENT

If a fracture is suspected of the lower extremity, carrying the athlete off the field or assisting with ambulation to prevent weightbearing on the injured extremity is necessary. A splint or immobilization device is utilized to protect the injured extremity from undue motion. Typically, it is best to immobilize on the field as far above and below the area in question as possible. A good rule of thumb is to immobilize a joint above and below the injured area. The athlete should be sent for confirmatory X-rays. Examples of basic extremity splinting will be presented at the end of the chapter.

FRACTURE EMERGENCIES

An open (compound) fracture is an orthopedic emergency, and the athlete should be transported to a hospital for immediate treatment, which includes thorough operative irrigation and removal (débridement) of dirt, debris, or foreign material (ie, clothing pieces); stabilization; and antibiotics by intravenous administration. Initial management of an open fracture is listed in Table 11-1.

Loss of circulation to a limb is uncommon, but it needs to be corrected as soon as possible. When severe deformity exists to a limb and the circulation is compromised, straight traction on the limb may reduce pressure on a blood vessel from a displaced bone end or remove a "kink" in the vessel from the angulated position of the limb. Traction should be applied gently, slowly, and in line with the limb; never should an attempt to forcibly reduce the fracture be performed. Documenting circulation before and after this maneuver is critical information for the treating emergency department to have. Also, transportation to the hospital should not be delayed in order to try and get circulation to return while the athlete is on the field. Splinting is then performed

---

Table 11-1
EMERGENCY MANAGEMENT OF AN OPEN FRACTURE

- Cover the wound with Betadine (iodine)- or alcohol-soaked gauze bandage.
- Immobilize the limb.
- Transfer the patient to the hospital immediately. (Infection risk increases if not treated within the first 6 hours!)

---

with the traction being held; this will improve the chances the limb will remain "straight" after splint application.

Compartment syndrome can occur following fracture due to rapid swelling in the closed compartments of the leg and forearm. The lower leg (below the knee) and forearm (elbow to hand) are the most common locations where a compartment syndrome can develop; however, it should never be assumed it cannot occur anywhere else (ie, thigh, foot, or hand). The classic signs of compartment syndrome are remembered as the "5 Ps": pain, pallor (whiteness), paresthesia (numbness or tingling), pulselessness, and paralysis.

Severe damage may have already occurred to the limb once symptoms progress to more noticeable symptoms that would cause an athlete to seek treatment. The pain with compartment syndrome is usually severe, unresponsive to splinting and medication, and out of proportion to what one might expect to see from an injury. Bandages or compression wraps can make symptoms worse and should be loosened; this alone sometimes relieves the pain. If the loosening of the bandage or wrap relieves the pain, it is likely that a full-blown compartment syndrome has not yet occurred. If there is any question, immediate transfer to the hospital is required. Surgery is usually the only treatment for this syndrome.

DISLOCATIONS

A dislocation is the most severe form of ligament and/or joint capsule injury. The normal relationship between the 2 bones forming the joint is lost; basically, the "ball is out of the socket."

EVALUATION

Dislocations can occur at any joint. There is an obvious injury in most cases and the individual may have heard a "pop" or felt the joint "slide" out of place. Pain is usually severe and motion is virtually impossible.

Attempts to passively range the joint are unsuccessful; there is a block to motion from the abnormal relationship of the 2 ends of the joint to one another. The ends are overlapping, creating a block to motion. The athlete is typically holding the injured limb to protect him- or herself from painful attempts at moving the joint (commonly known as *splinting*). A deformity is usually more obvious with a superficial joint, such as the fingers.

As with any extremity injury, careful evaluation of nerve function below the injury level is critical. Document all nerve function prior to any attempts at reducing the joint. Vascular status should similarly be evaluated and documented. The signs of nerve and vascular injury, as noted previously for fractures, apply to dislocations as well.

INITIAL TREATMENT

A trained member of the medical team can attempt a gentle reduction or "popping" the joint back in place. Forceful attempts to reduce the joint should never be attempted because there can be a tendon, ligament, or piece of bone trapped in the joint, preventing reduction. Also, a forceful reduction can cause a fracture or make an associated fracture worse. Always follow local protocol regarding attempted reduction of dislocations.

If the initial reduction attempt is successful, there will usually be a much more fluid motion to the joint and the athlete will be nearly pain free. In this scenario, the athlete can be placed in a splint or immobilizer (depending on the joint involved) and sent for X-rays that day or evening. It is important to always get X-rays to rule out a fracture and ensure there has been an adequate reduction. Often, an athlete can tell if the joint is reduced or not; when told by an individual that the joint is "not in," this should be taken seriously.

In the event that a trained and qualified person to reduce the joint is not available, the athlete should be transported to the local emergency room for X-rays and reduction there. Also, any signs of nerve or vascular injury require immediate transfer to the hospital, even if a successful reduction has been performed.

EMERGENCIES

As with fractures, any open dislocations require immediate attention. Also, any nerve or vascular injuries should be considered emergencies. As stated above, a joint that cannot be reduced should also be considered an emergency.

PRINCIPLES OF SPLINTING

Splinting of fractures, dislocations, or other extremity injuries has a number of benefits and should be included in the initial emergency management. Splinting benefits the injured athlete in the following ways:

* Reduces pain and swelling
* Prevents further blood vessel and nerve injury from sharp fracture ends
* Prevents sharp fracture ends from piercing the skin (turning a closed fracture to an open one)
* Decreases further contamination of open wounds

GENERAL PRINCIPLES

Sports emergency care personnel should follow these guidelines whenever splinting a fracture or dislocation:

* Remove clothing around the suspected injury to make sure there are no open wounds or deformities.
* Check pulse and nerve function below level of injury prior to splinting.
* Cover wounds with sterile dressing as noted previously (see Table 11-1).
* Splint should immobilize above and below area of injury.
* Pad splint well to avoid pressure points from rigid splints.
* Hold extremity immobile until splint hardens in desired position.
* If a deformity cannot be "straightened" by gentle, continuous traction, splint the limb in the position of deformity.

Table 11-2
SPLINTING MATERIALS

Splint Material	Padding Required	Water Required	Reusable	Heat Required
Plaster	Yes	Yes	No	No
Fiberglass	Yes	Yes	No	No
Aluminum	No	No	Often	No
Plastic	Sometimes	Sometimes	Yes	Yes
Pneumatic	No	No	Yes	No

MATERIALS

There are a variety of options when it comes to splinting, and all have their own pros and cons. It is beyond the scope of this chapter to critically analyze each type of splint, but general principles will be addressed. Splints come in plaster, fiberglass, metal (usually aluminum for easy molding), moldable thermoplastic material, and pneumatic (air splints). In addition, there are numerous preshaped splints; however, the "do-it-yourself" molding types usually are the most versatile. The advantage of prefabricated splints is they do not require water or heat to work. In general, most items can be used for a variety of extremity and joint injuries. The athletic trainer should sample several different splints and splinting materials to decide which he or she is most comfortable using. Proper preparation before an injury occurs will decrease the chance the athletic trainer is on the field with an emergency and does not have the proper tools. What is presented here is an example of different, available materials and is by no means all-inclusive. Table 11-2 provides some basic points on material types. Figure 11-4 shows examples of different materials commonly used.

The sports emergency care team should keep several different types and sizes of splinting material on hand. Cast padding of various sizes should be on hand for use when using plaster or fiberglass splints. Padding will decrease pressure from the splint and protect the skin. The padding, like splinting material, comes in a variety of sizes (typically 1 to 6 inches) in order to accommodate most joints and extremities. A bucket to fill with water is useful as well because plaster and fiberglass need to be wet in order to shape and to set or harden. A good pair of scissors to cut the material is essential as well. Gloves should be used when utilizing plaster and especially fiberglass to protect the user's hands. Several sizes of elastic bandages are required to hold the splint in place.

COMPLICATIONS OF SPLINTING

The major complication of splinting is a compartment syndrome. This is usually secondary to the cast padding or elastic bandage being wrapped too tightly or the application of a circumferential cast being applied too tightly. It is rarely necessary to apply a circumferential cast in the field, so this should not be a problem. As noted earlier, pain that is severe or out of proportion to what is expected is the first sign of an impending compartment syndrome. When an athlete complains of this kind of pain or tightness, it should raise a red flag. Simply loosening the elastic wrap will usually rapidly relieve the pain (within minutes). Avoiding the placement of cast padding circumferentially around the injured extremity will help to avoid this complication as well.

Figure 11-4. (A) SAM splint. Padded aluminum core for easy use and molding. (B) Different view of SAM splint. (C) Aluminum splints for small joint (finger) splinting. Padded and can be cut to fit better. Also, easily molded and can be secured with tape or elastic bandage. (D) Fiberglass material. Fiberglass, like plaster, requires water to harden or "set." Comes in variety of sizes from 1 to 6 inches, can literally be used to splint any joint or extremity. (E) Pneumatic splint. This is a Cramer Rapid Form Vacuum Immobilizer (Cramer Products Inc, Gardner, KS).

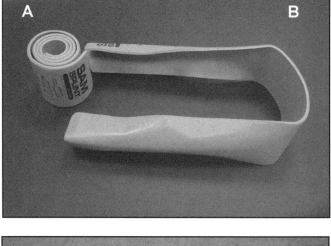

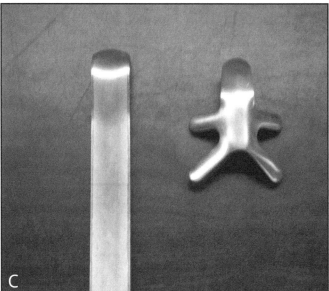

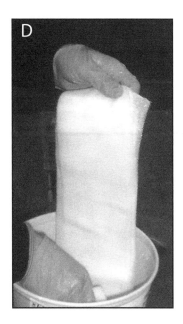

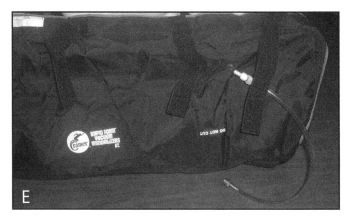

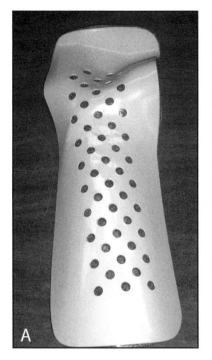

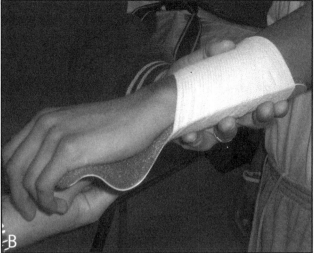

Figure 11-5. Wrist splint application.

Splinting by Extremity

Hand and Wrist

Prefabricated splints are easy to use and versatile for the majority of hand and finger injuries. They can often be used as protection and allow for functional return to athletic competition depending on the sport and the severity of the injury. Figure 11-5 shows examples of splints applied to the hand and wrist. The reader should realize that any plaster or fiberglass splint could be fashioned to work in the same way. Usually, the splint is applied to the volar (palm side) of the hand for hand and wrist injuries. The splint is applied to the hand and wrist area, and an elastic bandage is wrapped around the splint to hold it in place. When making a fresh splint from plaster or fiberglass, be careful to use enough padding to avoid pressure points and heat injury while the material hardens.

Splints such as the aluminum types shown in Figure 11-4C are good for isolated finger injuries. These finger splints are typically placed on the dorsal (opposite palm side) for finger splinting. This allows for comfort and possible continued use of the hand while the splint is worn.

Forearm and Elbow

It is often helpful to have the athlete lie down and an assistant hold his or her fingers for support. These splints need to include the elbow joint to provide the most stability and comfort. This type of splint is commonly referred to as a sugar-tong splint. A SAM splint (SAM Medical Products, Wilsonville, OR) is easy to use and easily molded for this application. In addition, it is reusable. However, any of these splints can be made out of simple plaster and/or fiberglass. Figure 11-6 shows an example of SAM splint application for a forearm injury. As shown in this example, including the hand improves comfort for forearm/elbow injuries because the muscles that move the wrist cross the elbow and insert or originate from the humerus.

Another useful splint for injuries to the forearm and elbow is the posterior splint. Again, this can be made of plaster, fiberglass, or from SAM splinting material. See Figure 11-7 for an example

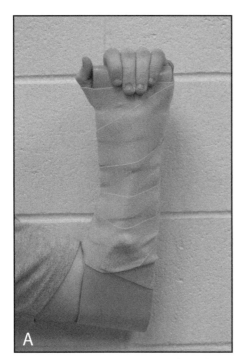 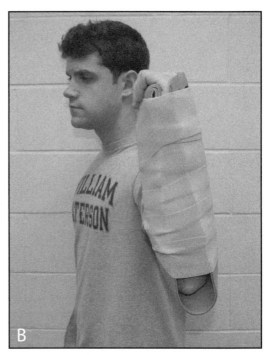

Figure 11-6. Immobilization of the forearm using a SAM splint.

of a posterior splint application utilizing plaster as the material. The cast padding is laid out to the appropriate length (based on the individual's arm length); the plaster is then laid out to be slightly smaller length than the padding. Usually 8 layers of plaster are utilized; too few layers make the splint weak, and too many layers can increase the risk of thermal injury. The plaster is placed in water and then back onto the padding; an additional layer of padding is placed on top, covering the plaster on both sides. The splint is held in place and wrapped with an elastic bandage.

Arm

Splinting suspected humerus fractures is basically the same as for elbow and forearm injuries, but the splint wraps around the elbow and the arm above. Also, a simple sling may be sufficient if no splinting material is available or for comfort to hold the arm while in a splint. A sling is usually all that is required for shoulder injuries because splinting the shoulder is difficult. The posterior splint (see Figure 11-7) can be used for this as well.

Thigh and Knee

Immobilizing the thigh can be difficult. In this scenario, a pneumatic splint may be the best splint to provide stability to a suspected femur fracture. Also, ligament sprains and fractures of the knee are well immobilized in these splints. If a deformity exists, it is helpful to have an assistant pull gentle traction from the foot to "straighten" the leg. Holding the leg in this position prior to applying the pneumatic brace or splint will increase the chances that the deformity will not return while in transport to the hospital. Figure 11-8 shows a Cramer Rapid Form Immobilizer being placed on a knee.

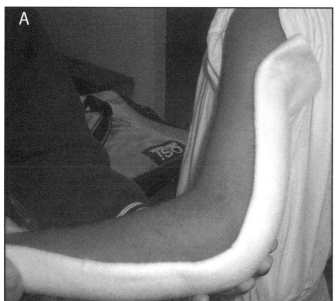

Figure 11-7. Elbow immobilization.

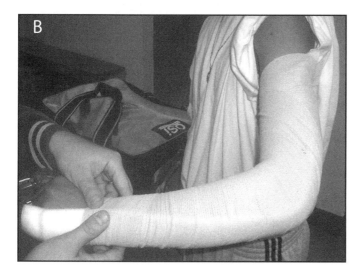

Leg, Ankle, and Foot

There are a variety of ways to splint this area. The vacuum splint in Figure 11-8 can work well for leg or tibia injuries, or the sugar-tong splint in Figure 11-6 can easily be made for a leg or ankle injury. The SAM splint, fiberglass, or plaster can all be used to make the splint. The posterior splint is simple and useful as well. This is basically the same as the splint shown in Figure 11-7 but adapted for the leg. A posterior leg splint utilizing fiberglass is shown in Figure 11-9. When applying a splint to the leg, the ankle should be held as close to neutral or a 90-degree angle as possible, as shown in Figure 11-9.

Figure 11-8. Vacuum splint application.

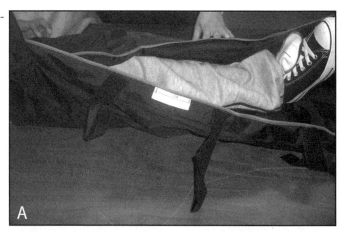

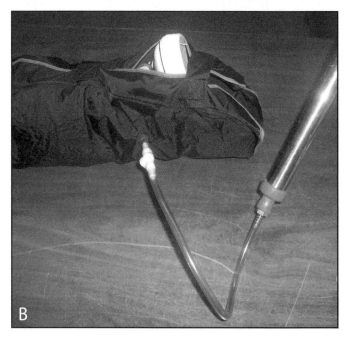

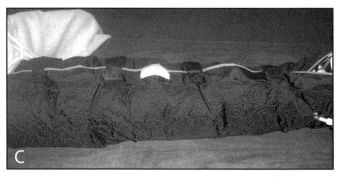

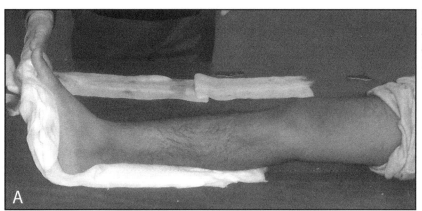

Figure 11-9. Splint application to the ankle and lower leg.

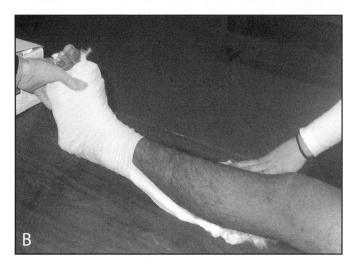

OPEN WOUNDS

An open wound is an injury in which the skin is interrupted, or broken, exposing the tissue underneath. The interruption can come from the outside such as with a laceration or from the inside such as when a fractured bone end tears outward through the skin. Sports emergency care personnel should be sure to observe body substance isolation and utilize personal protective equipment before treating any athlete with an open wound (Table 11-3).

TYPES OF OPEN WOUNDS

Abrasions and Lacerations

The classification of abrasions includes simple scrapes and scratches in which the outer layer of the skin is damaged but all layers are not penetrated. "Road rash," "mat burn," "floor burn," and skinned knees and elbows are examples of abrasions. There may be no detectable bleeding or only a minor ooze of blood from the capillary beds. The patient may be experiencing great pain, even if the injury is minor. The opportunity for infection is great because of dirt or other substances ground into the skin.

A laceration is a cut that can be either smooth (resembling an incision) or jagged. This type of wound is often caused by an object with a sharp edge, such as a piece of sharp metal or broken

> ## Table 11-3
> ## OPEN WOUND GENERAL TREATMENT GUIDELINES
>
> These guidelines are general guidelines; see each specific type of wound for more detailed guidelines.
> - Isolate the body substance.
> - Expose the wound.
> - Clean the wound surface. Simply remove large pieces of debris with a sterile dressing.
> - Control the bleeding. Start with direct pressure or direct pressure and elevation. When necessary, employ pressure. (A tourniquet is only to be used as a last resort!)
> - Treat for shock in cases of more serious wounds.
> - Wrap with a sterile dressing when available.
> - Bandage the dressing in place when bleeding has been controlled.
> - Check distal pulses.

glass. However, a laceration can also result from a severe blow or impact with a blunt object (ie, being punched or being struck by a hockey puck or ball). It may be difficult to determine the extent of damage in lacerations with rough edges because the damaged flaps of skin may hide damage to the underlying tissues. Obviously, deeper wounds will produce significant bleeding. However, bleeding may be partially controlled in some wounds by the natural retraction and constriction of the damaged blood vessels.

The first step in treating abrasions and lacerations is to reduce wound contamination. Bleeding from a large or deep laceration may be difficult to control. Applying direct pressure over the wound should always be the first method of bleeding control. Using direct pressure, followed by the application of a dressing and a pressure bandage, can control most wounds. In cases of more severe bleeding, an air-inflated splint or blood pressure cuff can be useful in the management of bleeding; however, great care must be taken to prevent further injury or complications that may arise from overinflation of the splint or cuff. A wound closure such as a butterfly-type bandage or Steri-Strips (3M, St. Paul, MN) can help keep wound ends together temporarily in severe lacerations. Pulses and motor and sensory functions should be checked distal to the injury. In cases when bleeding from lacerations cannot be controlled with the abovementioned treatment, the patient may require sutures, plastic surgery, and/or a tetanus shot, thus referral to a physician or hospital is required.

Puncture Wounds

Puncture wounds can be caused by objects that go undetected on playing fields or courts, such as nails, knives, splinters, or other sharp objects. The threat of contamination in a puncture wound is significant. A penetrating puncture wound can be shallow or deep. A perforating puncture wound has both an entrance wound and an exit wound. These wounds are not very common in sports as the most common example is a gunshot wound.

Use caution when treating puncture wounds. An object that appears to be embedded only in the skin may actually go all the way to the bone. In such cases, it is possible that the patient may not have serious pain due to either shock or damage to the nerves. Even an apparently moderate puncture wound may cause extensive internal injury with serious internal bleeding. What appears at first to be a simple, shallow puncture wound may be only part of a bigger, more severe injury. There also could be an exit wound that requires immediate care, so always be sure to evaluate for one.

A puncture wound may contain an impaled object. In sports, the object can be a piece of glass, a post, a sharp piece of metal, a javelin, or possibly even a wooden stick from a broken bat piercing any part of the body. Even though it is rare, the sports emergency care personnel may be confronted with a case where the impaled object is too long to make even emergency transport possible without shortening the object (ie, a javelin). In such cases, the sports emergency care personnel team must work together to determine what is the best direction to move in for the athlete/patient. In most cases, someone must hold the object, keeping it very stable, while it is gently sawed to the desired length. A fine-toothed saw with a rigid blade support should be used.

Never remove an impaled object. Doing so could cause further injury. The object may play a role in controlling the bleeding by acting as a barrier against severed blood vessels. Removal of the object may cause massive bleeding as well as further injury to nerves, muscles, and other soft tissues. Proceed as follows:

* Expose the wound area.

* Control bleeding with direct pressure, if possible.

* While the sports emergency care team stabilizes the object and controls bleeding, have another trained sports emergency care team member place several layers of bulky dressing around the injury so that the dressing surrounds the object on all sides. Continue placing dressings, pads, and other bulky materials around the wound until the object is as secure as possible. Once bandaged in place, the dressing will stabilize the object and exert downward pressure on the bleeding vessels.

* Secure the dressings in place.

* Care for shock.

* Position the patient to ensure minimal stress.

* Transport the patient to a medical facility as soon as possible.

Impaled objects in the cheek may be removed if they pose a threat to the airway. Remove the object by gently pulling it out in the direction that it entered the cheek. If this cannot be done easily, leave the object in place. Do not twist the object. If the second end of the object is impaled into a deeper structure, inhibiting you from seeing the second end, stabilize the object. Be prepared to control bleeding at the wound site from both inside and outside the mouth.

Treatment of an impaled object in the eye includes stabilizing the object using rolls of gauze or similar material. Stabilize the object on both sides. Place a cover over the uninjured eye to help reduce sympathetic eye movement.

Avulsion Wounds

Flaps of skin and tissues are torn loose or pulled off completely in an avulsion wound. When the tip of the nose is cut or torn off, this is an avulsion. The same applies to the external ear. An eye pulled out from its socket (extruded) is a form of an avulsion. The term *avulsed* is used in reporting the wound as in "avulsed eye" or an "avulsed ear." When tissue is avulsed, it is cut off from its oxygen supply and will die soon. In sports, the most common avulsions are a tooth avulsion, finger avulsion (in weight lifting), and ear avulsion.

Emergency care for avulsions is similar to that of other open wounds. Apply direct pressure using a sterile dressing. If the avulsed skin becomes detached, save the avulsed part by wrapping it in a dry, sterile gauze dressing secured in place by self-adherent roller bandage. Then place it in a plastic bag and send it to the hospital along with the athlete. Make sure to label the avulsed part with the following information: name of body part (and side), the patient's name and date, and the time the part was wrapped and bagged. The record should show the approximate time of the avulsion. Keep the part as cool as possible, without freezing it, by placing it in a cooler or any other available container so that it is on top of a cold pack or a sealed bag of ice. Do not use dry ice. Do not immerse the avulsed part in ice, cooled water, or saline. Label the container the same as the label used for the saved part.

Amputations

Amputations, although rare in sports, can occur. An amputation is when the fingers, toes, hands, feet, or limbs are completely severed from the body. Jagged skin and bone edges may be present, and there may be massive bleeding. Often, blood vessels retract, which limits bleeding from the wound site.

Treatment of amputations includes applying a pressure dressing over the distal edge of the amputation site. Pressure points may also be used to control the bleeding. A tourniquet should not be applied unless other methods used to control bleeding have failed. Wrap the amputated part in a sterile dressing and place it in a plastic bag. Place the bag in a cooler with ice. Do not bury the amputated part in the ice. Do not use dry ice to cool the part.

DENTAL EMERGENCIES

Dental emergencies are rarely life threatening but can be extremely painful. Rapid first aid care dramatically improves the outcome and can make it possible for a dentist to make permanent repairs. A victim with any kind of dental emergency should be referred to a dentist or oral surgeon for treatment as quickly as possible; many injuries can be repaired only within a relatively narrow window of time.

Management of Broken Tooth
(Sports Emergency Care Staff and Emergency Medical Services)

1. *Use a clean cloth and water to gently clean blood, dirt, and other debris away from the broken teeth; if there are still tooth fragments in the mouth, remove them to prevent choking.*
2. *If the jaw is not fractured, have the victim gently rinse the mouth with warm water to thoroughly clean the mouth. If you suspect that the jaw is fractured, stabilize the jaw by wrapping a bandage under the chin and over the top of the head; do not have the victim rinse the mouth with water.*
3. *Apply an ice pack to the victim's face over the broken tooth (teeth) to relieve pain and reduce swelling.*
4. *Transport to a dentist or oral surgeon.*

Oftentimes, knocked out teeth can be saved with proper emergency care and rapid treatment by a dentist. The ligament fibers necessary for successful reimplantation begin to die soon after the injury, so time is of the essence. A tooth can usually be successfully reimplanted if it is inserted back into the socket within 30 minutes. The odds of successful implantation decrease every minute the tooth remains out of the socket.

Management of an Avulsed Tooth
(Sports Emergency Care Staff and Emergency Medical Services)

A top priority in the case of a knocked-out tooth is finding the tooth and handling it properly. Never touch the root of tooth. Handle it only by the crown so you do not damage the ligament fibers necessary to save the tooth. Do not rinse the tooth unless you are reinserting it into the socket.

To treat the victim and tooth properly, follow these steps:

1. *Use a clean cloth and water to gently clean blood, dirt, and other debris away from the broken tooth; if there are still tooth fragments in the mouth, remove them to prevent choking.*
2. *If the jaw is not fractured, have the victim gently rinse the mouth with warm water to thoroughly clean the mouth. If you suspect that the jaw is fractured, stabilize the jaw by wrapping a bandage under the chin and over the top of the head; do not have the victim rinse the mouth with water.*
3. *Apply an ice pack to the victim's face over the broken tooth (teeth) to relieve pain and reduce swelling.*
4. *Transport to a dentist or oral surgeon.*

CONCLUSION

Management of fractures and dislocations on the field requires the careful inspection of the involved extremity, removing the athlete from further harm, splinting the injured extremity to protect the limb and provide comfort, then appropriate transfer to an emergency care center or hospital. Careful extremity assessment for open wounds, nerve or vascular injury, and deformity will avoid undue delays in transfer for appropriate care and give the athlete the best chance of avoiding complications from his or her injuries.

SUMMARY OF KEY POINTS

➡ Fractures, dislocations, and soft tissue injuries are among the most common injuries sustained in sports.

➡ The typical signs of a fracture are pain, swelling, and tenderness over the area. Movement of the extremity will aggravate the athlete's symptoms, and he or she cannot often bear weight on the lower extremity or move the upper extremity due to discomfort. Loss of function of the extremity is usually apparent.

➡ Assessment of an injured extremity includes a careful inspection of the limb, as well as assessment of vascular supply and nerve function.

➡ An open (compound) fracture is an orthopedic emergency, and the athlete should be sent to the hospital for immediate treatment.

➡ Compartment syndrome can occur following fracture due to rapid swelling in the closed compartments of the leg and forearm.

➡ A dislocation is the most severe form of ligament and/or joint capsule injury. The normal relationship between the 2 bones forming the joint is lost; basically, the "ball is out of the socket." As with any extremity injury, careful evaluation of nerve function below the injury level is critical.

➡ A trained member of the medical team can attempt a gentle reduction or "popping" the joint back in place. Forceful attempts to reduce the joint should never be attempted. Always follow local protocol regarding attempted reduction of dislocations.

➡ Splinting of fractures, dislocations, or other extremity injuries can reduce pain and swelling, prevent from further injury, and decrease further contamination of open wounds.

➡ Sports emergency care personnel should be sure to observe body substance isolation and utilize personal protective equipment before treating any athlete with an open wound.

➡ Never remove an impaled object. Doing so could cause further injury.

➡ For amputations or avulsed skin that becomes detached, save the avulsed part by wrapping it in a dry, sterile gauze dressing secured in place by self-adherent roller bandage and place it in a plastic bag. Keep the part as cool as possible, without freezing it, by placing it in a cooler or any other available container so that it is on top of a cold pack or a sealed bag of ice.

➡ Oftentimes, knocked out teeth can be saved with proper emergency care and rapid treatment by a dentist.

REVIEW QUESTIONS

1. Explain the difference between a simple fracture and a compound fracture.
2. What are the "5 Ps" that must be considered when assessing a patient with a possible case of compartment syndrome?
3. When applied properly, what are the benefits of splinting?
4. What would be the proper immediate care for a suspected femur fracture?
5. Describe proper care for an athlete with an amputation.

BIBLIOGRAPHY

Campbell JE. *Basic Trauma Life Support for the EMT-B and the First Responder.* 4th ed. Upper Saddle River, NJ: Pearson Prentice Hall; 2004.

Jenkins DB. *Organs and Organ Systems.* 8th ed. Philadelphia, PA: WB Saunders Co; 2002.

Karren KJ. *First Aid for Colleges and Universities.* 10th ed. New York, NY: Benjamin Cummings; 2012.

Limmer D, O'Keefe MF, Grant HD, Murray RH, Bergeron JD. *Emergency Care.* 11th ed. Upper Saddle River, NJ: Brady Books; 2009.

Sarwark J. *Essentials of Musculoskeletal Care.* 4th ed. Rosemont, IL: American Academy of Orthopaedic Surgeons; 2010.

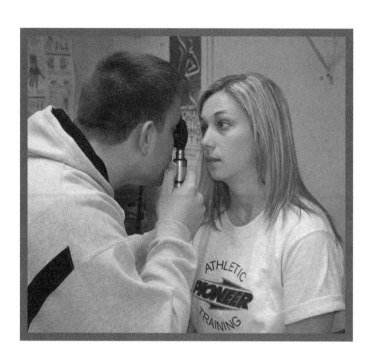

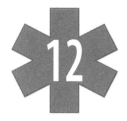

General Medical Emergencies

John L. Davis, MS, ATC

> *You are in the athletic training room at the end of the day when an athlete rushes in and asks if you have seen his teammate, Jim. He explains that while they were weight lifting, Jim suddenly began acting strange, slurring his speech, and staring into space.*
> *He tells you that when he asked Jim what was wrong, he got angry and ran away. As you search for him, you suddenly hear someone yell for help from the locker room. You enter to find Jim lying on the floor unconscious.*
> *What could it be? What would you do?*

When athletic trainers, coaches, and athletes think of injuries in athletics, they most often visualize the standard orthopedic problems that are most common in sports. When parents, administrators, the lay public, and other health care professionals think of injuries, they usually think of the more systemic, large-scale problems that call immediate attention to the field due to the need for quick response and transportation via an ambulance. Athletic trainers and other sports emergency care providers will need to work as a team to evaluate and provide quality and efficient emergency care to the injured athlete. The sports emergency care team needs to be well educated, practiced, and prepared for recognition and treatment of such conditions as shock, environmental emergencies (cold exposure and heat disorders), and other general medical conditions such as asthma, diabetes, and mononucleosis.

SHOCK: ORIENTATION TO ANATOMY AND PHYSIOLOGY

In many respects, the essence of what an athletic trainer does every day is to manage the blood flow of the athletes he or she treats. To treat an athlete for acute swelling, we put ice on a body

Rehberg RS.
Sports Emergency Care: A Team Approach,
Second Edition (pp 181-192).
© 2013 SLACK Incorporated.

part to slow blood flow. To improve blood flow after the initial swelling has stopped, we put heat on a body part to increase blood flow or use active exercise to get the blood flowing.

The body is an amazing machine, and it has the unique ability to adapt to different conditions, stresses, injuries, or illnesses. A simple understanding of the body's response to stress (injury) and how it adapts to intrinsic and extrinsic forces via changes in blood flow will help the sports emergency care provider tend to injured athletes more efficiently.

An explanation of the cardiovascular system starts with the idea that the system is made up of a container and its contents. The container is made of the muscular heart and the elastic vessels (arteries, veins, arterioles, venules, and capillaries). The contents of the system consist of the 12.6 pints (6 liters) of blood that the average adult has circulating through the body daily. Each part of the body gets a regular supply of blood. Blood flowing through the system is the method through which the body maintains its normal temperature (98.6°F [37°C]) and transport oxygen (O_2) and nutrients to each part of the body while removing waste products and carbon dioxide (CO_2).

SHOCK

Shock is defined as a syndrome in which the peripheral flow of blood is insufficient to return enough blood to the heart for normal function. Shock is the body's attempt to prioritize and maintain the vital organs. The normal circulation of blood (perfusion) and O_2 to organs and tissues of the body is compromised (hypoperfusion) during shock, depressing the body's vital functions. Think of shock as a basic defensive mechanism of the body.

Some tissues in the body are more sensitive to a lack of O_2 than others. For instance, brain tissue ischemia occurs when the brain has been deprived of O_2 for as little as 4 to 6 minutes. The heart muscle needs a constant supply of O_2, whereas the kidneys can survive 45 minutes without O_2 and skeletal muscles can last 2 hours.

Shock can occur as a result of many factors or stresses to the body. Every injury or medical condition to some extent causes a circulatory response and is influenced by the physical characteristics of the patient. Examples of some causative factors are trauma, drugs, poison, anoxia, hemorrhage, infection, dehydration, excessive heat, cold exposure, and choking or airway obstruction. The patient's age and general physical condition will go a long way in determining how severe a reaction the body exhibits.

There are many types of shock (Table 12-1), each caused by different factors. The body responds by creating a systemic shock in one of the following basic 3 ways:
1. Pump failure occurs when the heart is damaged in some way, such as in a myocardial infarction resulting from coronary artery blockage.
2. Pipe failure is caused when the blood vessels are injured in some way, such as when an athlete suffers a laceration or external bleeding associated with a compound fracture.
3. Fluid failure is caused when there is a general vasodilation or widening of the peripheral blood vessels due to a toxic reaction in the blood caused by some infection. Septic shock is an example of fluid failure.

The body will always respond to an injury or illness in one of the following 3 ways:
1. Changing the flow of blood by speeding up or slowing the rate of the heart.
2. Increasing (vasodilating) or decreasing (vasoconstricting) the size of the blood vessels locally or throughout the system.
3. Increasing or decreasing the amount of fluid content of blood in the system. (Blood has both a fluid [plasma] component and a solid [red and white blood cells and platelets] component.)

The sports emergency care provider must take these changes into consideration and respond to the signs and symptoms that the injured athlete's body presents.

Table 12-1
TYPES OF SHOCK

Type	Description	Cause
Anaphylactic	Allergic reaction to an allergen	Pipe failure
Cardiogenic	Conditions affecting the heart	Pump failure
Hypovolemic	Blood loss from bleeding	Pump failure
Metabolic	Fluid loss from vomiting, diarrhea, and urination	Fluid failure
Neurogenic	Vasodilation of peripheral blood vessels due to neurological injury	Pipe failure
Psychogenic	Vasodilation of peripheral blood vessels due to psychological response	Pipe failure
Septic	Vasodilation of peripheral blood vessels and blood leaking out of the blood vessels due to infection/toxins	Fluid failure

EXAMINATION

It is easy to understand how the body responds to an injury leading to shock if we follow a typical injury scenario and review how the body's vital signs and essential processes are affected. The vital signs are the signs and symptoms that you look for to give you clues to what is going on inside the body.

For example, an athlete suffers a compound fracture of his ankle playing soccer. The tibia and fibula are both fractured, and the distal portion of the tibia is protruding through the skin. There is significant bleeding due to a lacerated artery.

The heart responds initially to local bleeding by increasing the heart rate (rapid pulse). The athlete is also emotionally anxious, restless, and in severe pain due to the damage to the nervous system (restlessness, irritability, and anxiety). As the bleeding continues, the blood volume will drop as more blood is lost (pulse becomes rapid and weak and may become difficult to find; blood pressure subsequently decreases). The body will try to take fluid from other parts of the body to allow the production of more blood and increase the fluid portion of blood (excessive thirst). The body is now working hard to try and fight the injury. Breathing rate increases because there is a higher demand for O_2 at the injury site and throughout the body. To control the flow of blood and focus on the injured area and the vital internal organs, the peripheral blood vessels in areas other than the injury site will constrict. The skin will appear to be pale and cold to the touch. This will decrease the blood flow to uninjured areas while increasing it to areas under stress. In a further response, the body will start to sweat heavily (diaphoresis), leaving the skin moist and clammy. Some tissues in the body may be without O_2 for a period of time, so the body at some point will try to get O_2 to those body parts by rebalancing or equalizing the blood flow through all its parts by pulling blood from the vital organs. The vital organs are now without proper O_2 (further increasing breathing and pulse rate). O_2 is the key to function throughout the body. The vital organs will start to function poorly without O_2, and the brain—the controlling mechanism—will begin to be affected. The athlete will get lightheaded or feel as though he or she is about to faint. The pupils may have a dull, vacant look. As the cascade of poor function continues, the athlete will become drowsy, and he or she may become more restless. This level of consciousness will eventually suffer. The heart muscle

Table 12-2
SIGNS AND SYMPTOMS OF SHOCK

Vital Sign	Sign/Symptom
Heart rate	Decreasing (rapid then decreasing)
Pulse rate	Rapid and weak
Respiratory rate	Rapid and shallow
Skin color	Pale, blue, or gray
Skin temperature	Cool and moist (clammy)
Eyes	Dull, listless
Muscle function	Decreasing ability to control
Nausea/vomiting	Excessive thirst
Mental status	Lightheaded Restlessness, irritability, anxiety Drowsy, loss of consciousness

itself, which has been working extremely hard, will finally be affected as it gets deprived of O_2 and blood due to the compromised circulation. The heart rate and pulse will become increasingly faster and more irregular as the heart fights to keep itself and the body alive. The pulse will no longer be detectable.

The body fought to compensate for the severe blood loss by constantly changing the flow of blood through the body. In this example, the cascade of physiological events unfortunately resulted in this athlete entering into a severe state of shock.

MANAGEMENT AND TREATMENT

Sports emergency care providers must use their skills, experience, and knowledge to fully assess and determine the required care and treatment of injured athletes. Table 12-2 describes the signs and symptoms an injured athlete may exhibit during shock. Care of an athlete suspected of having shock or potentially experiencing shock should include the following steps:

* Do no further harm. Do not move the athlete and create additional injury.

* Assess CAB Sx3 (circulation, airway, and breathing, severe bleeding, shock, and spinal injury).

* Maintain an open airway, watch breathing, and control bleeding.

* Elevate lower extremities 12 inches (as long as there is not an upper body injury).

* A patient suffering a heart attack may be more comfortable in a semireclining position.

* Maintain the athlete's body heat (use blankets above and below the body if necessary).

* Reassure and calm the athlete and try to have him or her rest comfortably.

* Treat trauma to the body such as fractures or bleeding.

* Document and monitor vital signs.

* Limit fluids and food.

By correctly recognizing the signs and symptoms of shock, an emergency care provider will be able to assist the body in making natural adaptations. Once the athlete arrives at a hospital, more definitive care can be given to treat the condition that precipitated shock. Transfusions may be necessary for someone who lost a significant amount of blood. A patient who suffers from a cardiac-related episode may be given medication to help the damaged heart. A patient who suffers from a dilated vascular system will receive medication to constrict the blood vessels. An athlete with an orthopedic injury, such as a fracture, will be splinted, casted, or surgically treated to correct the problem.

GENERAL MEDICAL EMERGENCIES

There are several relatively common conditions that can create general medical emergencies that sports emergency care personnel must be prepared to address should they occur. Asthma, diabetes, and mononucleosis are conditions causing systemic problems if not treated correctly and quickly. Asthma and diabetes can both lead to death if not recognized immediately. As with the environmental disorders discussed in Chapter 13, prevention is the key to treatment. Pre-planning and awareness are necessary to avoid any first aid emergencies.

ASTHMA

Asthma is a chronic inflammatory lung disease that makes breathing difficult. When an attack occurs, the air passages will narrow and become congested to the point at which they function poorly, resulting in difficulty breathing.

History and Etiology

Asthma is a hyperresponse of the bronchial passages to various stimuli. It is thought of as an allergic reaction or response to allergens or triggers in the air. Triggers include allergies, mold, dust mites, pollen, smoke, animals, cold air, exercise, and respiratory infections. Children are most affected by asthma, but the incidence of asthma diagnosis is on the rise among all ages due to increased air pollution.

Examination

Asthma occurs when an allergic trigger causes the air passages to react in 3 interrelated ways. First, the muscles around the bronchi will spasm or vasoconstrict. The bronchi are the tubes connecting the trachea (windpipe) with the alveoli, which are deep inside the lungs. The alveoli, or air sacks, are where O_2 and CO_2 are exchanged in the blood. The second reaction is swelling inside the bronchial passages. Finally, a build-up of mucus occurs inside the passages. These 3 changes to the bronchi make them narrower and reduce the flow of O_2 into the body and the transfer of CO_2 out of the lungs.

The most common sign of asthma is wheezing, which is a hoarse, whistling sound made while exhaling. Wheezing occurs because air is trapped in the lungs. Other typical signs and symptoms of asthma are difficulty breathing, shortness of breath, tightness in the chest, restlessness while sleeping, coughing, difficulty talking, and inability to catch a breath after activity. If the condition is left unchecked or proves itself difficult to treat, severe respiratory distress and respiratory arrest can occur.

Management and Treatment

Asthma can occur at any age, but the treatment undertaken is usually based on the assumption that the condition is or will become chronic. Prevention is the key to management. Avoiding known triggers and the use of medications designed to open the air passages are the 2 best ways to treat this disorder. Medication comes in 2 forms—oral and inhaled. They can be used in combination or singularly to control asthmatic attacks. Inhaled medications have fewer side effects in general, but shorter durations of action. The following are 2 main types of asthma medication:

1. Quick relief or rescue medicines are designed to relieve symptoms after they start. These are known as *bronchodilators*. These medications open the bronchial tubes by relaxing muscle spasm in the walls of the tubes. In the event of an asthmatic attack, patients are encouraged to take puffs from the inhalers no more than 1 to 2 minutes apart. Do not use more often than recommended as overuse use can cause tachycardia.

2. Control medicines are designed to prevent the onset of asthma symptoms. Corticosteroids, either inhaled or oral, are examples of control medications.

It is very important for athletes to work with their doctors and learn the different medications designed to control and treat asthma. Athletic trainers and team physicians may need to re-evaluate if the condition worsens and/or the prescribed medication is not working effectively.

Special Considerations

Exercise-induced asthma (EIA) is a unique type of asthma that may be encountered by the athletic trainer. EIA is defined as bronchospasm caused by exercise. In this case, physical activity is the trigger for the asthmatic symptoms. It can occur in those with known asthma or crop up in athletes that have never suffered a normal asthma attack. The cause of EIA is still not well understood. There are medications designed to control EIA that are approved by various athletic bodies, such as the International Olympic Committee. Athletic trainers and their athletes should work with their team physicians and the family physicians to ensure that proper medication is being used by the competing athlete.

Acute Breathing Difficulties

Over the past 25 years, the number of asthma patients and individuals experiencing acute breathing episodes has increased.[1] Sports emergency care providers may encounter the following acute breathing difficulties:

* Athletes who experience an acute breathing episode with no history of asthma. The end result of the episode may or may not have asthma as the causative factor.

* Athletes who are known asthma sufferers but who do not have their medication with them.

* Athletes who have the wind knocked out of them.

* Athletes who have breathing difficulty related to physical trauma from an injury or as a byproduct of stress or anxiety issues the athlete may be experiencing.

The signs and symptoms an individual with acute breathing difficulties may display will be similar to those of asthma, such as wheezing, difficulty breathing or shortness of breath, tightness in the chest, coughing, difficulty talking, numbness in the hands and fingers, numb lips, dry mouth, and dizziness. The athlete may start panting or hyperventilating (breathing faster than normal) and disrupt the balance of O_2 and CO_2 in the body when trying to catch a breath.

Management and Treatment

First try to calm and reassure the athlete. Get the athlete in a comfortable position or a better posture position. Move him or her into a fresh air location. Work with the athlete to control his or her breathing rate and pattern. Have the athlete focus on following you as you demonstrate taking long, slow breaths in through the nose and long exhalations out through the month. Consider having the athlete breath into his or her cupped hands. What you are trying to accomplish is having the athlete regain voluntary control of his or her breathing. If a known asthma sufferer, try and get his or her medication from the athlete's locker, dorm, or parents.

It is of utmost importance to try and keep minor, nonemergency breathing difficulties from becoming major problems. Sports emergency care providers should continually monitor the athlete,

---

Table 12-3
SIGNS AND SYMPTOMS OF HYPOGLYCEMIA AND HYPERGLYCEMIA

Hypoglycemia
Sudden onset
Pale, cool, clammy skin
Mood changes, disorientation, confusion, or stupor
Unresponsiveness (late stages)

Hyperglycemia
Gradual onset
Flushed, warm, dry skin
Frequent urination
Fruity or sweet odor on breath
Irregular breathing
Drowsiness, disorientation, or stupor
Nausea, feeling and looking ill
Unresponsiveness (late stages)

---

assess his or her breathing rate, skin color, alertness, and mental function. Use a stethoscope to listen to the chest and the athlete's lung sounds. If the athlete's condition does not improve quickly or becomes serious, the health care provider should access 9-1-1 for emergency medical services (EMS) assistance and transport. Follow-up care is necessary to identify the cause; it is important for athletes, their parents, primary physicians, specialists, and the sports emergency care team to work together to control and treat asthma and all breathing disorders.

DIABETES

Diabetes mellitus is a disorder of carbohydrate metabolism resulting from inadequate production or utilization of insulin and inefficient use of blood sugar.

History and Etiology

Insulin is a hormone secreted by the pancreas. It is essential in the metabolism of glucose (simple sugar) and helps promote the storage of glucose in muscles and as glycogen in the liver. Insulin also helps control the transfer of glucose from the blood into skeletal and cardiac muscles. To function normally, the body cells need a proper balance of sugar and insulin. Diabetes can seriously affect the body in a variety of ways and contribute to other conditions such as blindness; kidney, heart, and tooth disease; and stroke.

Examination

Athletes with diabetes can compete if they are able to maintain blood sugar levels within normal limits. If the condition is not controlled properly, the athlete will have too much or too little sugar in the bloodstream. This imbalance will lead to a diabetic emergency. Symptoms for diabetic emergencies differ based on the type of imbalance.

There are 2 types of diabetes. In type 1, or insulin-dependent diabetes, the pancreas produces little or no insulin. This type of individual will need to monitor his or her blood sugar regularly and inject insulin several times a day. In type 2 diabetes (non–insulin-dependent diabetes), the body produces insulin, but either not enough or the cells do not use the insulin effectively. Type 2 diabetes is much more common than type 1. Most people with type 2 are able to regulate their blood sugar through diet and oral medication. There are 2 types of diabetic emergencies—hyperglycemia and hypoglycemia (Table 12-3).

When the level of insulin in the body is too low, the blood sugar levels will be too high and the athlete will suffer from hyperglycemia. In this condition, although there is enough glucose in the blood, it cannot be transported from the bloodstream. The cells in the body, needing food or glucose, will try to get energy from other stored foods, such as fats. Turning fat into energy is not efficient and will create a lot of waste products in the blood, and the athlete will become ill. This is called *diabetic ketoacidosis*. Signs and symptoms of diabetic ketoacidosis are hot, dry skin and a sweet, fruity breath odor. This can be mistaken for alcohol on the breath. A life-threatening condition known as *diabetic coma* may occur if diabetic ketoacidosis is not treated properly.

In hypoglycemia, the level of insulin in the body is too high and the glucose levels in the blood will be too low. Sugar is used up too fast. Left untreated, the athlete will develop insulin shock—another life-threatening condition.

Hypoglycemia and hyperglycemia have different causes and different symptoms (see Table 12-3).

Management and Treatment

Diabetes is not a reason for an individual to stop participating in athletics. In fact, exercise can help to control diabetes and increase insulin efficiency. However, the athlete needs to understand the necessary balance between diet and exercise. Regular monitoring of the blood sugar should be done with a glucose monitor.

Insulin injections may become a thing of the past as researchers look for and test new delivery methods. One promising delivery method that has already gained widespread acceptance, especially for athletes, is the insulin pump. The pump mimics the normal, regular release of insulin from the pancreas. The pump is not automatic; the user decides how much insulin will be given. These pumps weigh about 3 ounces, are about the size of a cell phone, and are worn on the belt or in the pocket. These units are computerized and programmed to give regular insulin 24 hours a day. The pumps have a small, flexible catheter tube with a fine needle on the end, which is inserted under the skin of the abdomen. The needle is normally taped in place. Frequent monitoring is still necessary to maintain the proper glucose and insulin balance. Specially designed and padded waist belts are available for use in athletic competition.

To treat an athlete experiencing a diabetic emergency, check for life-threatening conditions. If the athlete's past medical history is unknown, look for a medic alert tag or ask bystanders if they know if the athlete has diabetes. Most diabetic emergencies are hypoglycemic in nature. If the athlete is conscious, give him or her some form of sugar. Commercially available glucose paste is available for use and should be kept in every medical kit. Other alternatives such as cake icing, table sugar, candy, fruit juice, or soda will contain enough sugar to help restore a normal balance; however, do not give a victim food or drink if he or she is experiencing an altered state of consciousness. Glucose paste, cake icing, and table sugar can be placed under the tongue. If it is unclear whether the diabetic emergency is due to hypoglycemia or hyperglycemia, give sugar. If the sugar levels are low, recovery will be rapid. If they are too high, the additional sugar will not harm the athlete.

Prevention is key with athletes. Taking the time to review the condition with athletes with diabetes and their coaches may be very helpful. Consider reviewing the following items:

✳ Be sure the condition is properly documented on the preseason physical form and review the condition with the athlete so you are aware of his or her normal management plan.

✳ The diabetes should be well controlled before practice starts.

✳ Practices and games should be held at the same basic time of day and be about the same length.

✳ Have sugary snacks on hand to help balance out irregularities.

✳ Since the legs and arms will be used in activity, only give insulin injections in the abdomen.

✳ Be sure to maintain proper hydration. Remember that fluid is vitally important for all bodily functions.

❋ Be ready to test the athlete's blood glucose before and regularly during exercise.

❋ Regularly review the exercise plan and make adjustments.

Usually, most athletes with diabetes will be familiar with their condition and know how best to treat it. Ask for their help. If an individual is not feeling better after 5 minutes, call 9-1-1. Obviously, if he or she is unconscious, call 9-1-1 immediately, and do not give anything orally. Monitor and document vital signs until EMS arrives.

HYPONATREMIA

History and Etiology

Hyponatremia, often referred to as *water intoxication*, is a condition defined as having low plasma sodium (<130 mEq/L) and is caused by either ingesting too much fluid or excessive sodium losses due to sweating.

Examination

Signs and symptoms of hyponatremia include central nervous system dysfunction (ie, disorientation, seizures, or confusion), headache, nausea, and vomiting.[2] Victims of hyponatremia may also experience swelling of the extremities, pulmonary edema, and/or cerebral edema.[2] Hyponatremia often occurs in athletes participating in endurance or ultraendurance events but can occur whenever an athlete has consumed fluid in excess of their sweat rate, thereby diluting their plasma sodium levels below normal.

Management and Treatment

Prevention of hyponatremia is the best form of management of this condition, and can be accomplished by ensuring athletes know their individualized sweat rates and use a personalized hydration protocol as to avoid overhydration. Athletes suspected of hyponatremia should be treated through activation of EMS and immediate transport to a hospital.

EXERTIONAL SICKLING

History and Etiology

Exertional sickling is one of the top causes of death in athletes, and it occurs in individuals who have sickle cell trait. With exertion during exercise, and sometimes in conjunction with a warm environment, the athlete's blood cells begin to transform into a sickled shape, creating a "logjam in the blood vessels."[3] This can lead to ischemic rhabdomyolysis, hypoxemia, lactic acidosis, muscle hyperthermia, and red cell dehyration.[3,4]

Examination

Signs and symptoms of exertional sickling may consist of collapse (often within the first 30 minutes of intense exercise), fatigue, inability to continue exercise, and muscle pain with no visual muscle cramping as would be seen in a regular muscle cramp.[3] Exertional sickling is an "intensity syndrome," caused by high-intensity exercise in combination with the presence of the sickle cell trait.[4] Therefore, it is not an exertional heat illness but still a medical emergency that should be treated with activation of EMS, cessation of exercise, high-flow supplemental oxygen, and immediate transport to a hospital.

Management and Treatment

Prevention of exertional sickling is paramount. Screening of athletes to identify sickle cell trait is recommended, and members of the medical staff should be aware of which athletes have tested positive for sickle cell trait. Workouts and practice sessions should be modified by giving adequate rest breaks between sets or activities while monitoring the athlete closely. The athlete and coaching staff should also be aware if the sickle cell trait is present in order to better regulate the exercise regimen for the athlete so that the athlete is able to take breaks when needed.

MONONUCLEOSIS

Mononucleosis is a common infectious disease that can affect the liver, lymph nodes, and oral cavity.

History and Etiology

Mononucleosis is usually caused by the Epstein-Barr virus, a member of the herpes family of viruses. It gets its name from the traumatic increase in the number of white blood cells (mononuclear leukocytes) that are created when the Epstein-Barr virus infects the lymphatic system in the body. The lymphatic system is the complex disease-fighting system in the body and is made up of the following parts: bone marrow, spleen, thymus gland, lymph nodes, tonsils, and appendix.

The disease is mostly seen in adolescents and young adults aged 15 to 30 but can occur at any age. The disease is contracted through direct contact with saliva or mucus of an infected individual and is commonly transmitted by sharing food or drink containers or by kissing, giving its description as the "kissing disease." Some newly infected athletes may not have symptoms and may potentially spread the virus to others.

Examination

The incubation time for this disease is usually 2 to 7 weeks. The symptoms will last a few days to a couple of months, most often disappearing in 1 to 3 weeks. The signs and symptoms are rather vague and start with the athlete having a general fatigue or run-down feeling. This feeling may come and go. The person will feel he or she has a bad cold or the flu. Common additional symptoms include headache, chills, loss of appetite, and puffy eyes. As the athlete typically tries to fight through the disease, the symptoms will worsen, and he or she will experience swollen, tender glands, high fever, sore throat, and fatigue. The athlete will want to sleep often because he or she will never feel fully rested. The white blood cell count will be elevated and lymphatic system will be on full alert, with the spleen enlarged.

Athletes with these symptoms need to be referred to a medical professional for testing. An antibody blood test (monospot test) will be done to confirm the diagnosis and eliminate other possibilities.

Management and Treatment

There is no specific treatment for this disease. Basic treatment will be rest, taking acetaminophen or ibuprofen, and eating and drinking properly. This usually mild disease will run its course in a few weeks. The sore throat will be at the worst during days 3 to 5, gradually improving by day 10. The fever may last 2 weeks. The athlete once diagnosed should stay away from practice and school until the fever goes away and he or she feels more rested. The athlete will be encouraged not to push it or try to rush the process. The glands may stay swollen for almost 1 month.

Special Considerations

Sports emergency care personnel must be concerned about athletes with mononucleosis because of the enlarged spleen and the increased chance of rupturing it during activity. A splenic rupture is a medical emergency and can be life threatening (see Chapter 10 for more details). Contact sports and heavy lifting should be avoided. Return-to-play considerations must be made after an ultrasound test is done to ensure the spleen has returned to normal size and the white blood cell count has returned to somewhat normal levels.

Summary of Key Points

➡ Shock is defined as a syndrome in which the peripheral flow of blood is insufficient to return enough blood to the heart for normal function. Shock is the body's attempt to prioritize and maintain the vital organs.

➡ Sports emergency care providers must use their skills, experience, and knowledge to fully assess and determine the required care and treatment of injured athletes.

➡ By correctly recognizing the signs and symptoms of shock, an emergency care provider will be able to assist the body in making natural adaptations.

➡ Asthma is a chronic inflammatory lung disease that makes breathing difficult. When an attack occurs, the air passages will narrow and become congested to the point at which they function poorly, resulting in difficulty breathing. The most common sign of asthma is wheezing, which is a hoarse, whistling sound made while exhaling.

➡ Prevention is the key to managing asthma.

➡ EIA is a unique type of asthma caused by exercise.

➡ Diabetes mellitus is a disorder of carbohydrate metabolism resulting from inadequate production or utilization of insulin and inefficient use of blood sugar.

➡ Mononucleosis is a common infectious disease that can affect the liver, lymph nodes, and oral cavity. The disease is mostly seen in adolescents and young adults aged 15 to 30 but can occur at any age. The disease is contracted through direct contact with saliva or mucus of an infected individual and is commonly transmitted by sharing food or drink containers or by kissing, giving its description as the "kissing disease." Some newly infected athletes may not have symptoms and may potentially spread the virus to others.

Review Questions

1. Explain in detail what occurs when an athlete is in shock.
2. What is the proper care for shock in an ill or injured athlete?
3. Describe the proper management of an acute asthma attack.
4. What are the 2 diabetic emergencies that an athlete might experience? Describe in detail.
5. Why could an athlete who suffers from mononucleosis be at risk for serious injury?

References

1. Centers for Disease Control and Prevention. Behavioral Risk Factor Surveillance System (BRFSS) prevalence data. http://www.cdc.gov/asthma/brfss/07/current/tablec1.htm. Accessed June 17, 2009.
2. Binkley HM, Beckett J, Casa DJ, Kleiner DM, Plummer PE. National Athletic Trainers' Association position statement: exertional heat illnesses. *J Athl Train.* 2002;37(3):329-343.
3. Anderson S, Eichner ER. National Athletic Trainers' Association consensus statement: sickle cell trait and the athlete. http://www.nata.org/sites/default/files/SickleCellTraitAndTheAthlete.pdf. Accessed September 30, 2012.
4. Eichner ER. Pearls and pitfalls: exertional sickling. *Curr Sports Med Rep.* 2010;9(1):3-4.

Bibliography

American Diabetes Association. About insulin pumps http://www.diabetes.org/living-with-diabetes/treatment-and-care/medication/insulin/insulin-pumps.html. Accessed September 30, 2012.

American Red Cross. Emergency Response. Yardley, PA: Staywell; 2001.

American Red Cross. *Responding to Emergency.* Yardley, PA: Staywell; 2000.

Cerny F, Burton H. *Exercise Physiology for Health Care Professionals.* Champaign, IL: Human Kinetics Publishers; 2001.

Magee D. *Orthopedic Physical Assessment*. 2nd ed. Philadelphia, PA: WB Saunders Co; 1992.

McArdle W, Katch F, Katch V. *Sports and Exercise Nutrition*. Baltimore, MD: Lippincott Williams and Wilkins; 1999.

Miller M, Weiler J, Baker R, Collins J, D'Alonzo G. National Athletic Trainers' Association position statement: management of asthma in athletes. *J Athl Train*. 2005;40(3):224-245.

National Safety Council. *First Aid and CPR*. 4th ed. Sudbury, MA: Jones and Bartlett Publishers; 2000.

Papazian R. On the teen scene: being a sport with exercise-induced asthma. Food and Drug Administration, Publication No. 94-1217.

Perrin D, ed. *Assessment of Athletic Injuries*. Champaign, IL: Human Kinetics Publishers; 2000.

Starkey C. *Athletic Training and Sports Medicine*. 4th ed. Sudbury, MA: Jones and Bartlett Publishers; 2006.

Starkey C, Ryan J. *Evaluation of Orthopedic and Athletic Injuries*. 2nd ed. Philadelphia, PA: FA Davis; 2002.

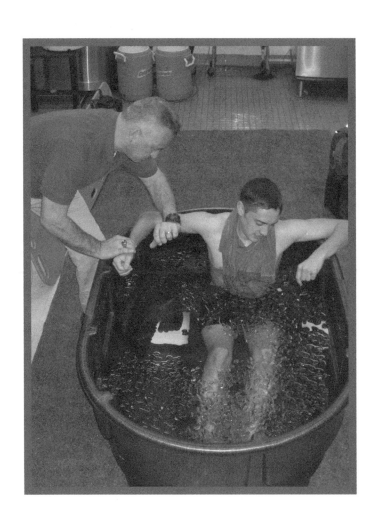

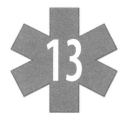

Environmental Emergencies

Rebecca M. Lopez, PhD, ATC, CSCS

> *You are providing medical coverage of a college track meet on a very hot, humid day. During the 3200-meter men's race, one of the athletes suddenly stops running and walks off the track. As you walk toward him, you notice that his skin is flushed, and he is breathing heavily. Before you get to the athlete, he suddenly collapses, and you arrive to find him unconscious.*
> *What's going on? What should you do?*

Aside from the normal stresses the human body encounters during exercise, some environmental conditions can further add stress to exercising individuals. Exercising individuals can usually adapt to the environment, however, at times the stressor exceeds the body's ability to maintain homeostasis and results in distress. According to Hans Selye's General Adaptation Syndrome (GAS), the body's response to stress consists of 3 stages: alarm, resistance, and exhaustion.[1] Based on Selye's GAS principle, the body is initially alarmed by a new stressor but can then adapt to this stressor after being continually exposed to it. Depending on the duration of this exposure to stress, the body may either continue to adapt via physiological changes or be unable to continue to adapt and succumb to the stressor. It is important to note that a person's reaction to a stressor is individualized; therefore, a group of individuals may react differently to the same stressor.[2] Education is key to preventing medical emergencies that may result from environmental stressors, such as the cold, heat, altitude, or lightning.

THERMAL PHYSIOLOGY

Humans are homeotherms, able to regulate their body temperature and maintain homeostasis, regardless of the external temperature. However, the balance between the amount of heat lost and

Rehberg RS.
Sports Emergency Care: A Team Approach,
Second Edition (pp 195-208).
© 2013 SLACK Incorporated.

heat gained can be off-centered due to variety of factors. Heat can be gained or lost via different mechanisms such as conduction, convection, radiation, and evaporation. Heat transfer occurs from the warmer object to the cooler object.[3] Conduction consists of heat gained or lost from with an object (ie, an ice bag sitting on a hot metal bleacher). Convection is the loss or gain of heat via the movement of air or fluid (water) against the skin's surface including wind, fanning, or being immersed in cold water. Radiation is the energy transfer from higher to lower energy surfaces via electromagnetic radiation, such as the sun's radiant heat reflecting off of a track onto the running athlete. The heat balance equation[4] demonstrates these avenues through which the body can gain or lose heat:

S = M − (± Work) ± E ± R ± C ± K

S represents heat storage, M represents metabolic heat production, E represents evaporation, R represents radiation, C represents convection, and lastly, K represents heat lost or gained via conduction.[4]

Various factors, such as exercise intensity, environment, playing surface, and equipment, can affect the amount of heat lost or gained as well as the avenues through which this occurs. The hypothalamus in our brains acts as a thermostat, altering various physiological responses in order to maintain normal body temperature (98.6°F). During exercise, it is common for body temperature to be slightly elevated in response to the increased metabolic demands. In attempts to prevent dangerously elevated temperatures during exercise, our body effectively loses heat via various mechanisms, such as peripheral vasodilation for dissipation of heat through the skin and the sweating mechanism, whereby sweat production is increased and the evaporation of that sweat from the skin results in body cooling. However, if the air is saturated with water due to high humidity, the sweat on the skin's surface is not evaporated and the amount of heat lost through sweating is diminished. The body must then rely on other mechanisms of heat loss (namely convection and radiation).[2] Decreased exposure of the skin's surface, such as when wearing a football uniform or other protective clothing, may also preclude sweat loss via evaporation; in these circumstances, the body must also rely on other means to dissipate heat.

EXERTIONAL HEAT ILLNESS

The term *exertional heat illness* can refer to a few conditions that can occur while individuals exercise in the heat, as their name implies. The conditions include heat cramps, heat syncope, heat exhaustion, and exertional heat stroke (EHS). While it is important for certified athletic trainers and other clinicians to be aware of the prevention, recognition, and management of these conditions, only one of these—EHS—is a medical emergency that could potentially result in death. Nonetheless, all of the exertional heat illnesses are discussed here in order to properly differentiate the causes, recognition, and treatment of these conditions.

EXERCISE HEAT CRAMPS

The topic of muscle cramps has been one of great debate in recent years. While some prefer the term *exercise-associated muscle cramps*, others refer to them as *heat cramps*.[5] The terminology is important because it describes the actual cause of the muscle cramp, and therefore, the means by which to prevent and/or treat them once they occur. For the sake of this chapter's focus on environmental conditions, heat cramps will refer to the involuntary muscle cramps in the lower extremity musculature (most commonly the gastrocnemius) that usually occur while exercising in the heat. Although the exact cause may be unclear, heat cramps often occur due to muscle fatigue, fluid losses, and most importantly, loss of electrolytes.[6] Those who tend to be salty sweaters, with large sodium and chloride losses in their sweat, may be more predisposed to heat cramps.[5,7] For athletes who know they are prone to cramping, adding some salty snacks to their diet, such as pretzels or canned soup, may be helpful in preventing the onset of cramps. Adding about ¼ teaspoon of table salt into a 32-ounce sports drink may also be helpful. Once heat cramps occur, treatment consists of removing the athlete from activity as well as light stretching. Replacing lost fluid with sodium-containing fluids is key, though carbohydrate-electrolyte solutions often do not contain enough sodium to replace the amount lost in sweat. Adding some table salt to a sports drink will be more beneficial than ingesting water or a sports drink alone.

HEAT SYNCOPE

Heat syncope, often referred to as *orthostatic dizziness*, may occur when an individual is exposed to high environmental temperatures.[3] Activities that require standing for long periods of time or immediate cessation of an activity while exercising in the heat may cause heat syncope due to peripheral vasodilation, postural pooling or blood, or diminished venous return.[3] Lack of heat acclimatization, engaging in activities such as marching band, or standing in formation for the military may result in heat syncope. Treatment for heat syncope involves ruling out other life-threatening conditions (ie, cardiac, heat stroke, or exertional sickling), then moving the victim to a cooler area, monitoring vital signs, and elevating the legs above the level of the head.[3] If dehydration may have caused the heat syncope, rehydrate orally if possible.

EXERTIONAL HEAT EXHAUSTION

Exertional heat exhaustion has been defined as the inability to continue exercising due to cardiovascular insufficiency, often while exercising in a hot, humid environment.[3,8] An athlete experiencing heat exhaustion may often present with weakness, nausea, pallor, vomiting, and chills. The athlete often feels faint and dizzy but has no central nervous system (CNS) dysfunction and may have a slightly elevated temperature (<104°F) but within normal limits for an individual exercising in the heat. Some of the causes of heat exhaustion include exercising in the heat combined with dehydration, sodium losses, and energy depletion.[3]

Prevention of exertional heat exhaustion can be achieved by ensuring athletes have been gradually acclimatized to the heat and are properly hydrated prior to activity in the heat. Educating athletes about their individualized sweat rates, a balanced diet, and adequate sleep can go a long way in the prevention of heat exhaustion. Once EHS has been ruled out, treatment of heat exhaustion includes the removal of excess equipment and/or clothing, moving the athlete to a cooler area, and rehydration, if possible. Cold ice towels can also be placed over the athlete's head and neck area. Symptoms of heat exhaustion usually resolve fairly quickly; however, if the athlete's symptoms do not improve or if they worsen after 15 to 30 minutes, activate emergency medical services (EMS).

EXERTIONAL HEAT STROKE

EHS is a potentially fatal exertional heat illness consisting of exercise-induced hyperthermia (>104°F to 105°F) and altered mental status. It occurs when an exercising individual has greater heat gains than heat losses and the individual is unable to continue exercise, often collapsing. A recent retrospective analysis of American football deaths found that from 1980 to 2009 there were 58 documented deaths related to hyperthermia during American football in the United States.[9] Although there are EHS deaths every year, clinical research has shown that death from EHS can be prevented with early recognition and the appropriate treatment. Signs and symptoms of EHS may include confusion; combativeness; unconsciousness or other similar signs of CNS dysfunction; dizziness; vomiting; diarrhea; hot, wet, or dry skin; and a rectal temperature of greater than 104°F. A misconception regarding EHS in athletes is that the victim's skin will be hot and dry; however, when an EHS victim collapses, he or she will often still be sweating

Table 13-1
DISPELLING MYTHS ABOUT EXERTIONAL HEAT STROKE

Myth	Fact
The athlete is still sweating so it must not be EHS.	In most cases of EHS, the athlete will still be sweating and have hot, wet skin.[13,30]
There is a continuum of heat illnesses where someone will develop heat exhaustion before it progresses to EHS.	EHS can occur suddenly without heat exhaustion or warning signs that the athlete is about to collapse.
Tympanic, temporal, or oral thermometers can be used to diagnose EHS.	The only valid and reliable temperature devices that should be used with exercising individuals are rectal thermometers or ingestible thermistors.[10]
Cold water immersion is dangerous and can lead to shock, cardiac arrest, or increased hyperthermia.	Cold water immersion has resulted in survival from EHS in 100% of cases, particularly when initiated immediately after collapse.
Immediately sending an athlete with EHS to the emergency room is the best treatment.	Initiating aggressive cooling before an athlete is transported to the ER is best. Not doing so may result in delayed cooling and potentially death for the athlete. "Cool first, transport second."[12,13,30]
Death from EHS may not always be preventable.	With a rapid diagnosis and rapid and aggressive cooling, death from EHS is preventable.[12,30]

(Table 13-1). Another misconception held by some clinicians is that assessing body temperature axillary, orally, tympanically, or temporally can be used to diagnose EHS. Rectal thermometry is the most valid and reliable temperature measure in exercising individuals, particularly in an emergency setting.[10] Although gastrointestinal thermistors are also reliable in this setting, the athletes would have had to ingest it approximately 4 to 5 hours prior to taking a reading; a rectal temperature is the most practical method and should be used to either diagnose or rule out EHS in a collapsed athlete.

If an athlete collapses and/or has signs of CNS dysfunction along with hyperthermia, EHS is the likely diagnosis (Figure 13-1). Prompt, aggressive cooling via cold-water immersion should be initiated and EMS activated. It is important to note that the EHS victim should be cooled prior to being transported to the hospital (see Table 13-1), as it is vital to bring the core temperature below 104°F as soon as possible to prevent multisystem organ failure and death.[3,11-13] The athlete should be cooled until core temperature reaches 102°F, then continuously monitored until EMS arrives. Should cold-water immersion not be available, the athletic trainer or other health care professional should try any other means of aggressive cooling, such as rotating ice cold towels, dousing the athlete with ice and water, or using a hose or locker room shower to cool the athlete. It should also be noted that the cooling rate of ice bags over peripheral arteries is ineffective in rapidly cooling the athlete; any of the other aggressive cooling strategies mentioned should be used to ensure survival.[14,15] Cold

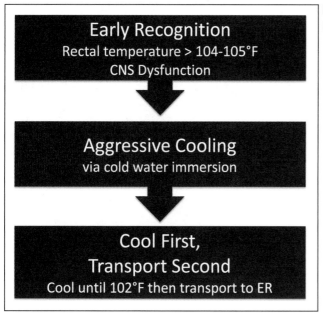

Figure 13-1. Preventing death from EHS.

Early Recognition
Rectal temperature > 104-105°F
CNS Dysfunction

Aggressive Cooling
via cold water immersion

Cool First,
Transport Second
Cool until 102°F then transport to ER

water immersion has had a 100% survival rate when used on actual EHS victims.[12,15] As seen in Figures 13-2 and 13-3, having a cold tub with ice and water readily available prior to an EHS episode is essential for athletic trainers to be ready to effectively treat a victim of EHS.

Although prevention of death from EHS is possible with proper recognition and aggressive cooling, one may not always prevent EHS from occurring. However, there are a few important preventative measures that athletic trainers, coaches, and athletes can take to attempt to minimize the onset of EHS.

EHS is a multifactorial phenomenon. A combination of intrinsic and/or extrinsic factors may lead the athlete to have an excess of metabolic heat production and a reduction in the ability to rid the body of heat. Some of the intrinsic factors include having a fever or other illness, lack of acclimatization, lack of sleep, poor physical fitness and/or body composition, dehydration, and overzealousness.[3,16] Extrinsic factors leading to EHS may include a high wet bulb globe temperature (>81°F), wearing excess equipment, improper work-to-rest ratios, and lack of access to fluids. Athletic trainers and others in the emergency sports care team who may be responsible for ensuring the safety of athletes should take these predisposing risk factors into account to prevent EHS in the athletic setting by ensuring there is a proper heat acclimatization process at the beginning of every sport season, making sure athletes who may be ill are kept out of practice, allowing rehydration and rest breaks, as well as other steps to limit risk.

COLD INJURIES

Competitive athletes often do not let the elements stop them from engaging in physical activities that may predispose them to a cold injury. Adventurous activities (ie, hiking and trail running) and snow-based sports (ie, cross country skiing and snowboarding) may place athletes in danger of a cold injury if the proper precautions are not taken. When exposed to a cold environment, the body must make physiological adjustments in order to preserve metabolic heat.[2] In order to maintain homeostasis, the body adjusts physiologically through peripheral vasoconstriction to decrease heat loss and shivering to increase metabolic heat production.[2]

Figure 13-2. Cold water tub.

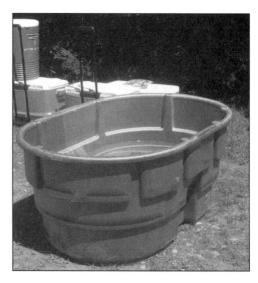

Figure 13-3. Medical tent ready for EHS victims.

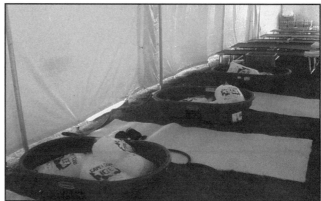

The following physiological factors play a role in whether or not the body will be able to maintain homeostasis[2,17]:

* Air temperature

* Air moisture

* Air movement

* The duration of cold exposure

In cold environments, the human body loses or gains heat in the same manner as in a hot environment—through convection, conduction, radiation, and evaporation. The convective effects of cold temperatures combined with air movement (commonly referred to as *wind chill*) across the skin's surface account for a significant amount of heat loss.[2] Figure 13-4 depicts the combined effects of cold air temperatures and wind.[18] Similarly, the combination of cold air and water (ie, water immersion or wet clothing) can be even more dangerous because it can cool the body at a faster rate than air of the same exact temperature.[2]

Therefore, athletic trainers and other health care providers need to be aware of the environmental conditions in order to educate athletes and coaches on proper clothing, adjustments to practices or game times, and other preventative measures in order to keep exercising individuals safe from the environment.

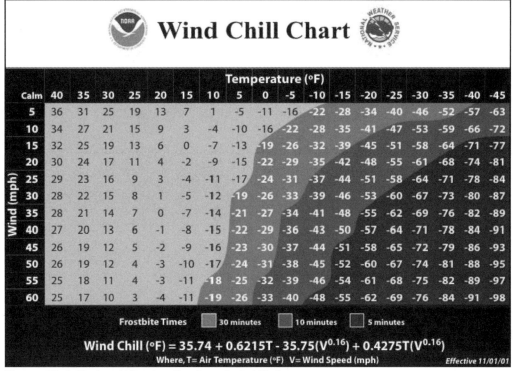

Figure 13-4. National Weather Service wind chill chart.

The National Athletic Trainers' Association (NATA) position statement[18] on environmental cold injuries defines the following 3 classifications of cold injuries:

1. Hypothermia
2. Freezing injuries of the extremities
3. Nonfreezing injuries of the extremities

It is imperative for health care providers to be aware of the differences between these conditions in order to be able to properly recognize and treat a victim of a cold injury.

HYPOTHERMIA

Hypothermia, defined as a decrease in body temperature below 95°F,[18] is a potentially fatal condition resulting from exposure to cold conditions. Hypothermia can be classified based on below normal body temperature as mild (95°F to 98.6°F), moderate (90°F to 94°F), or severe (<90°F). Signs and symptoms may include shivering, fine motor skill impairment, apathy, and a rectal temperature below normal (<98.6°F).[18,19] With more dangerous levels of hypothermia, the decreased core body temperature may result in impaired gross motor skills and altered mental status, such as slurred speech or unconsciousness. Having a valid temperature assessment with hypothermia is just as important as with heat stroke because the severity of the hypothermia will dictate the appropriate the treatment and course of action. Figure 13-5 demonstrates the appropriate course of action to successfully treat a victim of hypothermia.

If the athlete is unconscious or showing other signs of altered mental status, EMS should be activated immediately and a primary survey of vital signs initiated. If possible, carefully move the hypothermic victim to a warmer area and remove any wet clothes. The victim should be covered with dry, warm clothing or blankets and given warm fluids to drink (only if conscious and able to

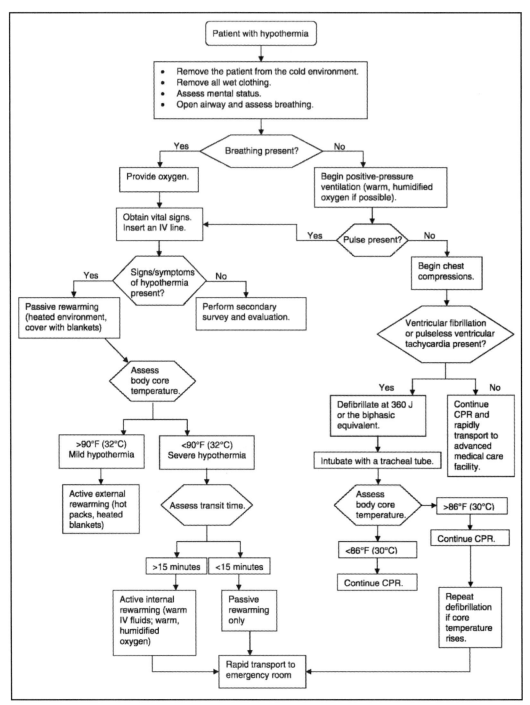

Figure 13-5. Algorithm for treating hypothermia. (Reprinted with permission from Cappaert TA, Stone JA, Castellani JW, Krause BA, Smith D, Stephens BA. NATA position statement on environmental cold injuries. *J Athl Train*. 2008;43[6]:640-658.)

do so on his or her own). If warming with heat packs or external heaters, only apply heat to the chest, axilla, trunk, and groin; applying warmth to the extremities may cause peripheral vasodilation and result in a hypothermic drop in the core.[18] Caution should also be taken when warming the victim so that the method (heater, blanket, or water immersion) is not so hot that it could burn the victim.[2] Because frostbite may be present as well, avoid massaging the victim's tissues, as this can cause further harm.[18] Continuous monitoring of vital signs and warming should occur until the victim is transported to the hospital.

FROSTBITE AND FROSTNIP

Frostbite is the freezing of body tissues resulting from overexposure to a cold, dry environment and is considered a medical emergency.[18] Frostbite occurs when the tissue temperature is below 32°F.[19] Frostbite can range in severity from mild, where superficial skin and subcutaneous tissues are frozen, to the most severe, which results in the freezing of deeper tissues including muscles, tendons, and bone.[18] Frostbite commonly occurs in exposed skin, such as the nose and ears, but is also common in the hands and feet due to the peripheral vasoconstriction that transpires with the threat of hypothermia. In an attempt to prevent a decrease in core body temperature, there is a decrease in the blood flow to the periphery, resulting in the freezing of the tissues of the extremities (usually toes and fingers) that are overexposed to the cold. Frostnip, a precursor to frostbite, is a mild cold injury usually resulting when the skin is exposed to cold and windy conditions.[18] Frostnip results in the freezing of only superficial skin that may cause cold sensitivity in the future but serious injury.

Superficial and deep frostbite may both present with edema, redness, or gray mottled skin. To differentiate between the 2, check for tissue stiffness and complaints of temporary tingling or burning that indicates superficial frostbite; if the tissue will not rebound and the victim experiences numbness, this may be more severe frostbite.[18] Treatment of frostbite includes ruling out hypothermia to determine the most appropriate course of action.

NONFREEZING COLD INJURIES

Trench foot and chilblains are the most common nonfreezing cold injuries and occur when tissues are exposed to cold, wet conditions.[19] An individual is at risk for trench foot when tissues are exposed to cold, wet conditions between 32°F to 60°F for more prolonged periods of time (ie, wearing wet socks and shoes continuously between 12 hours to 4 days).[19] Chilblains, also known as *pernio*, is a more superficial injury that can occur with damp or wet socks after only a few hours of exposure (1 to 5 hours, <60°F).[18,19]

Trench foot, also referred to as *immersion foot*, is characterized by burning, numbness, pain or sensitivity, cyanotic or blotchy skin, and swelling of the foot.[18,19] This condition can result in nerve and blood vessel damage, and peripheral pulses may be absent.[2,18] Although this condition is not likely to occur with athletes, individuals participating in ultraendurance events, hiking, or similar prolonged activities may be at risk and should take some preventative measures. Athletes engaging in these prolonged activities, where their feet may be wet or constantly sweating for prolonged times, should be instructed to change into dry socks frequently (at least 2 to 3 times a day) and use moisture-wicking socks.[18,19]

Chilblains is a superficial cold injury resulting from cold-induced vasocontriction that causes localized cell ischemia and an inflammatory response.[2,18] Chilblain will present with reddish areas or small erythematous papules on the skin (usually around the ears, face, or other exposed areas).[18] These lesions can be itchy, painful, and/or swollen; however, there is no lasting effect from chilblains.[19] Treatment involves removing the cold, wet clothing; washing and drying the area; and elevating the area when the extremities are involved. Warm the affected area by applying dry blankets. During this time, no rubbing or massaging of the affected area should be applied; the victim should be monitored for the return of normal circulation and sensation to the area.[18]

ALTITUDE

Many athletes may not be exposed to the stress of high altitude on a regular basis, but athletic trainers and others providing medical care to athletes should be aware of the physiological effects of altitude and how to prevent a potentially fatal situation. High altitude has been defined as elevations over 4921 feet (1500 meters).[20] With increases in altitude there is a decline in barometric pressure (hypobaria) along with a decrease in the partial pressure of oxygen (hypoxia).[21] Hypoxic conditions result in the body not being able to meet the demands of oxygen utilization in cells.[2] This becomes increasingly more difficult and taxing on homeostasis when an individual is exercising and metabolic needs are increased. If the body is not able to adapt to these conditions, this stressor to the body's metabolism may lead to deleterious effects for those unaccustomed to the hypobaric environment. The effects can range from mild (sluggishness or a headache) to more severe, potentially fatal situations (cerebral or pulmonary edema).[2] Certain pre-existing conditions, such as sickle cell trait, may place some athletes at additional risk when traveling to compete or exercise at a higher altitude.[22]

The term *high-altitude illness* refers to 3 conditions that occur as a result of acute exposure to hypobaric hypoxia.[20] These conditions are preventable through altitude acclimatization, though they can still occur in mountain climbers who make too rapid of an ascent.[20] High-altitude illnesses include the following:

* Acute mountain sickness (AMS)

* High-altitude cerebral edema (HACE)

* High-altitude pulmonary edema (HAPE)

Of these 3, AMS is the mildest, while HACE and HAPE are potentially fatal conditions that must be recognized and treated early to prevent a catastrophic event. AMS and HACE are considered "cerebral syndromes" in that their clinical characteristics are related to the brain.[20] The symptoms of AMS can be incapacitating to the point where an individual may not be able to complete a planned activity. Symptoms of AMS include headache, nausea, irritability, loss of appetite, decreased urine output, lightheadedness, and vomiting.[2] In some cases, symptoms may be experienced as early as 1 hour upon arrival to high altitude, but begin after 6 to 10 hours.[20] The symptoms reach their peak in 24 to 48 hours, but should subside after a few days.[2] Therefore, if an athlete is competing in an event in high altitude, plan to arrive days before the event in order to gradually acclimatize and possibly prevent AMS.

Treatment for AMS may be dependent on the particular situation, such as if the individual is planning further ascent, if there is a history of altitude illness, and the severity of symptoms.[20] Halting the ascent (or descending, if possible), supplemental oxygen, hyperbaric therapy, and medications such as acetazolamide (125 to 250 mg by mouth twice a day) and dexamethasone (4 mg every 6 hours) have been shown to alleviate the symptoms of AMS.[2,20]

If AMS is not treated properly or the individual continues a rapid ascent, AMS may develop into HACE, a life-threatening condition. Progression from AMS to HACE usually takes about 3 days but has been known to occur in as little as 12 hours.[2] The most common symptoms of HACE include deterioration in mental status or level of consciousness (such as confusion, bizarre behavior, or coma) and ataxia (loss of gross motor function).[2,20] Treatment for HACE consists of immediate descent, supplemental oxygen, hyperbaric therapy if possible, and dexamethasone (8 mg intravenously/intramuscularly/by mouth initially then 4 mg every 6 hours).[20]

Prevention of AMS and HACE consists of having climbers follow a graded ascent, sleeping at lower elevations, consuming a diet of more than 70% of calories from carbohydrates, and performing mild exercise to aid with acclimatization.[2]

HAPE, like HACE, is also a life-threatening condition that occurs in individuals, usually climbers, who are unacclimatized to high altitude and who ascend too rapidly. The onset usually takes a few hours to ensue, however, once present, the individual's condition may deteriorate rapidly; early diagnosis and treatment are the key to survival for HAPE patients. Symptoms of HAPE include dyspnea at rest; tachycardia; rales; cyanosis; white, pink, or yellow frothy sputum; and exercise limitation.[2,20,23] Treatment for HAPE consists of supplemental oxygen, descent of greater than 500 to 1000 meters as soon as possible, hyperbaric therapy (if oxygen is not available), and in some cases, medications such as nifedipine (10 mg by mouth) and inhaled beta-agonists such as albuterol may be given.[20] Preventative measures for HAPE are similar to those of AMS and HACE and may include slowly ascending, sleeping at low altitudes, and acetazolamide prior to climbing.[2]

These 3 high-altitude illnesses are more prevalent for those individuals partaking in climbing expeditions and may not be such a high risk for other types of athletes. However, it is important to note that when athletes travel for competitions to areas of a higher altitude than they are accustomed to, they may be susceptible to some altitude sickness symptoms. Furthermore, other pre-existing conditions, such as having sickle cell trait, may predispose an athlete to a dangerous situation. For example, in 2007, a National Football League football player experienced a medical emergency when playing in Denver, Colorado, due to complications from his sickle cell trait and being in high altitude.[22] The risk of hypoxia with altitude and sickle cell trait when combined with physical exertion may lead to a life-threatening situation. Therefore, when traveling to a location at high altitude, it is imperative for the athletic trainer and other medical staff to be aware of their athletes' medical history and any pre-existing condition that may be exacerbated by the hyperbaric-hypoxic environment seen with altitude.

LIGHTNING SAFETY

To date in 2012, there have already been 28 lightning fatalities in 16 states, with Florida leading the nation with 5.[24] The National Weather Service has shown similar numbers in previous years as 2011 had 26 fatalities in 18 states and Guam, 2010 had 29 fatalities in 19 states, and 2009 had 34 fatalities in 22 states and Puerto Rico.[24] These lightning strikes have occurred while people were engaged in various activities including baseball, fishing, walking, jogging, and attending other sporting events.[24] The highest incidence of lightning fatalities occurred in June, July, and August. Physically active individuals and those that help organize athletic events should be aware of safety guidelines and develop guidelines to help prevent a lightning catastrophe.

Education is key to ensuring lightning safety. Unfortunately, many individuals are misinformed about lighting and oftentimes are not aware of the appropriate course of action to take during a thunderstorm.[25] Table 13-2 contains lighting facts to staying safe in a storm. It is also imperative for athletic organizations to have a lightning safety policy in place. This ensures that athletic trainers, coaches, administrators, or those individuals in charge of organizing athletic events and/or athletic facilities will have the knowledge on the prevention of lighting injuries as well as proper management should a lightning strike occur.

The lightning safety policy should include a few key components. One of the most important components is identifying who will the making the call to suspend the activity.[25,26] The person chosen for this responsibility may vary by setting. For example, a certified athletic trainer may be given this responsibility at one school while other settings may have the school principle, coach, or referee in charge of making the call to remove individuals from the field during a thunderstorm. The safety guidelines should also have suggested locations that may serve as safe shelters in the event of a thunderstorm. The safest location would be a grounded, frequently inhabited building,[25] such as the school building, if moving athletes from the school's field. Avoid seeking shelter in dugouts, golf carts, under trees, and picnic shelters.[26] Unfortunately, in the athletic or recreational setting, people seek these unsafe areas as shelter from lightning storms. Having a set

Table 13-2
LIGHTNING FACTS

- Lightning often strikes 3 miles from the center of the storm. Sometimes lightning bolts can strike 10 to 15 miles away from the storm. If you are caught in a storm, don't lie flat on the ground. Keep moving toward a safe shelter or assume the lightning-safe position (ie, crouched on the ground, weight on balls of the feet, feet together, head lowered, and ears covered).[24,25]

- Height, pointy shape, and isolation are main factors to avoid during a thunderstorm as these are the objects most likely to get struck by a lightning bolt.

- Metal does not attract lightning; however, it is a good conductor of electricity so avoid contact with metal objects including fences and metal bleachers.

Adapted from National Weather Lightning Safety. http://www.lightningsafety.noaa.gov.

policy that explains the safest locations to seek shelter as well as information on when an activity should be suspended due to lightning and when the activity can resume is essential to assist athletic trainers, coaches, athletes, and others in knowing when it is safe for individuals to be outside. The 30-30 rule, explained in the next section, is often incorporated into lightning safety guidelines. Some lightning safety guidelines recommend seeking shelter as soon as lightning is seen or thunder is heard[27]; the National Weather Service's lightning safety guidelines include the phrase "when thunder roars, go indoors."[24]

THE 30-30 RULE

The 30-30 rule is used to determine 2 factors: when individuals should seek shelter due to a lightning storm and when it is safe for an activity to resume following a storm. The first "30" refers to the number of seconds between when one sees a lightning bolt and hears the ensuing thunder (commonly referred to as *flash-to-bang*). When the flash-to-bang is 30 seconds or less, individuals should seek shelter immediately. The second "30" refers to when it is safe to resume an activity after a storm. After seeking safe shelter, individuals should wait 30 minutes from the last lightning bolt seen or thunder heard before resuming activity. Therefore, if after 20 minutes of going indoors another lightning bolt is seen or thunder is heard, the clock restarts and individuals should wait at least 30 minutes before resuming activity (assuming this was the last lightning bolt seen). However, recent guidelines are moving away from the 30-30 rule and toward seeking shelter immediately once lightning is seen or thunder is heard.[27]

CARE OF A LIGHTNING-STRIKE VICTIM

A common myth regarding lightning strikes is that other individuals can get electrocuted if they come into contact with a lightning-strike victim, when, in fact, this is not true.[24] The scene may be unsafe if there is a chance that others in the area may also be struck by lightning, but it is safe to touch the victim and chances of survival are greatest when immediate medical care is given.[26] A lightning strike usually results in apnea and asystole, therefore, immediate care should include activation of EMS, moving the victim to a safe area, and evaluating and treating for respiratory and cardiac arrest.[25] Once the victim has a stable pulse and respirations, treat for shock and evaluate and treat for burns and/or fractures.[25]

SUMMARY OF KEY POINTS

➡ Although the exact cause may be unclear, heat cramps often occur with muscle fatigue, fluid losses, and most importantly, loss of electrolytes.

➡ Heat syncope, often referred to as orthostatic dizziness, may occur when an individual is exposed to high environmental temperatures.

➡ Exertional heat exhaustion has been defined as the inability to continue exercising due to cardiovascular insufficiency, often while exercising in a hot, humid environment

➡ Prevention of exertional heat exhaustion can be achieved by ensuring athletes have been gradually acclimatized to the heat and are properly hydrated prior to activity in the heat.

➡ EHS is a potentially fatal exertional heat illness consisting of exercise-induced hyperthermia (>104°F to 105°F) and altered mental status. The athlete should be cooled until core temperature reaches 102°F then continuously monitored until EMS arrives. Cold water immersion has had a 100% survival rate when used on actual EHS victims.[12,15]

➡ Hypothermia, defined as a decrease in body temperature below 95°F,[18] is a potentially fatal condition resulting from exposure to cold conditions.

➡ Frostbite is the freezing of body tissues resulting from overexposure to a cold, dry environment and is considered a medical emergency.[18]

➡ Trench foot and chilblains are the most common nonfreezing cold injuries and occur when tissues are exposed to cold, wet conditions. An individual is at risk for trench foot when tissues are exposed to cold, wet conditions between 32°F to 60°F for more prolonged periods of time.

➡ High-altitude illnesses, including AMS, HACE, and HAPE, occur as a result of acute exposure to hypobaric hypoxia.

➡ The 30-30 rule is used to determine 2 factors: when individuals should seek shelter due to a lightning storm and when it is safe for an activity to resume following a storm.

REVIEW QUESTIONS

1. Describe the differences between exertional heat exhaustion and EHS.
2. Describe the proper immediate care for EHS.
3. Describe the proper care for frostbite.
4. What are the 3 conditions that result from hypobaric hypoxia?
5. What is the 30-30 rule? Why is it important?

REFERENCES

1. Perdrizet GA. Hans Selye and beyond: responses to stress. *Cell Stress Chaperones.* 1997;2(4):214-219.
2. Armstrong LE. *Performing in Extreme Environments.* Champaign, IL: Human Kinetics; 2000.
3. Binkley HM, Beckett J, Casa DJ, Kleiner DM, Plummer PE. National Athletic Trainers' Association position statement: exertional heat illnesses. *J Athl Train.* 2002;37(3):329-343.
4. Castellani JW. Physiology of heat stress. In: Armstrong LE, ed. *Exertional Heat Illnesses.* Champaign, IL: Human Kinetics; 2003:1-15.
5. Bergeron MF. Exertional heat cramps: recovery and return to play. *J Sport Rehabil.* 2007;16(3):190-196.
6. Casa DJ, Almquist J, Anderson S. Inter-Association Task Force on Exertional Heat Illnesses consensus statement. *NATA News.* 2003;June:329-343.
7. Bergeron MF. Heat cramps: fluid and electrolyte challenges during tennis in the heat. *J Sci Med Sport.* 2003;6(1):19-27.
8. Armstrong LE, ed. *Exertional Heat Illnesses.* Champaign, IL: Human Kinetics; 2003.
9. Grundstein AJ, Ramseyer C, Zhao F, et al. A retrospective analysis of American football hyperthermia deaths in the United States. *Int J Biometeorol.* 2012;56(1):11-20.

10. Casa DJ, Becker SM, Ganio MS, et al. Validity of devices that assess body temperature during outdoor exercise in the heat. *J Athl Train.* 2007;42(3):333-342.

11. Lopez RM, Casa DJ, McDermott BP, Stearns RL, Armstrong LE, Maresh CM. Exertional heat stroke in the athletic setting: a review of the literature. *Athletic Training & Sports Health Care.* 2011;3(4):189-200.

12. Casa DJ, Anderson JM, Armstrong LE, Maresh CM. Survival strategy: acute treatment of exertional heat stroke. *Strength Cond Res.* 2006;20(3):462.

13. Armstrong LE, Casa DJ, Millard-Stafford M, Moran DS, Pyne SW, Roberts WO. American College of Sports Medicine position stand. Exertional heat illness during training and competition. *Med Sci Sports Exerc.* 2007;39(3):556-572.

14. Casa DJ, McDermott BP, Lee EC, Yeargin SW, Armstrong LE, Maresh CM. Cold water immersion: the gold standard for exertional heat stroke treatment. *Exerc Sport Sci Rev.* 2007;35(3):141-149.

15. McDermott BP, Casa DJ, Ganio MS, et al. Acute whole-body cooling for exercise-induced hyperthermia: a systematic review. *J Athl Train.* 2009;44(2):84-93.

16. Rav-Acha M, Hadad E, Epstein Y, Heled Y, Moran DS. Fatal exertional heat stroke: a case series. *Am J Med Sci.* 2004;328(2):84-87.

17. Folk GE Jr, Riedesel ML, Thrift DL. *Principles of Integrative Environmental Physiology.* Lanham, MD: Austin & Winfield Publishers; 1998.

18. Cappaert TA, Stone JA, Castellani JW, Krause BA, Smith D, Stephens BA. National Athletic Trainers' Association position statement: environmental cold injuries. *J Athl Train.* 2008;43(6):640-658.

19. Castellani JW, Young AJ, Ducharme MB, Giesbrecht GG, Glickman E, Sallis RE. American College of Sports Medicine position stand: prevention of cold injuries during exercise. *Med Sci Sports Exerc.* 2006;38(11):2012-2029.

20. Gallagher SA, Hackett PH. High-altitude illness. *Emerg Med Clin North Am.* 2004;22(2):329-355, viii.

21. Imray C, Wright A, Subudhi A, Roach R. Acute mountain sickness: pathophysiology, prevention, and treatment. *Prog Cardiovasc Dis.* 2010;52(6):467-484.

22. Altitude could preclude Clark's playing. http://sports.espn.go.com/nfl/news/story?id=4617421. Accessed June 23, 2011.

23. Zhou Q. Standardization of methods for early diagnosis and on-site treatment of high-altitude pulmonary edema. *Pulm Med.* 2011;2011:190648.

24. National Weather Lightning Safety. http://www.lightningsafety.noaa.gov. Accessed July 11, 2011.

25. Walsh KM, Bennett B, Cooper MA, Holle RL, Kithil R, Lopez RE. National athletic trainers' association position statement: lightning safety for athletics and recreation. *J Athl Train.* 2000;35(4):471-477.

26. Zimmermann C, Cooper MA, Holle RL. Lightning safety guidelines. *Ann Emerg Med.* 2002;39(6):660-664.

27. Walsh KM. *Emerging Position Statements: Lightning Safety for Athletics and Recreation.* Presented at the National Athletic Trainers' Association Annual Meeting. New Orleans, LA, June 20, 2011.

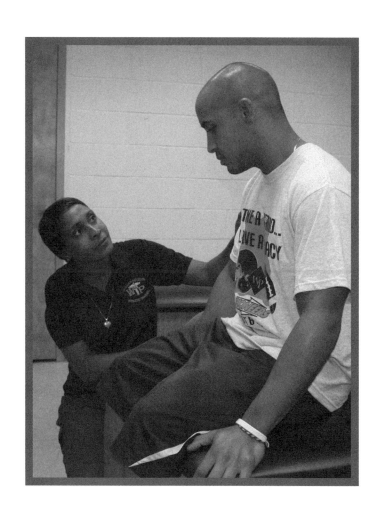

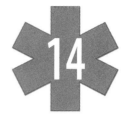

Managing
Mental Health Emergencies

Eileen Lubeck, PsyD

> *As you close up and prepare to leave after a long day's work, one of your athletes comes to you and tells you she is very concerned about her teammate, who is in the locker room. She tells you that her teammate has been acting differently lately and has made some strange comments. She tells you that she thinks her teammate may be considering suicide, and pleads with you to help.*
> *What do you do? What do you say?*

There are situations in which members of a sports emergency care team may find themselves confronted with a mental health emergency. Although these may be somewhat different in nature than the medical emergencies that the sports emergency care team is accustomed to managing, the basic principle for good management of these situations is the same. That is, preparation is the key to a good outcome. In this case, preparation involves awareness of the potential situations one might face while working with student athletes, education about some of the basic skills needed to address individuals who may be in crisis, and knowledge of the available resources so that assistance can be obtained as quickly as possible.

The 2 significant mental health emergencies a sports emergency care team may face are situations in which a student athlete becomes psychiatrically unstable and situations in which an athlete dies or becomes critically injured and the sports emergency care team must manage the emotional impact of that event on the remainder of the team. Before these situations are discussed in detail, it is useful to delineate some practical communication and relationship-building skills that, if utilized, will enable a treatment provider to be prepared long before an emergency arises.

Rehberg RS.
Sports Emergency Care: A Team Approach,
Second Edition (pp 211-218).
© 2013 SLACK Incorporated.

THE UNIQUE RELATIONSHIP WITH ATHLETES

Members of a sports emergency care team are in a position to have a close relationship with the athletes they treat. Developing trust within that relationship is critical so that the athlete feels he or she can seek out assistance from the treatment provider when needed. The provider needs to establish that trust so that the athlete will be forthright about any medical symptoms he or she is experiencing. This will enable the provider to accurately assess and treat an injury and to make appropriate decisions about readiness for play or not. In situations where an athlete is spending a considerable amount of time with a treatment provider, the individuals are likely to get to know one another on a deeper level, and the relationship may develop to the point where other issues are being discussed.

ACTIVE LISTENING

In order to help an athlete feel as if he or she is being heard and can trust the treatment provider, it can be helpful for the sports emergency care personnel to be skilled in active listening techniques. Active listening, which is based on the concepts of empathy and attending to others described by Rogers,[1] involves utilizing both verbal and nonverbal modes of communication to demonstrate attention and understanding to the other. Nonverbal strategies utilized in active listening involve maintaining eye contact, establishing the appropriate amount of personal space between both people, and taking a stance that conveys a sense of openness to the speaker such as placing one's arms down at the sides rather than having them folded across one's chest. Verbal strategies utilized in active listening involve paraphrasing and summarizing what the speaker has said to ensure that the content has been accurately understood.[2]

MAINTAINING APPROPRIATE BOUNDARIES

The development of a relationship between an athlete and a provider who are working closely together is not unusual. It can contribute to a comfort level that facilitates the work that is being done to help the athlete heal. It is vital, however, for sports emergency care personnel to always remain mindful of both the power and the limits of that relationship. Although the relationship may feel quite close, it is still a professional relationship, and it is the responsibility of the treatment provider to uphold professional boundaries at all times. Again, it is not unusual for athletes to begin discussing other personal issues with the treatment provider. The potential problem with this is that the treatment provider can easily find him- or herself in a situation where the athlete has shared something that is worrisome and indicates some level of risk to the athlete or to someone else. It is, therefore, vitally important for the treatment provider to recognize one's own limitations in providing care to an athlete and to know other professionals to whom they can refer athletes if the topics of conversation are outside the bounds of the athletic trainer's area of knowledge and training. One example is a situation in which an athlete reveals eating-disordered behavior that is beyond the treatment provider's skill level. Recognizing the need to refer the athlete to a treatment team that involves a nutritionist, mental health professional, and medical professional who can order and monitor lab work is likely to lead to the best possible outcome for the athlete.

It is also critically important that a sports emergency care professional never agree to keep secrets that may be shared by an athlete. It is very easy for well-meaning professionals to make this mistake because of the hope that the athletes with whom they are working will trust them and be open about their problems. The risk here is that even those with the best intentions can find themselves in situations where the secret involves someone's well-being and the treatment provider is then in a position to either violate that trust or keep the secret and feel stuck in an overwhelming and uncertain predicament, unable to manage the situation alone. An example of this is a situation in which an athlete shares contemplations of suicide. One can see how treatment providers who have agreed to keep such a secret will quickly feel in over their heads and at a loss for how to proceed in managing that situation. It is far better to let an athlete know that you cannot remain confidential about issues that jeopardize someone's safety but that you can promise to get help for that athlete and treat the information shared as delicately as possible. Often people agree to keep secrets for fear that if they do not promise to do so then the person who has something to confide will decide not to share it. The potential risks of agreeing to keep a secret are too high, so it is far better to be honest about the limits and let that person decide.

SUICIDE PREVENTION

Having some basic knowledge about suicide and suicide prevention is critical to be adequately prepared for a potential mental health emergency. Whether working with athletes at the high school, college, or professional level, suicide is a real concern. In the United States, suicide is the third leading cause of death for individuals in the 15- to 24-year-old age group and the second leading cause of death for individuals in the 25- to 34-year-old age group.[3] It is not uncommon for individuals who are contemplating suicide to show signs of distress that people around them can pick up on, especially if they know what to look for. While members of a sports emergency care team would never be expected to know how to counsel a suicidal person, they could potentially be close enough to the athlete to recognize the warning signs and assist in getting the athlete the appropriate care. There are multiple suicide prevention training programs, often referred to as *gatekeeper training*, that are specifically geared toward teaching people on the front lines how to intervene. Gatekeepers, such as coaches and athletic trainers, are likely to be among the first people to recognize a problem. If such a training program is offered, it is highly recommended that members of a sports emergency care team avail themselves of that opportunity. A list of gatekeeper training programs can be found on the Suicide Prevention Resource Center Web site under the Best Practices Registry for Suicide Prevention.[4]

In the event that one has not had training on suicide prevention, there are still some key pieces of information that would be useful to know in order to be prepared to intervene. The American Association of Suicidology has delineated a 2-tiered model for responding to warning signs for suicide.[5] The creation of the 2-tiered model has been viewed as a useful system for laypeople and individuals who serve as first responders.[6] There are several warning signs of suicide on the first tier that should be responded to immediately by calling 9-1-1 or by calling the National Suicide Prevention Lifeline (1-800-273-TALK [8255]). These include the following:

* Suicidal threats either expressed directly, such as "I want to die," or indirectly, such as "It doesn't really matter what happens, I'm not going to be around much longer."

* Seeking out a weapon or other means of killing oneself.

* Someone talking or writing about dying, death, or suicide, especially in situations that are out of context or out of the ordinary for the individual. This can be in academic papers, letters, notes, and online sites or other electronic means.

In addition, on the second tier, there are indications that someone is distressed and may need referral to a mental health professional even if the need for intervention is not emergent.[5] These include the following:

* Depression characterized by sadness, apathy, expressions of hopelessness and despair, dramatic weight change, or mood changes that can include an improvement in mood following a period of despair.

* Social isolation.

* Nervousness, agitation, or irritability.

* Significant change in hygiene.

* Increased alcohol/drug use or other reckless behavior.
* Extreme anger.
* Insomnia or excessive sleep.

Once someone suspects that an individual may be contemplating suicide, the only way to know for sure is to ask the question directly. Many people buy into the myth that talking about suicide may give someone the idea to attempt suicide even if the person was not previously suicidal. This simply is not accurate.[7] It is important to ask whether the person is thinking of "suicide" or "killing him- or herself" and to do so with those specific words. Although the person asking the question may be uncomfortable with the topic, it is vital to avoid using other, less direct, language so as not to cause any confusion about what question is being asked.[8] In situations where an athlete indicates feeling suicidal, the sports emergency care team must get help immediately. The topic of resources and referrals will be addressed later in this chapter, but it should noted that the National Suicide Prevention Lifeline, 1-800-273-TALK (8255) can provide assistance with referrals even in situations when the suicide threat is not imminent.

ATHLETE BECOMES PSYCHIATRICALLY ILL

In addition to suicidal crises, an athlete can experience a period of psychiatric instability that warrants intervention on an emergency basis. The onset of bipolar disorder and first episodes of psychosis in schizophrenia and other chronic psychiatric conditions typically occur in the early 20s to mid 30s.[9,10] It is also not atypical for some symptoms of significant mental illness to appear more than a year before the full manifestation of the illness emerges.[11] One can see why sports emergency care personnel who are working with athletes at an age where they are vulnerable to the development of mental illness would need to be prepared in the event that a psychiatric emergency arises. Once a problem has been detected, there may be some reluctance to call for help. Reasons for this may include lack of knowledge regarding the specific nature of the illness, uncertainty about the resources available, especially if the athlete becomes ill while traveling to an away game in an unfamiliar area, and discomfort in calling attention to the problem due to the stigma still associated with mental health issues. Another barrier to getting help might be reluctance to get the athlete in trouble in instances where it is suspected that the psychiatric instability has been caused by substance use. There have been instances where coaches and training staff have been very far from home when an athlete became ill and, rather than take him or her to a nearby emergency room, they have opted to try to manage the situation on their own until they can get the athlete back to family and familiar treatment settings. This has included staying awake all night to monitor the athlete and traveling home on a bus or an airplane with the ill person. The risks in doing this are tremendous because psychiatrically ill people can be unpredictable and the emergency can quickly escalate to the point where containment in a safe place (ie, hospital) and medication may be warranted to stabilize the individual. Despite the aforementioned barriers, it is imperative for sports emergency care personnel to take the psychiatrically ill athlete to the nearest emergency room without delay. In addition to suicidal ideation, which has been previously discussed, signs of significant distress include, but are not limited to, strange or unusual behavior that induces fear, violent ideation, bizarre speech, nervousness, agitation, irritability, marked changes in personal hygiene, social isolation or withdrawal, inability to control anger, and paranoia.

DEATH/CATASTROPHIC ILLNESS OF AN ATHLETE

Unfortunately, there are situations in which an athlete dies or becomes seriously injured in either a practice or game situation, or in an unrelated event such as a motor vehicle accident. The sports emergency care personnel may have to attend to the mental health needs of other individuals on the team once the initial emergency has concluded. Teammates spend an inordinate amount of time together in an environment that can be very close-knit. The members of the team, including the coaching staff, may have a difficult time coping with a significant tragedy, and the sports emergency care personnel should have a postvention plan in place before an emergency arises. *Postvention* is a term "used to describe prevention measures implemented after a crisis or traumatic event to reduce the risk to those who have witnessed or been affected by the tragedy."[12p6] In the case of a tragedy that affects a team, sports emergency care personnel need to make themselves available in such a way that communicates their readiness to help, if needed. They need to help the team understand that it is not uncommon for tragedy to bring about reactions in the remaining players and staff and that they will assist with any feelings or concerns that arise as a result. They should be prepared to monitor the reactions of the remaining team members and be prepared to intervene with appropriate action if someone displays signs of significant distress. It is also important for providers to be able to quickly call upon grief counselors who can provide needed support and implement psychological first aid.

PSYCHOLOGICAL FIRST AID

Psychological first aid is a mental health intervention that has historically been utilized to assist with recovery after significant events such as large-scale natural disasters and terrorist attacks, but it is also deemed valuable for use following crises that affect individuals or smaller groups of people.[13] "Psychological First Aid is designed to reduce the initial distress caused by traumatic events and to foster short- and long-term adaptive functioning and coping."[14p96] It is an intervention that is most often delivered by mental health professionals who are called in to field settings to assist in the aftermath of a tragic event, but nonmental health workers can also be trained to provide psychological first aid.[15] Sports emergency care personnel and emergency medical services (EMS) workers may be able to join community response teams and avail themselves of the specific training needed to deliver psychological first aid directly. Even if sports emergency care personnel are not going to be trained to deliver the intervention themselves, it is highly recommended that providers read the *Psychological First Aid Field Operations Guide* available on the National Child Traumatic Stress Network Web site (www.nctsn.org/sites/default/files/pfa/english/1-psyfirstaid_final_complete_manual.pdf) in order to familiarize themselves with the model.

SELF-CARE FOR SPORTS EMERGENCY CARE PROFESSIONALS

It is vital for anyone in a helping profession to practice self-care skills so as to preserve one's own well-being while taking care of others. This can be especially important when recently faced with managing a trying emergency and may be even more critical when a provider who is not necessarily trained in mental health issues has been faced with an unfamiliar psychiatric emergency. Good self-care includes taking care of the physical self by getting enough rest, eating a well-balanced diet, and finding time for exercise, but it also includes taking care of emotional health. This involves finding balance between work and home life and incorporating healthy forms of recreation and time with loved ones. It is also essential for providers to recognize that they will have their own emotional responses to a trying or traumatic experience and that it is key to acknowledge those feelings and access sources of support for processing those feelings such as a trusted supervisor or colleague or perhaps a personal therapist. The *Psychological First Aid Field Operations Guide* includes a section on self-care for providers that contains suggestions that would be useful to implement even if one is not dealing with a tragic event.[14]

RESOURCES AND REFERRALS

As has been emphasized throughout this book, good preparation by everyone can help handle an emergency situation and have a significant impact on the outcome of the emergency itself. A critical component of good preparation for mental health emergencies is knowing the resources available in advance. At the very least, the members of the sports emergency care team should know mental health professionals with whom they can consult if they are concerned about an athlete and want to make a referral for treatment. This would go beyond simply knowing the name of the school counselor, for example. Good preparation would entail cultivating working relationships with relevant mental health professionals so as to facilitate care, when needed. If the sports emergency care team is working in a setting where there are already protocols in place for managing mental health emergencies, such as on a college campus, it would behoove them to know what those protocols are. It would also be important to know which hospitals in the area manage mental health emergencies or have mobile screening teams that can assess a mental health emergency on-site. In situations where an emergency occurs when a team is traveling, the sports emergency care team would obviously not know about available resources, but they can ask the personnel at the competition site for this information and providers can always call 9-1-1 for assistance, regardless of location. Someone who is acutely psychiatrically ill while at an away competition should always be taken to the nearest emergency room for evaluation, rather than attempt to get the athlete home. Finally, it would be helpful to know, in advance, how to access individuals in the area who are trained in psychological first aid in the event that the team faces a tragic event and requires this kind of an intervention. Many counties or states have organized disaster response teams that can be utilized if needed. A simple Internet search for local disaster mental health teams should yield the needed information. Additionally, response teams can be located through the American Psychological Association's Disaster Response Network or through the American Red Cross Disaster Mental Health Services.[13]

SUMMARY OF KEY POINTS

➡ The 2 significant mental health emergencies a sports emergency care team may face are situations in which a student athlete becomes psychiatrically unstable and situations in which an athlete dies or becomes critically injured and the sports emergency care team must manage the emotional impact of that on the remainder of the team.

➡ Active listening, which is based on the concepts of empathy and attending to others, involves utilizing both verbal and nonverbal modes of communication to demonstrate to the other that he or she is being attended to and understood.

➡ It is critically important that a sports emergency care professional never agree to keep secrets that may be shared by an athlete.

➡ Whether working with athletes at the high school, college, or professional level, suicide is a real concern. In the United States, suicide is the third leading cause of death for individuals in the 15- to 24-year-old age group and the second leading cause of death for individuals in the 25- to 34-year-old age group.

➡ It is not uncommon for individuals who are contemplating suicide to show signs of distress that people around them can pick up on, especially if they know what to look for.

➡ Once someone suspects that an individual may be contemplating suicide, the only way to know for sure is to ask the question directly, using specific words.

➡ An athlete can experience a period of psychiatric instability that warrants intervention on an emergency basis. The onset of bipolar disorder and first episodes of psychosis in schizophrenia and other chronic psychiatric conditions typically occur in the age range between the early 20s and mid 30s.

Table 14-1

SUMMARY OF RESOURCES

- National Suicide Prevention Lifeline: 1-800-273-TALK (8255)
- Suicide Prevention Resource Center Web site: www.sprc.org. Search this site to find Best Practices Registry for Suicide Prevention, a list of gatekeeper trainings, and other helpful information pertaining to the topic of suicide prevention
- *Psychological First Aid Field Operations Guide* located on the National Child Traumatic Stress Network Web site: www.nctsn.org/sites/default/files/pfa/english/1-psyfirstaid_final_complete_manual.pdf
- Search American Psychological Association's Disaster Response Network or the American Red Cross Disaster Mental Health Services to access local disaster response teams

---

➡ Postvention is a term "used to describe prevention measures implemented after a crisis or traumatic event to reduce the risk to those who have witnessed or been affected by the tragedy."[12p6]

➡ Psychological first aid is a mental health intervention that has historically been utilized to assist with recovery after significant events such as large-scale natural disasters and terrorist attacks, but it is also deemed valuable for use following crises that affect individuals or smaller groups of people.

➡ It is vital for anyone in a helping profession to practice self-care skills so as to preserve one's own well-being while taking care of others.

➡ A critical component of good preparation for mental health emergencies is knowing the resources available in advance. See Table 14-1 for a summary of resources described in this chapter.

REVIEW QUESTIONS

1. Describe some of the warning signs of suicide.
2. What does it mean to maintain appropriate boundaries? Why is it important?
3. Describe the concept of "postvention."
4. What are some of the signs of significant distress?
5. Why are self-care skills essential for every sports emergency care provider?

REFERENCES

1. Rogers C. *Client-Centered Therapy: Its Current Practice, Implications, and Theory.* Boston, MA: Houghton Mifflin; 1951.
2. Robertson K. Active listening: more than just paying attention. *Aust Fam Physician.* 2005;34(12):1053-1055.
3. Web-based Injury Statistics Query and Reporting System (WISQARS). Centers for Disease Control and Prevention, National Center for Injury Prevention and Control. http://www.cdc.gov/injury/wisqars. Updated 2007. Accessed August 2, 2011.
4. Best Practices Registry (BPR) for Suicide Prevention. Suicide Prevention Resource Center. www2.sprc.org/category/bpr-gatekeeper/yes. Accessed July 27, 2011.

5. American Association of Suicidology. Understanding and helping the suicidal individual. http://www.suicidology. org/c/document_library/get_file?folderId=232&name=DLFE-30.pdf. Accessed July 27, 2011.

6. Rudd M, Berman A, Joiner T Jr, et al. Warning signs for suicide: theory, research, and clinical applications. *Suicide Life Threat Behav.* 2006;36(3):255-262.

7. Bertini K. *Understanding and Preventing Suicide.* Westport, CT: Praeger; 2009.

8. Syracuse University Counseling Center. *Campus Connect: Suicide Prevention Training for Gatekeepers.* Syracuse, NY: Author; 2006.

9. Tondo L, Lepri B, Cruz N, Baldessarini RJ. Age at onset in 3014 Sardinian bipolar and major depressive disorder patients. *Acta Psychiatr Scand.* 2010;121(6):446-452.

10. Kaplan HI, Sadock BJ. Schizophrenia. In: Kaplan, HI, Sadock, BJ, eds. *Synopsis of Psychiatry.* 8th ed. Baltimore, MD: Lippincott Williams and Wilkins; 1998:456-491.

11. Haas GL, Sweeney JA. Premorbid and onset features of first-episode schizophrenia. *Schizophr Bull.* 1992;18(3):373-386.

12. National Center for Mental Health Promotion and Youth Violence Prevention. How schools can prevent suicide. http://www.promoteprevent.org/publications/prevention-briefs/how-schools-can-prevent-suicide Accessed October 18, 2012.

13. Vernberg E, Steinberg A, Jacobs A, et al. Innovations in disaster mental health: psychological first aid. *Prof Psychol: Res Pr.* 2008;39(4):381-388.

14. Brymer M, Layne C, Jacobs A, et al. *Psychological First Aid Field Operations Guide.* 2nd ed. Los Angeles, CA: National Child Traumatic Stress Network and National Center for PTSD; 2006.

15. Everly G Jr, Flynn B. Principles and practical procedures for acute psychological first aid training for personnel without mental health experience. *Int J Emerg Ment Health.* 2006;8(2):93-100.

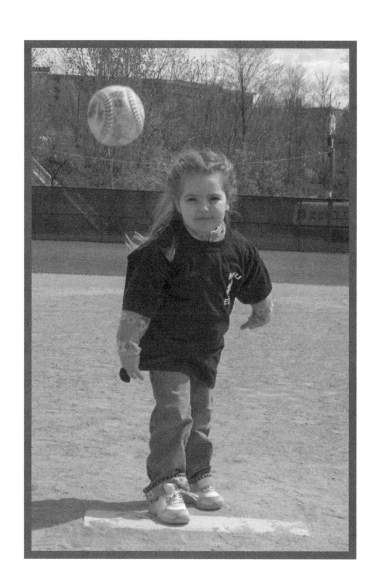

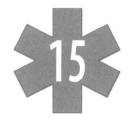

Emergency Care Considerations for the Pediatric and Youth Athlete

Jeff G. Konin, PhD, ATC, PT, FACSM, FNATA and
Rebecca M. Lopez, PhD, ATC, CSCS

There has been a significant increase in the number of youths participating in organized and recreational sports over the past 15 years.[1] In particular, a dramatic rise has been seen in the number of youths participating in such sports as softball, Pop Warner Football, and soccer. As such, both the overall number of injuries and the severity of these injuries have grown in volume.[2,3] The increases in participation and injury rates have been attributed to a number of factors, including but not limited to, the federal government's passing of Title IX legislation allowing for greater equality for female athletic participation; an increased level of interest for certain youth sports such as soccer; increased media coverage of sports such as gymnastics, skating, tennis, and swimming; and a greater-than-ever emphasis on competition driven by year-round desires to improve skill and conditioning levels for hopes of obtaining collegiate-level scholarships to offset the cost of a college education.[3] A recent study examining the emergence of female high school flag football found that flag football had an injury rate per 1000 exposures to be 1.13 for practices and 5.58 for competitions; this was found to be the second highest injury rate for female sports after soccer.[4] According to recent data reported by the national Safe Kids Campaign, from 2001 through 2009, approximately 1,770,000 children aged 14 years sought emergency medical care for a sports-related injury, many the potential result of parents being unsure of how to determine the seriousness of an injury or illness.[5-7] Furthermore, children aged 5 to 14 years account for nearly 40% of all sports-related injuries treated in hospital emergency departments.[7] Boys aged 10 to 14 years are twice as likely as girls of the same age to be treated in a hospital emergency room for a sports-related injury and are also more likely than girls to suffer from multiple injuries simultaneously.

Professional medical care is absent at the majority of organized youth sporting activities. With few exceptions, such as national, tournament-like events (eg, Little League World Series) and high schools that may employ certified athletic trainers, emergency medical care is often managed impromptu, without any advanced planning, and by a coach or parent who is most comfortable aiding and assisting an injured individual, though this person may not be medically credentialed or qualified in any such manner to provide formal care. A recent survey of high school coaches in South Dakota found that 89% of them were responsible for giving immediate medical care to their injured athletes at practices and 75% held this same responsibility for games.[8] Of about 250 respondents, less than 50% of these coaches held current cardiopulmonary resuscitation (CPR)

Rehberg RS.
Sports Emergency Care: A Team Approach,
Second Edition (pp 221-238).
© 2013 SLACK Incorporated.

certifications and 80% strongly agreed that they needed more injury management education.[8] Similarly, a recent survey of Florida high school athletic directors who had football at their schools reported that 71% (n = 129) had an emergency technician or paramedic working football games and most had an emergency medical technician, a physician, and/or certified athletic trainer at the games; however, despite having football at their schools, 34% of the athletic directors reported having no medical coverage at all.[9] While the "Good Samaritan" approach is appreciated, it does not reflect the optimal standard of care. More importantly, it could potentially lead to more harmful and/or mishandled circumstances.[10,11] Outside of organized sporting events for today's youth, the involvement with higher risk activities via the use of trampolines, in-lines skates, and other activities has also spawned an increase in traumatic injuries to children, oftentimes without any parental supervision, leading to nontreatment or a delay in the treatment of medical emergencies.

One should not be too naïve to recognize that providing on-site professional medical care at all youth sporting events regardless of the level of competition is solely an issue of cost. However, this fact should not mislead the public into realizing that the risk and severity of injuries sustained by children is of less importance than those sustained by adults. In fact, in many cases, the risk, prevalence, and severity are of greater concern given the immaturity of a child's anatomical features and underdevelopment of certain vital organs. Given the predicted continual growth identified with youth sport involvement, it would behoove parents and others to adapt improved guidelines for emergency care of traumatic-type injuries to children.

PREVENTION OF YOUTH SPORT EMERGENCIES

Much debate exists within the medical community as to whether or not injuries can actually be prevented, let alone acute traumatic and unpredictable types of injuries. Despite the lack of evidence, the majority of medical professionals believe that there are some common sense prevention measures that can be taken in an effort to identify potential risk factors for injury and illness among children participating in sports.

PREPARTICIPATION PHYSICAL EXAMINATIONS

Several professional associations have teamed together to identify the preparticipation physical examination (PPPE) as the gold standard for assessment (Table 15-1).[12] The purpose of the PPPE is to provide for a more sports-specific assessment of an individual, not to replace the standard physical examination performed by a physician during a typical and routine office visit. Depending upon the approach, a single physician can perform such an assessment or a multitude of individuals can collaborate in a team-like manner and perform a station-based PPPE. Lombardo first described the PPPE in 1994, identifying the following reasons for performing a PPPE, and later others endorsed a similar evidence-based approach to the PPPE[13-15]:

❋ To gather baseline data for future reference

❋ To detect manageable medical conditions that may interfere with sports participation

❋ To determine whether there are contraindications to participation

❋ To serve as a limited general health screening

❋ To fulfill legal requirements

Table 15-2 identifies components recommended as portions of a standardized examination.[16-18]

It is suggested that an examination be performed within 6 weeks of the beginning of participation. This would allow for both recent medical conditions to be identified and present with ample time to perform any further medical and/or laboratory tests with definitive results and findings prior to the start of an athlete's participation time frame.[18]

Table 15-1
MEDICAL ORGANIZATIONS ESTABLISHING A CONSENSUS STATEMENT REGARDING THE PREPARTICIPATION PHYSICAL EVALUATION AS THE GOLD STANDARD FOR SCREENING

- American Academy of Family Physicians
- American Academy of Pediatrics
- American College of Sports Medicine
- American Medical Society for Sports Medicine
- American Orthopaedic Society for Sports Medicine
- American Osteopathic Academy of Sports Medicine

Table 15-2
RECOMMENDED PORTIONS OF A STANDARDIZED EXAMINATION

Medical history questionnaire	Blood pressure
General appearance	Cardiovascular
Vision	Neurological
Respiratory	Musculoskeletal
Abdominal/genitourinary	History of heat illness/intolerance
Integumentary	Sickle cell trait
Weight and height	

In today's world, some form of PPPE appears to be the standard acceptance of clearance prior to formal organized participation. However, some in the medical profession question whether or not certain aspects of the examination are worth performing since they yield such low prevalence rates of findings.[19] Numerous musculoskeletal findings that could be classified as "deficits" or perhaps "non-normative" have not been demonstrated to be the causative factor of any eventual catastrophic or even mild injury. Magnes et al[20] reported on 10,540 preseason evaluations on children between the ages of 10 to 19 years over a 5-year period and found that overall 47 (0.4%) failed the exam, 18 (0.2%) had hypertension, 6 (0.06%) presented with blindness, 5 (0.06%) were absent a testicle, and 4 (0.05%) had postconcussion symptoms. With such small numbers of conditions being identified, the resources of time and money are questioned as to their worth in performing such lengthy exams.

Best[19] feels as though the PPPE has minimal effect on overall mortality and morbidity associated with sport participation and that no standard PPPE exists whereby a true consensus is found. Furthermore, Best states that there is no clear consensus on who should perform the PPPE, and that in fact a proper medical history may be more effective than the clinical exam itself.[19] On the other hand, Drezner and Corrado[21] have found that approximately 1 in 500 athletes may have an occult cardiovascular condition. Due to this risk of sudden cardiac death, a cardiovascular screening and the integration of an electrocardiogram screening may be warranted.

In 2006, Briskin et al[22] concluded that among highly active female adolescent dancers, a history of compromised bone quality was significantly associated with a predictive finding of a stress fracture. This finding is suggestive of dual-emission X-ray absorptiometry scanning when working with this population as a means of proactively recognizing if lower bone mineral density is present. A proactive approach may prevent more significant and complicated acute fractures that take longer to heal and may ultimately impact long-term athletic activity.

Some sudden death conditions resulting from athletic participation appear to be undetectable during a PPPE. For example, according to Maron et al,[23] 1 in 10 sudden deaths in young people are associated with sports; 158 deaths occurred between 1985 to 1995, of which 24 (15%) were attributable to noncardiovascular causes. Of the 134 remaining, 120 deaths were in males and due to a variety of causes of which the most common was hypertrophic cardiomyopathy; 115 of the 158 had a PPPE, but only 4 were suspected of having cardiovascular disease and in only one was the lesion identified correctly.[5]

The American Academy of Pediatrics[5] has identified certain medical conditions that can be used to determine if participation would create an increased risk of injury or adversely affect the medical condition itself. While the list may not be all-inclusive since circumstances vary, this type of information is found to be valuable during a PPPE when determining the status of sports participation eligibility (Table 15-3). These decisions are oftentimes not black and white, and in fact may be quite complex and challenging. An exam should not only include written criteria that are identified as suggested guidelines, but also clinical expertise of the physician, recommendations of other expert physicians, the current health status of the athlete, the specific sport, and the athlete's position and its inherent risks, among other considerations. The American College of Sports Medicine[24] recently adopted a new medical screening tool to be used as a PPPE that was developed in collaboration with itself, the American Academy of Family Physicians, American Medical Society for Sports Medicine, American Orthopaedic Society for Sports Medicine, and American Osteopathic Academy of Sports Medicine.

FIELD SAFETY

Unfortunately, many injuries that are preventable are the result of poor field conditions. Traumatic injuries can be the result of carelessness in maintaining a safe playing environment. In general, field safety is an area of prevention that can be practiced by all parties involved with youth sports, including parents, coaches, and community recreational employees. A systematic approach should be taken and documented on a regular basis to assess the safety status of all playing surfaces and equipment. Some of the items to be considered as possibly leading to a higher incidence of injury risk include the following:

❋ Uneven playing surfaces

❋ Surfaces with greater than normal friction (ie, old hardwood courts)

❋ Slippery playing surfaces (ie, fields with puddles) (Figure 15-1)

❋ Improper lighting for night events

❋ Irrigation systems not completely buried (Figure 15-2)

❋ Baseball dugouts without proper protection from hit balls

❋ Fences that surround fields with protruding parts

❋ Goal posts and other fixed apparatus that are not properly protected with padding

Table 15-3

Medical Conditions Requiring Potential Further Inquiry Prior to Allowing Sports Participation

- Atlantoaxial injury
- Bleeding disorders
- Cardiovascular disease
- Cerebral palsy
- Congenital heart disease
- Diabetes mellitus
- Diarrhea
- Dysrhythmia
- Eating disorders (anorexia nervosa, bulimia)
- Fever
- Heart murmur
- Heat illness
- Hepatitis
- Human immunodeficiency virus infection
- Hypertension
- Hyponatremia
- Kidney disease
- Liver disease
- Malignant neoplasm
- Musculoskeletal disorders
- Neurological disorders (concussion, epilepsy)
- Obesity
- Organ transplant recipient
- Ovary (absence of one)
- Respiratory conditions (asthma, upper respiratory infection)
- Sickle cell trait
- Skin disorders (boils, herpes simplex, impetigo, scabies, molluscum contagiosum)
- Spleen enlargement
- Testicle (undescending or absence of one)
- Visual deficits (loss of an eye, detached retina)

Figure 15-1. A neighborhood playground with puddles that could lead to children slipping and getting hurt.

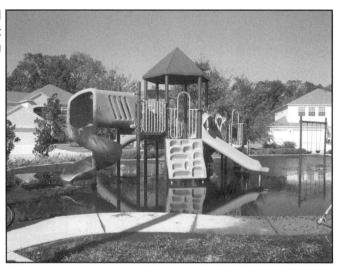

Figure 15-2. An example of a sprinkler head at a ball field that is not properly maintained for safety precautions.

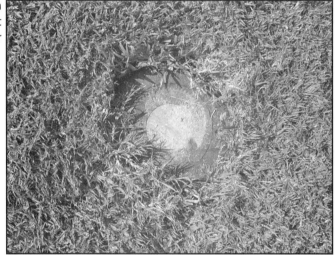

EQUIPMENT SAFETY

All equipment that is used, and especially that reissued on an annual basis as part of a recreational or organized program, should be carefully inspected and repaired as needed and according to any standards or guidelines that may exist. This may include helmets, baseball bats, gloves, pads, braces, and masks. Protective equipment serves numerous functions according to Konin and McCue[25] and therefore should be kept in current functioning order. These functions include, but are not limited to, absorbing forces, limiting anatomical movements, supporting joint structures and musculotendinous structures, enhancing proprioceptive feedback, and securing protective pads.[25] In general, any equipment issued or reissued should be properly fitted and sized, specifically helmets for sports such as football and ice hockey and shoulder pads for football, ice hockey, and lacrosse.[16] Loose-fitting helmets and shoulder pads can lead to a greater impact of forces sustained through direct contact, potentially leading to more serious injuries. In particular as it relates to younger children and those playing a sport for the first time, feedback regarding poor-fitting braces, pads, or helmets may not be accurate (Figure 15-3). Thus, individuals with

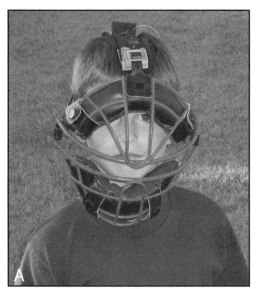
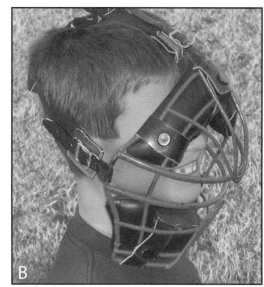

Figure 15-3. Example of an improperly fitted facemask for baseball that is too big for the size of the child.

knowledge on proper equipment fitting should be involved with appropriate equipment issuing and regular maintenance. Young athletes should also be educated on the use of protective equipment for "extreme" sports such as in-line skating, snowboarding, and skateboarding. A survey of 333 adolescents[26] who participate in these activities reported wearing less protective equipment than what is recommended; discomfort and perceived lack of need for this equipment were the most common reasons for not wearing the recommended protective equipment. Recently, some sports/events have placed an emphasis on certain pieces of protective equipment as both a response from adverse experiences and/or data demonstrating a high incidence of specific injuries. These include pole vault, lacrosse, field hockey, football, baseball, and soccer. Mouth guards in particular have been a common protective piece of equipment for athletes in many sports that have gained recent popularity with emphasis of use.

POLE VAULT

As a result of the potential risk associated with awkward and unprepared landings, even some possibly beyond the limits of the protective matted landing cushion, helmets have now been designed specifically for vaulters. These helmets are composed of a carbon and e-glass composite shell and weigh about as much or less than a standard bicycle helmet. In addition, the vault box is now made with a "soft box" soft cushion inner lining to further pad the athlete's landing.

WOMEN'S LACROSSE

Effective January 1, 2005, the sport of women's lacrosse at the intercollegiate level mandated the use of protective eyewear. This was the result of a rash of eye and facial injuries, and thus established the goal of prevention of rare but catastrophic eye injuries. Lacrosse associations within the United States have been proactive in educating youth athletes on how to obtain eyewear that has been proven and tested to sustain such forces. The most current standard, ASTM F803-03, states that protective eyewear should withstand forces generated by a ball traveling 45 miles per hour for youth play and 60 miles per hour for adult play (high school and older). In women's lacrosse, eyewear must meet the current ASTM specification standard, and US Lacrosse must receive independent confirmation from a third party testing facility that is recommended by the Protective Eyewear Certification Council (PECC) and meets the American Association of Laboratory Accreditation standards.[27]

MEN'S LACROSSE

Men's lacrosse, though a contact sport by nature, has gone relatively unscathed with respect to catastrophic injuries until recently. As a result of a rash of deaths related to commotio cordis, 4 of which involved men's lacrosse players over the past 5 years, a summit discussing the condition was formed that included representatives from US Lacrosse, National Athletic Trainers' Association (NATA), National Collegiate Athletic Association (NCAA), the American College of Sports Medicine, the American Medical Society for Sports Medicine, and youth baseball equipment manufacturers.[24-28] To date, discussion has surrounded the weight (5 ounce) and material (rubber) of the ball, the speed at which the ball travels (up to 90 mph), and the time frame whereby blunt trauma to the heart can lead to ventricular fibrillation (20-millisecond window). An emphasis on research in this area has been established, and the use of good preparation that includes effective emergency action plans with an on-site automated external defibrillator (AED) is now considered the standard of care for this arena. The National Federation of State High School Associations (NFHS) also recently made some rule changes in an effort to minimize injuries. Some of these changes included removing the ability of a player to check with or to the head. Furthermore, if a player is exhibiting signs, symptoms, or behaviors consistent with a concussion, that player will be removed from the game and may not return to play until cleared by "an appropriate health care professional."[28]

FIELD HOCKEY

Recently, collaboration has occurred between the NCAA Field Hockey Committee and equipment manufacturers to develop eyewear that will promote extended views while providing for optimal protection. As products are developed from research and collaboration at the professional and intercollegiate levels, these same pieces of equipment will be designed for children to afford them the same level of safety as their adult counterparts. The NFHS recently released a memorandum[29] regarding a new rule stating that the protective eyewear for field hockey players must meet the current ASTM standard (ASTM F2713-09).

FOOTBALL

Tinted face shields have become a trend for many athletes in the sport of football. However, complaints have been leveled against these nontransparent, or nonclear, shields because it is difficult to see another player's eyes behind them. This posed concerns for both medical personnel as well as football players themselves when playing against one another. As a result, the *NCAA Football Rules and Interpretations Handbook, 2009-2010*[30] lists tinted eye shields under illegal equipment and therefore cannot be worn in intercollegiate football games.

The American Academy of Pediatrics[5] in 2004 issued advice pertaining to protective eyewear for young athletes. A summary of the points includes the following:

* All children are encouraged to wear appropriate eye protection if participating in a sport that poses a risk of eye injury.

* Proper fit is essential.

* Three-mm polycarbonate lenses should be used for children with narrow faces who cannot fit well in goggles.

✴ Goggles approved by the American National Standards Institute are considered to be of the gold standard.

✴ Wearing contact lenses offers no protection in and of itself.

✴ Functional athletes with one eye should wear protection.

The PECC also exists to test for standards in eyewear. Eyewear approved in the laboratory for adults is considered acceptable for youth as well. Currently, no guidelines exist for eyeglass wearers, and goggles are not designed to cover standard eyeglasses.[31] With respect to actual competitions, game officials only assess that eyewear is worn; they do not have the capability to assess if appropriate standard eyewear protection is being used. Parents, coaches, and medical providers must take the responsibility to ensure that appropriate protection is being implemented. The recent findings[32,33] of reported orofacial injuries seen in children's sports will continue to place this issue at the forefront of those involved with caring for such traumatic incidents.

BASEBALL

The sport of baseball is also entertaining discussion regarding catastrophic injuries that could potentially occur. Though rare, commotio cordis is also a concern, especially to the individual playing the catcher position. At ball speeds of 40 mph, the risk of commotio cordis is greatest, and when the speeds increase, the risk decreases. However, the 40 mph speed is closely related to the speeds seen with Little League throwers. Recommendations[34] have been made to include using baseballs with softer core insides as well as using thermoplast-molded chest protectors. This concern as it relates to baseball has not yet received the same level of attention as it has with lacrosse.

SOCCER

The sport of soccer has not experienced a wave of catastrophic injuries despite its growing popularity throughout the world. However, it has not gone without some discussion regarding ways to reduce the number of serious head injuries experienced when colliding with the goal posts as well as from direct player-to-player contact. Questions have been raised as to whether or not goal posts should be changed from wood and metal to vinyl or padded. Currently, the main issue appears to be related to safety versus cost. That is, are there enough catastrophic head injuries that warrant a mandate that will cost millions of dollars to change the equipment? Published reports[16] of Injury Surveillance Systems show very low incidence of the need to justify such a change at this time.

MOUTH GUARDS

Protective mouth guards are an important piece of equipment for anyone exposed to the risk of contact or collision to the facial area (Figure 15-4).[16] This includes not only sports such as football and wrestling but also basketball and soccer, in which someone's elbow may accidentally hit another player in the mouth, and ice hockey, field hockey, and lacrosse, where a ball traveling at high speeds can hit a player in the mouth. Various forms of mouth guards exist, ranging from the standard shelf-stocked to the custom fitted and formed types. As one would expect, more protection is afforded with the mouth guards that are custom formed. Although mouth guards are viewed as an effective way of preventing and/or reducing the severity of dental injuries, whether or not they actually help prevent concussions is controversial.[35,36]

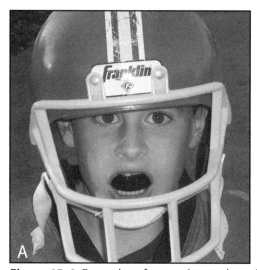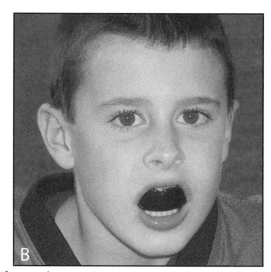

Figure 15-4. Examples of a mouth guard used for youth sports.

SPORTING RULES

While some catastrophic and acute emergency-like injuries are not preventable and are unfortunately accepted as part of sport participation, others can be prevented through rule changes. Of greatest note is in the sport of football, where the rules related to tackling, specifically the avoidance of "spearing" and head-to-head contact, have been implemented at all levels of play.[16] Various levels of competition, including the National Football League, have begun to strongly enforce rules to prevent football players from hitting defenseless opponents in the head or neck, as well as prohibiting hits delivered by an opponent with his helmet against any part of a defenseless player's body.[37]

In all sports, league officials and referees have taken a stronger stance against flagrant play and unsportsmanlike conduct in an effort to prevent unnecessary severe injuries. This vigilance against such play not only prevents immediate injury, but potentially long-term complications and recurrent inappropriate behavior.

Little League baseball has implemented rules that relate to limiting the number of pitches a child can throw in any given day and week. This is not likely designed to prevent an acute emergency but rather long-term, upper extremity damage at a young age that may develop through chronic overuse.[38] Though the rules have good intentions, honest enforcement and the fact that many children nowadays play simultaneously in multiple leagues with no method of monitoring the number of overall throws in a given time frame pose difficulty in actual quantitative interventions. At this time, no episodes of acute emergencies such as fractures or dislocations related to excessive throwing in a child have been reported.

PHYSICAL AND PSYCHOLOGICAL IMMATURITY

Medical emergencies can occur to children in slightly different ways than they do with adults for a variety of reasons. Children's bodies are still growing and their coordination is still developing, and therefore, their physical and emotional maturity levels are not on par with those of an adult. Prior to puberty, girls and boys are likely to experience the same risk of sports injuries. However, during puberty, boys will experience a greater number of injuries and more severe injuries than girls. The American Academy of Pediatrics[5] recommends that late-developing youths avoid contact sports until their bodies have developmentally "caught up" to the body size of their peers because children and adolescents who are less developed than a more mature child or adolescent of the same age and weight are at increased risk of injury. When adolescents are participating in a contact or collision sport but are physiologically at different stages of development, the coaches or certified athletic trainer are responsible for avoiding dangerous match-ups to ensure athlete safety.

In general, young children may not be able to accurately assess the risks associated with participating in certain sports. They are lacking in various aspects of physical maturity, such as having slightly less developed coordination skills, slower reaction times, and less accuracy as it relates to movement patterns. Imbalances in muscular development can lead to muscle strains and avulsion-type fractures. As such, sports that involve greater levels of contact, collision, or even sudden, rapid movements tend to pose a greater risk of injury. Those who are just beginning to partake in a sport for the first time are also more susceptible to injury, especially one of greater magnitude as a result of the lack of knowledge and awareness of the sport.

Anatomically, a child is at greater risk of physical injury merely due to the fact that aspects of his or her musculoskeletal system are not yet fully developed. Children who sustain fractures that involve immature growth plates will need to be assessed carefully to determine the extent of the injury. In some cases, such fractures can be treated conservatively, and healing will occur rather quickly without a high percentage of potential complications. On the other hand, if a significant disruption occurs to an immature growth plate, more aggressive intervention may be needed to secure adequate circulation in an attempt to prevent premature closure. It is important to identify such situations as early as possible so as to not compromise any potential outcome.[39-42] Ideally, the presence of a certified athletic trainer at youth sporting events is essential for the proper recognition and management of severe musculoskeletal injuries.

Thoracic wall injuries are commonplace among pediatric and adolescent children. In fact, Sartorelli and Vane[43] identify thoracic trauma as the second leading cause of death in children, behind brain injuries. Although these types of injuries are not seen as often in children as they are in adults, they remain a source of morbidity and mortality.[44] The compliant chest wall of children affords far more opportunistic injuries such as pulmonary contusions and rib fractures.[43] In addition, children's thoracic wall anatomy and physiology differ from that of an adult with respect to pulmonary function, residual capacity, blood volume, chest wall and spinal soft tissue mobility, and cardiac function.[44] Neve et al[45] have shown that both lung and thoracic development occur during and until the end of puberty in the adolescent male; conversely, in adolescent females, lung development is almost finished following menarche.

Traumatic abdominal wall herniations have been described in the literature[46-52] more commonly as of late, with an emphasis on the etiology coming from a bicycle accident and the subsequent force of the abdominal wall hitting the handlebars (Figure 15-5). Children as young as 7 years old have suffered intra-abdominal injuries, in many cases surgical intervention was required.[51,52] Similar types of injuries have also been reported in children under the age of 17 years taking part in alpine skiing activities, particularly trauma to the kidneys.[53] Storsved and Rieger[54] described a case of a congenital solitary kidney (renal agenesis) in a 17-year-old offensive lineman who landed on his backside while participating in the sport of football. The youth presented with typical findings such as pain in the lower back and gluteal region, radiating pain down the leg, and shortness of breath. A computed tomography scan revealed a hematoma without renal abnormality and the absence of a right kidney. Renal agenesis is very rare and no evidence exists regarding the risk of return to a sport, particularly one such as football.

Identifying physical injuries in a child, especially those of an emergent nature, can oftentimes be a challenge because children do not always possess the psychological maturity to accurately convey their perceived levels of pain and discomfort. It is not uncommon for a child to actually

Figure 15-5. The position of the handlebars on a child's bike are such that any sudden stop of the bike would propel a child forward with the handlebars pushing up against the chest and abdominal wall area.

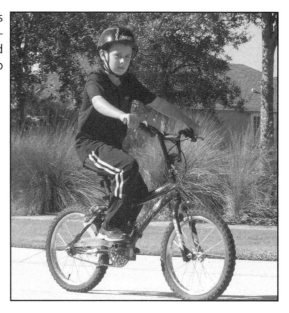

sustain a fracture and complain of pain, but the parent or coach writes it off as anything from a simple bruise to a growing pain. The same child only hours later may even be playing actively in the backyard with a fractured arm or leg. It is only several days later that the fracture is identified. Furthermore, referral patterns from injuries to internal organs may not be identified or accurately reported by a child. Another area of recent concern is symptoms reported by a child following a concussion and how accurate the subjective history may be. A head injury sustained by a child may in fact be more severe than that suffered by an adult due to the ongoing neurocognitive development of the child's brain.[55,56] This is an area of research that is in its infancy. However, these physiological differences in the younger concussed athlete have led to more conservative guidelines for the treatment and return to play of the child and adolescent athlete.[57] A recent consensus statement[57] recommends that regardless of the level of competition, a child or adolescent athlete who suffered a concussion should not return to play on the same day as the injury. An interesting finding that has been reported by Broshek et al[58] is that following a sustained concussion, female athletes tend to have significantly greater declines in both simple and complex reaction times when compared to baseline testing prior to the concussion. This same work found that females report more symptoms postconcussion than males of similar circumstances. In fact, females were found to be nearly 1.7 times more cognitively impaired than males following a concussion. One should keep this in mind and not always consider such reporting of a greater number of symptoms as a magnified result related to a more severe injury.

It is important to mention that along with the physical immaturity associated with identifying children's injuries, there is also psychological immaturity as well. Part of this rests on the shoulders of a child who has not yet formulated adult-like thought processes, and yet another part of the blame falls on overzealous parents. Parents may put added pressures on their children to not only participate, but in fact to succeed in sports at high levels. Children participate in recreational teams, travel teams, and other organized forms of competition year round, and sometimes participate on more than one team simultaneously. This has led to an abundance of overuse injuries from the physiological perspective, but also feelings of burn-out, disinterest, and even withdrawal from a child who is being pushed to play without an adequate level of self-enjoyment. A recent study[59] examining the prevalence of overtraining in elite young athletes found an incidence rate of ~20% to 30%, with potentially higher rates in individual sport athletes, females, and those competing at

---

Table 15-4

COMPONENTS OF A WELL-DESIGNED EMERGENCY ACTION PLAN

- Purpose of plan (eg, goals and objectives)
- Personnel involved (eg, ATC, EMT, MD, first responders)
- Role of various personnel (eg, MD, EMT, ATC)
- Preferred methods of communication (eg, land line phone, cell phone, walkie-talkie)
- Necessary equipment available (eg, AED, splints)
- Preferred methods of transportation (eg, ambulance, personal vehicle)
- Coverage plans (eg, on-site, on-call)
- Emergency contact information (eg, ATC, EMT, MD, police)
- Procedural methods for various circumstances (eg, unforeseen evacuations)
- Geographical and textual maps and directions
- Environmental policies (eg, lightning, heat)
- Planned written collaborative procedures with local hospital (eg, helmet removal)

---

the highest levels. Participation as the result of external pressures can lead to a child not paying attention to detail and ultimately can be the cause of a potentially dangerous situation, resulting in a severe injury.

A recent NATA position statement[60] on the prevention of pediatric overuse injuries suggests the following:

※ There is a need to improve injury surveillance in youth sports in order to enhance prevention and treatment of these injuries.

※ PPPE and injury surveillance systems can be used together in order to link PPPE findings with ways to prevent injury in the pediatric athletic population.

※ Youth sport coaches should have certifications or credentials regarding youth sport safety, knowledge of proper skill technique, and the knowledge to monitor for overuse injuries.

※ Pediatric athletes should avoid taking part in more than 16 to 20 hours of vigorous activity per week to avoid overuse injury.

EMERGENCY ACTION PLANS

Injuries of an emergency type are unavoidable; they will occur due to the very nature of athletic and activity participation. From anaphylactic reactions as the result of a bee sting to being hit in the head with a pitched ball, it is critical to have a plan in place to manage such concerning situations. An emergency action plan (EAP), though standardized in nature, must be developed by vested individuals and relate specifically to a venue and its geographical surroundings.

An EAP should be developed, reviewed, and revised by individuals familiar with the venues of play, administrators, medical personnel, coaches, parents, legal counsel, and others who have keen awareness to detail. Table 15-4 includes a list of items to consider when drafting such a plan. According to the NATA position statement[61] on emergency planning in athletics, implementation of the EAP should include putting the EAP in writing, educating all parties involved in the EAP,

Figure 15-6. A rare, on-the-field clinical examination of an acute injury being performed on a child by a certified athletic trainer at a youth sporting event.

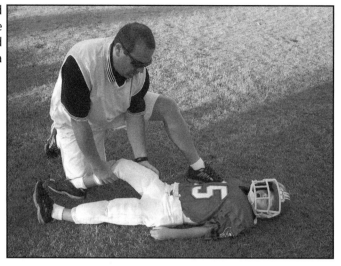

and rehearsing the procedures in the EAP. The EAP should be rehearsed on a scheduled basis and at all times when new personnel, coaching staff, or others are involved in leadership roles. Components of the plan should also involve a minimal skill set expectation, with coaches and league officials being certified in CPR and the use of AED at minimum. Written copies of the plan should be disseminated to anyone involved with expectations of intervening in an emergency situation, and the plan should be posted in plain sight and in legible format for those present to identify with in the case of an emergency.

Lastly, parents and coaches should possess additional awareness of how to respond to emergencies involving children with a higher risk of injury. For example, if a child playing youth soccer is diabetic, then coaches of that team should have knowledge of this condition and at minimum know how to recognize and respond to warning signs of a diabetic coma or insulin shock. A good prevention plan can have a tremendous impact on properly managing emergency situations.

Today, all professional and college/university sports medicine programs have documented and implemented various forms of an EAP. However, the same approach for recreational, organized, and community youth sporting events lags significantly behind (Figure 15-6). Examples of well-designed EAPs can be found on university sports medicine Web sites and can serve as a basis of development for youth sport venue emergency action planning.[62,63] If a sports team or league is not able to have adequate medical coverage at events, at the very least it should consult with a medical professional for assistance with an EAP and how to best prevent or be prepared for an emergency; however, having an EAP with no medical professional on-site may result in misdiagnosis or improper care when the duty to care for an injured athlete is left to an untrained coach or parent.[64] A high school football coach was recently arrested and then acquitted after one of his athletes experienced exertional heat stroke and later died as a result of improper care at the school. This case suggests that perhaps coaches are not able to provide the appropriate medical care that an athlete may require in an emergency situation.[65]

CONCLUSION

Properly planned preventive measures are key to avoiding many traumatic injuries that may occur to children. Understanding of the rules of the sport; safe, contemporary, and properly fitting equipment; PPPEs; and a collaborative EAP all contribute to a safe youth sport environment. The general immediate care of emergencies for pediatrics and adolescents is handled no differently than it is for adults. The appropriate first aid assessment and required cardiopulmonary function should be assessed, stabilization of structures should occur when needed, and triage to a facility of care as soon as possible are key. Considerations for management of these injuries may differ once the primary vital signs are stable, so that long-term complications may be minimized or eliminated.

SUMMARY OF KEY POINTS

➡ There has been a significant increase in the number of youths participating in organized and recreational sports over the past decade, and the overall number of injuries and the severity of these injuries have grown in volume.

➡ Despite the lack of evidence, the majority of medical professionals believe that there are some common sense prevention measures that can be taken in an effort to identify potential risk factors for injury and illness among children participating in sports.

➡ The purpose of the PPPE is to provide for a more sports-specific assessment of an individual, not to replace the standard physical examination performed by a physician during a typical and routine office visit.

➡ Many injuries that are preventable are the result of poor field conditions.

➡ All equipment that is used, and especially that reissued on an annual basis as part of a recreational or organized program, should be carefully inspected and repaired as needed and according to any standards or guidelines that may exist.

➡ While some catastrophic and acute emergency-like injuries are not preventable and are unfortunately accepted as part of sport participation, others can be prevented through rule changes.

➡ Medical emergencies can occur to children in slightly different ways than they do with adults for a variety of reasons. Children's bodies are still growing and their coordination is still developing, and therefore, their physical and emotional maturity levels are not on par with those of an adult.

➡ Anatomically, a child is at greater risk of physical injury merely due to the fact that aspects of his or her musculoskeletal system are not yet fully developed.

➡ Thoracic wall injuries are commonplace among pediatric and adolescent children, and some research indicates thoracic wall injuries as the second leading cause of death in children, behind brain injuries.

➡ An area of recent concern is symptoms reported by a child following a concussion and how accurate the subjective history may be. A head injury sustained by a child may in fact be more severe than that suffered by an adult due to the ongoing neurocognitive development of the child's brain.

➡ EAPs should be developed, reviewed, and revised by individuals familiar with the venues of play, administrators, medical personnel, coaches, parents, legal counsel, and others who have keen awareness to detail.

REVIEW QUESTIONS

1. Why are PPPEs so important? Explain in detail.
2. Name some field safety concerns that can lead to a higher risk of injury.
3. Anatomically, why are children at greater risk of physical injury than adults?
4. How can sporting rules help decrease the incidence of injury in youth athletes?
5. Explain in detail best practices that can decrease the chances for injury in youth sports.

REFERENCES

1.   SNews. *2006* Participation trends in fitness, sports and outdoor activities. http://www.snewsnet.com/cgi-bin/snews/05751.html. Accessed July 3, 2006.

2.   Methodist Hospital System. Important sports safety for the entire family. http://www.methodisthealth.com. Accessed July 3, 2006.

3.   Lindskog D. Increase in adult-type injuries among children and adolescents. http://www.ynhh.org/healthlink/pediatrics. Accessed July 3, 2006.

4.   Graulich I, Konin J, Morris BJ, Liller K. *Flag Football: An Emerging Sport for Female Athletes.* Tampa, FL: AAHPERD; 2009.

5.   Committee on Sports Medicine and Fitness. American Academy of Pediatrics policy statement on medical conditions affecting sport participation. *Pediatrics.* 2001;107(5):1205-1209.

6.   Ingersoll CD, Sitler M, Mickalide AD, Taft AR. A national survey of parents' knowledge, attitudes and self-reported behaviors concerning sports safety. *J Athl Train.* 2001;36:S73.

7.   Safe Kids USA. Sports and recreation safety. http://www.safekids.org/safety-basics/safety-resources-by-risk-area/sports-and-recreation/. Accessed October 10, 2012.

8.   Cross PS, Karges JR, Adamson AJ, Arnold MR, Meier CM, Hood JE. Assessing the need for knowledge on injury management among high school athletic coaches in South Dakota. *S D Med.* 2010;63(7):241-245.

9.   Konin J, Morris B, Liller K, Carey A, Coris E, Pescasio M. Status of medical coverage for high school football games in Florida. *Athletic Training & Sports Health Care.* 2011;3(5):226-229.

10. Allard RH. Legal aspects of sports injuries [Dutch]. *Ned Tijdschr Tandheelkd.* 2005;112(5):184-187.

11. Pearsall AW, Kovaleski JE, Madanagopal SG. Medicolegal issues affecting sports medicine practitioners. *Clin Orthop Relat Res.* 2005;(433):50-57.

12. American College of Sports Medicine, American Academy of Family Physicians, American Academy of Pediatrics, American Medical Society for Sports Medicine, American Orthopaedic Society for Sports Medicine, the American Osteopathic Academy of Sports Medicine. *Pre-participation Physical Evaluation.* 3rd ed. Minneapolis, MN: McGraw-Hill Co; 2004.

13. Lombardo JA. Pre-participation physical evaluation. *Prim Care.* 1984;11(1):3-21.

14. Lombardo JA, Badolato SK. The preparticipation physical examination. *Clin Cornerstone.* 2001;3(5):10-25.

15. Smith DM, Lombardo JA, Robinson JB. The preparticipation evaluation. *Prim Care.* 1991;18(4):777-807.

16. *National Collegiate Athletic Association Sports Medicine Handbook.* Indianapolis, IN: National Collegiate Athletic Association; 2004.

17. Kurowski K, Chandran S. The preparticipation athletic evaluation. http://www.aafp.org/afp/20000501/2683.html. Accessed July 3, 2006.

18. Mick TM, Dimeff RJ. What kind of physical examination does a young athlete need before participating sports? *Cleve Clin J Med.* 2004;71(7):587-597.

19. Best TM. The preparticipation evaluation: an opportunity for change and consensus. *Clin J Sport Med.* 2004;14(3):107-108.

20. Magnes SA, Henderson MM, Hunter SC. What conditions limit sport participation: experience with 10,540 athletes. *Phys Sportsmed.* 1992;20(3):143-158.

21. Drezner J, Corrado D. Is there evidence for recommending electrocardiogram as part of the pre-participation examination? *Clin J Sport Med.* 2011;21(1):18-24.

22. Briskin SM, Stanford A, Davis JH, Congeni J, Loud KJ. Identification of stress fracture risk factors in female college dance majors. Presented at: 53rd Annual Meeting of the American College of Sports Medicine; May 31–June 4, 2006; Denver, CO.

23. Maron BJ, Shirani J, Poliac LC, Mathenge R, Roberts WC, Mueller FO. Sudden death in young competitive athletes. Clinical, demographic, and pathological profiles. *JAMA.* 1996;276(3):199-204.

24. Athletes, physicians urge adoption of new medical screening tool: survey shows nearly unanimous support for the preparticipation evaluations. American College of Sports Medicine; 2010. http://www.acsm.org/about-acsm/media-room/acsm-in-the-news/2011/08/01/athletes-physicians-urge-adoption-of-new-medical-screening-tool. Accessed May 18, 2011.

25. Konin J, McCue FC, eds. Taping, bracing, and strapping. In: Wilk KE, Andres JR, eds. *The Athlete's Shoulder.* New York, NY: Churchill Livingstone; 1994.

26. Young "extreme" athletes underuse protective equipment. American College of Sports Medicine News Release. www.acsm.org/publications. July 1, 2005. Accessed May 18, 2011.

27. US Lacrosse. Approved eyewear list. http://www.uslacrosse.org/UtilityNav/AboutTheSport/SportsScienceandSafety/ApprovedEyewearList.aspx. Accessed October 10, 2012.

28. Summers K. High school boys lacrosse rules changes seek to minimize risk of injury: National Federation of State High School Associations. August 18, 2010. http://www.nfhs.org/content.aspx?id=4173. Accessed May 18, 2011.

29. Hopkins BE. Statement on various types of protective eyewear for field hockey. National Federation of State High School Associations, 2011. www.nfhs.org/Workarea/DownloadAsset.aspx?id=5244. Accessed November 27, 2012.

30. NCAA Football Rules and Interpretations Handbook, 2009-2010. http://www.ncaapublications.com/p-3926-2009-10-ncaa-football-rules-and-interpretations-2-year-publication.aspx. Accessed October 10, 2012.

31. Vinger PF, Parver L, Alfaro DV 3rd, Woods T, Abrams BS. Shatter resistance of spectacle lenses. *JAMA*. 1997;277(2):142-144.

32. Gordy FM, Eklund NP, DeBall S. Oral trauma in an urban emergency department. *J Dent Child (Chic)* 2004;71(1):14-16.

33. Ranalli DN, Demas PN. Orofacial injuries from sport: preventive measures for sports medicine. *Sports Med*. 2002;32(7):409-418.

34. Weinstock J, Maron BJ, Song C, Mane PP, Estes NA 3rd, Link MS. Failure of commercially available chest wall protectors to prevent sudden cardiac death induced by chest wall blows in an experimental model of commotio cordis. *Pediatrics*. 2006;117(4):e656-e662.

35. Benson BW, Hamilton GM, Meeuwisse WH, McCrory P, Dvorak J. Is protective equipment useful in preventing concussion? A systematic review of the literature. *Br J Sports Med*. 2009;43(suppl 1):i56-i67.

36. Maeda Y, Kumamoto D, Yagi K, Ikebe K. Effectiveness and fabrication of mouthguards. *Dent Traumatol*. 2009;25(6):556-564.

37. League's Official Player Safety Rules. NFL News. November 30, 2010. http://www.nfl.com/news/story/09000d5d81c8823a/article/leagues-official-player-safety-rules. Accessed May 19, 2011.

38. Salvo JP, Rizio L 3rd, Zvijac JE, Uribe JW, Hechtman KS. Avulsion fracture of the ulnar sublime tubercle in overhead throwing athletes. *Am J Sports Med*. 2002;30(3):426-431.

39. Brown JH, DeLuca SA. Growth plate injuries: Salter-Harris classification. *Am Fam Physician*. 1992;46(4):1180-1184.

40. Chen FS, Diaz VA, Loebenberg M, Rosen JE. Shoulder and elbow injuries in the skeletally immature athlete. *J Am Acad Orthop Surg*. 2005;13(3):172-185.

41. Lalonde KA, Letts M. Traumatic growth arrest of the distal tibia: a clinical and radiographic review. *Can J Surg*. 2005;48(2):143-147.

42. Vaquero J, Vidal C, Cubillo A. Intra-articular traumatic disorders of the knee in children and adolescents. *Clin Orthop Relat Res*. 2005;(432):97-106.

43. Sartorelli KH, Vane DW. The diagnosis and management of children with blunt injury of the chest. *Semin Pediatr Surg*. 2004;13(2):98-105.

44. Bliss D, Silen M. Pediatric thoracic trauma. *Crit Care Med*. 2002;30(suppl 11):S409-S415.

45. Neve V, Girard F, Flahault A, Boule M. Lung and thorax development during adolescence: relationship with pubertal status. *Eur Respir J*. 2002;20(5):1292-1298.

46. Chen HY, Sheu MH, Tseng LM. Bicycle-handlebar hernia: a rare traumatic abdominal wall hernia. *J Chin Med Assoc*. 2005;68(6):283-285.

47. Erez I, Lazar L, Gutermacher M, Katz S. Abdominal injuries caused by bicycle handlebars. *Eur J Surg*. 2001;167(5):331-333.

48. Goliath J, Mittal V, McDonough J. Traumatic handlebar hernia: a rare abdominal wall hernia. *J Pediatr Surg*. 2004;39(10):e20-e22.

49. Kubota A, Shono J, Yonekura T, et al. Handlebar hernia: case report and review of pediatric cases. *Pediatr Surg Int*. 1999;15(5-6):411-412.

50. Linuma Y, Yamazaki Y, Hirose Y, et al. A case of traumatic abdominal wall hernia that could not be identified until exploratory laparoscopy was performed. *Pediatr Surg Int*. 2005;21(1):54-57.

51. Mancel B, Aslam A. Traumatic abdominal wall hernia: an unusual bicycle handlebar injury. *Pediatr Surg Int*. 2003;19(11):746-747.

52. Nadler EP, Potoka DA, Shultz BL, Morrison KE, Ford HR, Gaines BA. The high morbidity associated with handlebar injuries in children. *J Trauma*. 2005;58(6):1171-1174.

53. Radmayr C, Oswald J, Muller E, Holtl L, Bartsch G. Blunt renal trauma in children: 26 years clinical experience in an alpine region. *Eur Urol*. 2002;42(3):297-300.

54. Storsved JR, Rieger M. Acute kidney injury in a high school football player. *J Athl Train*. 2005;41(2):S74.

55. Rocchi G, Caroli E, Raco A, Salvati M, Delfini R. Traumatic epidural hematoma in children. *J Child Neurol*. 2005;20(7):569-572.

56. Patel DR, Shivdasani V, Baker RJ. Management of sport-related concussion in young athletes. *Sports Med*. 2005;35(8):671-684.

57. McCrory P, Meeuwisse W, Johnston K, et al. Consensus statement on concussion in sport: the Third International Conference on Concussion in Sport held in Zurich, November 2008. *J Athl Train*. 2009;44(4):434-448.

58. Broshek DJ, Kaushik T, Freeman J, Erlanger D, Webbe F, Barth JT. Sex differences in outcomes following sports-related concussion. *J Neurosurg*. 2005;102(5):856-863.

59. Winsley R, Matos N. Overtraining and elite young athletes. *Med Sport Sci*. 2011;56:97-105.

60. Valovich McLeod TC, Decoster LC, Loud KJ, et al. National Athletic Trainers' Association position statement: prevention of pediatric overuse injuries. *J Athl Train*. 2011;46(2):206-220.

61. Anderson J, Courson R, McLoda T. National Athletic Trainers' Association position statement: emergency planning in athletics. *J Athl Train*. 2002;37(1):99-104.

62. JMU Emergency Action Plan. James Madison University Sports Medicine. http://www.jmusports.com/ViewArticle.dbml?DB_OEM_ID=14400&ATCLID=777727. Accessed July 3, 2006.

63. Information for visiting teams: emergency action plans. University of Georgia Sports Medicine. http://georgiadogs.collegesports.com/sports-med/visiting-teams.html#track. Accessed July 3, 2006.

64. Pagnotta KD, Mazerolle SM, Casa DJ. Exertional heat stroke and emergency issues in high school sport. *J Strength Cond Res.* 2010;24(7):1707-1709.

65. Casa DJ, Pagnotta KD, Pinkus DE, Mazerolle SM. Should coaches be in charge of care for medical emergencies in high school sport? *Athletic Training & Sports Health Care.* 2009;1(4):144-146.

Financial Disclosures

Casey Christy has no financial or proprietary interest in the materials presented herein.

Ron Courson has no financial or proprietary interest in the materials presented herein.

John L. Davis has no financial or proprietary interest in the materials presented herein.

Dr. Jeff G. Konin has no financial or proprietary interest in the materials presented herein.

Dr. Rebecca M. Lopez has no financial or proprietary interest in the materials presented herein.

Dr. Eileen Lubeck has no financial or proprietary interest in the materials presented herein.

Dr. David A. Middlemas has no financial or proprietary interest in the materials presented herein.

Michael A. Prybicien has no financial or proprietary interest in the materials presented herein.

Dr. Robb S. Rehberg has no financial or proprietary interest in the materials presented herein.

Dr. Louis Rizio has no financial or proprietary interest in the materials presented herein.

Index

abdomen
    anatomy of, 144–145
    guarding, 149, 151
    organs of, 144–145
    palpation of, 149–150
    quadrants of, 144
    rebound tenderness of, 149
    wall herniations in youth athletes, 231
abdominal injuries, 143, 158
    avoiding, 145–146
    changing diagnostic signs of, 146–147
    clinically relevant anatomy in, 144–145
    common, 152–157
    emergency care of, 152, 154–155
    evaluation and recognition of, 146–150
    hollow organ, 151–152
    referred pain in, 148
    solid organ, 150–151
    structured interview for, 153
    with thoracic injuries, 132
abdominal pain
    digestive problems causing, 155–156
    evaluation of, 153–155
    in girls and women, 157
    hepatitis in, 157
    reducing likelihood of, 154
abdominopelvic cavity, anatomy of, 144–145
abrasions, 173–174
absence (petit mal) seizures, 104, 105
acetaminophen
    for concussion-related headache, 122
    for mononucleosis, 190
acetazolamide, for high-altitude illness, 205
active listening, 212, 217
acute abdomen, emergency care of, 154–155
advanced airway devices, 41–42
advanced emergency medical technicians (AEMTs), 8–9
airway
    anatomy of, 37–38
    assessment of, 23
        in loss of consciousness, 97
    establishing, 38–39
        adjuncts in, 39–45
    management of, 37
        in cervical spine injuries, 66
    obstruction of with thoracic injury, 133
airway adjuncts, 12
albuterol, for high-altitude illness, 205
allergic triggers, asthma, 185
allergies, in SAMPLE history, 26

altitude, 204–205
ambulances, 13
American Red Cross Disaster Mental Health Services, 216, 217
amnesia
    anterograde, 115
        testing for, 118
    retrograde, 115
    types of, 98–99, 115
amputations, 176, 178
angina pectoris, 54
aortic rupture, traumatic, 55
aortic valve defects, 56
appendicitis, 156
appendix, inflamed or infected, 156
arenas, emergency action planning for, 14
arm, splinting of, 170
arrhythmias, cardiac, 56
assessment, 19
    approaching athlete in, 20–22
    diagnostic signs in, 30–32
    head-to-toe, 27
    history and physical examination in, 24–26
    initial, 22–24
    for loss of consciousness, 96–100
    mechanism of injury in, 19–20
    obtaining additional information in, 26–27
    rapid trauma, 27
    rule of 100 in, 32–33
    vital signs in, 27–30
asthma, 185, 191
    acute breathing difficulties in, 186–187
    examination for, 185
    exercise-induced, 186, 191
    history and etiology of, 185
    management and treatment of, 185–186
    special considerations in, 186
athlete
    active listening to, 212
    approaching for assessment, 20–22
    death and catastrophic illness of, 214–215
    down and motionless, 96, 97
    in emergency planning, 10
    maintaining appropriate boundaries with, 212–213
    pediatric and youth, emergency care for, 221–235
athletic trainers, 3
    approaching injured athlete, 21
    in emergency care team, 8
    trailing the team, 20
athletic training students, 10
athletics staff, 10

auscultation, of blood pressure, 30–31
automated external defibrillators (AEDs), 13, 228
AVPU scale, 22
avulsion wounds, 175–176
axial loading mechanism, 60–62

backboards, 12
    for spinal injuries, 73
bag-valve mask, 45
Balance Error Scoring System (BESS), 119, 125
balance testing, for traumatic brain injury, 119
baseball equipment safety, 229
bleeding
    assessing in head trauma, 102
    internal, in abdominopelvic injuries, 148–194, 152
    intracranial, 109–110, 113–114
        with traumatic brain injury, 122–124
    severe
        assessment of, 23
        in cervical spine injuries, 68–69
blood, 21
    sugar levels of in diabetes, 187–188
blood flow, managing, 181–182
blood pressure
    initial assessment of, 30–31
    Rule of 100 of, 32–33
blood vessel disorders, 56
Bloodborne Pathogens Standard, Occupational Safety
    and Health Administration, 21
Board of Certification, Inc, 8
bone, anatomy of, 161–162
bone mineral density, preparticipation testing of, 224
boundaries, maintaining appropriate, 212–213
bowel sounds assessment, 154
brain
    anatomy of, 110–111
    traumatic injury of, 126–127
        academic accommodations for, 122, 123
        in asymptomatic athlete, 122
        catastrophic, 122–124
        categories of, 109–110
        changing awareness of, 109
        chronic, 124
        clinically relevant anatomy of, 110–111
        concussion in, 111–112
        consciousness assessment in, 99
        diffuse and focal, 111
        evaluation of, 114–120
        home care for, 120–122
        intracranial bleeding in, 113–114
        mechanisms of, 111
        physician referral for, 120
        red flags for, 114
        return to play after, 124–126
        signs and symptom evaluation for, 115–118
brainstem, 110
breathing
    acute difficulties of, 186–187
    assessment of, 23, 42–44
        in cervical spine injuries, 66–68
        with loss of consciousness, 97
    clinically relevant anatomy in, 37–38
    compromised, 37
    managing emergencies in, 46–48
    supporting, 45–46
        oxygen administration in, 46–48
bronchial tree injury, 136–137
bronchodilators, 186

CAB Sx3 algorithm, 22–24
    for loss of consciousness, 97
    for spinal injury, 64, 68
capillary refill, 31–32

cardiac tamponade, 55
cardiomyopathy, hypertrophic, 53
cardiopulmonary resuscitation (CPR)
    in cervical spine injuries, 69
    coaching staff training in, 9
    in initial assessment, 23
    in traumatic brain injury, 114
cardiovascular system, 182
    function of in cervical spine injuries, 68
    medical emergencies of, 51, 57
        angina pectoris, 54
        cardiac arrhythmias, 56
        cardiac tamponade, 55
        chest pain assessment in, 52
        clinically relevant anatomy in, 51–52
        myocardial contusion, 56
        myocardial infarction, 54
        myocarditis, 56
        stroke, 55
        sudden cardiac arrest, 53–54
        syncope, 56
        traumatic aortic rupture, 55
        valve and blood vessel disorders, 56
carotid pulse, in cervical spine injuries, 68
cartilage, 162
cerebellum, 110
cerebrospinal fluid, 111
cerebrum, 110
    contusions of, 109, 114
cervical immobilization device, 74
cervical lordosis, normal, 61
cervical spine injuries (CSIs), 59–60
    acute management of, 64–70
    axial loading mechanism in, 60–62
    head-down contact and, 62
    hyperflexion, 61
    initial assessment of, 65–70
    protocol for protective equipment removal in, 87–89
chest cavity, 132
chest injury, signs and symptoms of, 133
chest pain
    assessment of, 52
    common causes of, 52
    with pneumothorax, 134
chest wall trauma, 138
chilblains, 203–204
children, physical and psychological immaturity of,
    230–233
cholecystitis, 156
circulation assessment, 22–23
    in cervical spine injuries, 66
    for loss of consciousness, 97
climbing, high-altitude illness and, 204–205
coaching staff, 9
cognitive testing, in traumatic brain injury, 115–118
cold injuries, 199–203
    nonfreezing, 203–204
cold-water immersion, 198–199, 200
coma, 101–102
    diabetic, 188
CombiTube, 41–42
commotio cordis, 53
communications equipment, 12–13
compartment syndrome, 165, 167, 177
computed tomography, for spinal injuries, 86–87
concussion, 109–110, 111
    home care for, 120–122
    information on, 121
    physician referral for, 120
    recover and graded exercise program log for, 126
    recovery rate for, 125
    return to play after, 124–126
    signs and symptoms of, 111–112, 121

concussion laws, 109
consciousness. *See also* unconsciousness
    levels of
        after traumatic brain injury, 115
        assessing, 22, 97–99
    loss of, 96, 106
        assessment of, 96–100
        understanding causes of, 100–103
cooling strategies, 198–199, 200
coordination testing, for traumatic brain injury, 119–120
corticosteroids, for asthma, 186
costochondral separation/dislocation, 138
CPR mask, 12, 45
crackles, 138
cranial nerve function assessment, 118–119
crutches, 13

decerebrate posturing, 99, 100
decorticate posturing, 99, 100
dehydration, in heat exhaustion, 197
dental emergencies, 176–177, 178
diabetes mellitus, 187, 191
    examination for, 187–188
    history and etiology of, 187
    management and treatment of, 188–189
diagnostic signs
    significant, 31–32
    vital, 27–30
diagnostic tools, 13
diaphragm, 132
    tears in, 137
diaphyseal bone, 162
diencephalon, 110
digestive organs, 144
digestive problems, 155–156
disaster resources, 216–217
Disaster Response Network, American Psychological Association, 216, 217
dislocations, 177–178
    emergencies, 166
    evaluation of, 165
    initial treatment of, 166
    splinting of, 166–172
disorientation, 101
diverticula, 156
diverticulitis, 156
dyspepsia, 155–156
dyspnea, with pneumothorax, 134

ectopic pregnancy, 157
education, in emergency planning, 16
educators, 4
elbow, splinting of, 169–171
emergency action plan (EAP), 7, 8, 14
    for different venues, 14
    equipment for, 11–13
    evaluating and education in, 16
    personnel involved in, 8–10
    rehearsal in, 14
    rules for, 10–11
    sample, 15
    for spinal injuries, 63–64
    for youth and pediatric sports, 233–234
emergency care team, personnel of, 7–8
emergency medical responders (EMRs), 8
emergency medical services (EMS)
    for head trauma, 102
    for unconscious or incoherent athlete, 97
emergency medical services personnel, 3–4
    protocols for, 11
    self-care for, 215
    training of, 8–9
emergency medical technicians (EMTs), 8–9

EMT-Basic: National Standard Curriculum, 11
encephalopathy, chronic traumatic, 124
endotracheal tube, 41–42
environmental emergencies, 195
    altitude related, 204–205
    exertional heat illness, 196–204
    lightning related, 205–206
    thermal physiology and, 195–196
environmental stress, 195
epidural hematoma, 109, 113
epilepsy, 104
    causing seizures, 103
    participation in sports with, 105–106
EpiPens, 13
epiphyseal bone, 161–162
Epstein-Barr virus, 190
equipment
    for emergency medical care, 11–13
    safety of for youth athletes, 225–229
esophageal injury, 137
evacuation helicopter, 13
evaluation, in emergency planning, 16
exertional heat illness, 196–204
exertional sickling, 189–190

face shields, tinted, 228
facemask
    components of, 75–76
    removal of
        in spinal injuries, 74–85
        tools for, 13, 77–85
female athletics, greater equality for, 221
field hockey safety, 228
field safety, for youth athletes, 224–226
finger-to-nose test, 119–120
first responders. *See* emergency medical responders (EMRs)
flail chest, 135–136
football safety equipment, 228–229
forearm, splinting of, 169–171
fractures, 177–178
    clinically relevant anatomy of, 161–163
    emergencies, 164–165
    evaluation of, 163–164
    initial treatment of, 164
    open, 164–165
    rib, 135–136, 138
    splinting of, 166–172
    sternal, 137
    thoracic spine, 138–139
frostbite, 203
frostnip, 203

gallbladder, inflamed, 156
gallstones, 156
gastroesophageal reflux disease (GERD), 155–156
gatekeeper training, 213
General Adaptation Syndrome (GAS), 195
genitalia, injuries to, 151–152
Glasgow Coma Scale, 98
glucagon, 13
glucose levels, in diabetes, 187–188
glucose paste, for diabetes, 188
grand mal seizures, 103, 104
groin injuries, 151

hand, splinting of, 169–170
head and neck immobilization, 64
head-down contact, 62
head injuries
    causing seizures, 103
    evaluation process for, 114
    of down athlete, 114

in sideline and office, 115–120
signs and symptoms of, 121
unconsciousness after, 102
head-tilt chin-lift, 24, 39
headache
concussion-related, 122
post-traumatic, 125
prolonged post-traumatic, 125
heart, anatomy of, 51–52
heart valve defects, 56
heat balance equation, 196
heat cramps, exercise-associated, 196–197
heat exhaustion, exertional, 197
heat illness, stupor in, 101
heat stroke, exertional, 197–199
heat syncope, 197
heat transfer, 196
helmet removal, in spinal injuries, 87–88
hemothorax, 131
massive, 135–136
hepatitis, 157
high-altitude cerebral edema (HACE), 204–205
high-altitude pulmonary edema (HAPE), 204–205
homeostasis, 195–196
in cold environment, 199–200
hospital staff, in sports emergency care team, 9
hyperbaric therapy, 205
hyperglycemia, 187–188
signs and symptoms of, 187
stupor in, 101
hyperthermia, exercise-induced, 197–199
hypoglycemia, 187, 188
hyponatremia, 189
hypothalamus, 110
hypothermia, 32, 201–203
hypoxia, altitude and, 205

ibuprofen, for mononucleosis, 190
imaging techniques, for spinal injuries, 86–87
immaturity, physical and psychological, 230–233
immersion foot, 203
immobilization
for dislocation, 166
of fracture, 164
for spinal injuries, 64, 70–74
with splint, 168–173
for traumatic brain injury, 120
impalement, 152, 175
infectious materials, minimizing exposure to, 21
inhalers, 13
injury, mechanism of, 19–20
injury/illness, events leading to, 26
insulin, 13
for diabetes, 188
secretion of, 187
insulin shock, 101
Inter-Association Task Force for Appropriate Care of
the Spine-Injured Athlete recommendations, 11
Inter-Association Task Force for Emergency
Preparedness and Management of Sudden
Cardiac Arrest in High School and College
Athletic Programs, 53–54
intercostal muscles, contusion of, 138
intestinal gas pain, 156
intracerebral hemorrhage, 114
irritable bowel syndrome, 156

jaw thrust
in airway management, 39
modified, 24
joints
anatomy of, 162
dislocation of, 165–166

Kehr's sign, 148
ketoacidosis, diabetic, 188
kidney stones, 157
kidneys, 144, 145
injuries to, 150–151
kissing disease, 190
knee, splinting of, 170–172

lacerations, 173–174
lacrosse safety
men's, 228
women's, 227–228
laryngeal mask airway (LMA), 41–42
last oral intake, in SAMPLE history, 26
life support training, 8–9
lifesaving medications, 13
ligaments, 162, 163
lightning
care of victims of, 206
facts about, 206
safety procedures for, 205–206
30-30 rule in, 206
Little League rules, 230
liver, 144, 145
injuries to, 150
log-roll technique, 71–72
Long QT syndrome, 56
loop strap fasteners, 77–80
lungs, 132
bruising of, 136, 138

magnetic resonance imaging, for spinal injuries, 86–87
McBurney's point, 156
mediastinum, 132
medical emergencies
general, 181–191
preparing for, 7–17
medical history, 26
medications, in SAMPLE history, 26
memory assessment, 115
memory loss, 98–99. See also amnesia
meninges, 110–111
menstrual cycle, abdominal pain in, 157
mental health emergencies, 211
death/catastrophic illness and, 214–215
psychiatric illness in, 214
psychological first aid in, 215
relationship with athletes in, 212–213
resources and referrals for, 216–217
self-care for professionals in, 215
suicide, 213–214
mitral valve defects, 56
mononucleosis, 190, 191
motor nerves, 110
mountain sickness, acute, 204–205
mouth guards, 229–230
mouth injury, protective equipment for, 21
muscle cramps, exercise-associated, 196–197
muscles, thoracic, 132
myocardial contusion, 56
myocardial infarction, 54
myocarditis, 56

nasopharyngeal airway, 41
National Athletic Trainers' Association, acute spinal
injury management statement of, 60, 63
National Child Traumatic Stress Network Web site, 215
National Emergency Medical Technicians Education
Standards, 9, 11
National Football League, rule enforcement by, 230
National Suicide Prevention Lifeline, 213–214, 217
neurocognitve testing, 124
nonresponsiveness, 96, 97

open wounds, 173
    treatment guidelines for, 174
    types of, 173–176
OPQRST assessment, 26–27
organs
    hollow, 144–145
        injuries of, 149, 151–152
    solid, 145
        injuries of, 150–151
orientation evaluation, 115
oropharyngeal airway, 39–41
orthostatic dizziness, 197
overhydration, 189
oxygen administration, 46–48
    for high-altitude illness, 205
    for tracheal or bronchial tree injury, 137
oxygen systems, therapeutic versus emergency, 47

pain
    chest, 52
    onset and duration of, 26–27
    provocation/palliation of, 26
    quality of, 27
    region/radiation of, 27
    severity of, 27
palpation, of blood pressure, 30–31
paramedics, 8–9
patient history, in traumatic brain injury, 115
pediatric athletes
    emergency care for, 221–235
    physical and psychological immaturity of, 230–233
pelvic injuries, 150–152, 158
    avoiding, 145–146
    clinically relevant anatomy of, 144–145
    common medical emergencies in, 152–157
pelvis
    anatomy of, 144–145
    hollow organs of, 151–152
    solid organs of, 150–151
peritoneum, 144
peritonitis, 149, 151
personal protective equipment, 21
physical examination
    in abdominal injuries, 149–150
    preparticipation, for youth athletes, 222–224, 233
        medical conditions requiring, 224–225
physician referral, for traumatic brain injury, 120
physicians, in sports emergency care team, 9
pleura, 131
pneumothorax, 131
    management of, 135
    with rib fractures or contusions, 138
    signs of, 135
    spontaneous, 134–135
    tension, 133–134, 135
pole vault safety, 227
postictal period, 104
PREPARE acronym, 7, 14
    for spinal injury management, 63–64
preparticipation physical examination, 222–225, 233
pressure dressings, 175, 176
protective equipment
    for abdominal region, 146
    removal of
        in emergency department, 87–89
        in spinal injuries, 70
protective eyewear, 228–229
protocol, emergency, 10–11
psychiatric illness, 214
psychological first aid, 215, 217
Psychological First Aid Field Operations Guide, 215, 217
psychological immaturity, in youth athletes, 230–233
pulmonary contusion, 137

pulse
    in initial assessment, 28–29
    in spinal injuries, 68
pulse oximetry, 31
puncture wounds, 174–175

radial pulse, in cervical spine injuries, 68
radiographic plain film, for spinal injuries, 86
rales, 44
referred pain patterns, 148
rehearsal, 14
    of spinal injury management, 63–64
reproductive organs, 144, 145
    injuries to, 151–152
respiration
    in cervical spine injuries, 66–67
    initial assessment of, 30
respiratory compromise, in hemothorax, 135
respiratory distress
    with diaphragmatic tears, 137
    with flail chest, 136
respiratory rate, resting, 43
resuscitation equipment, 13
reticular activating system, 110
return to play
    after traumatic brain injury, 124–126
    testing tools for, 124–125
Revolution fastener, 82–85
rhonchi, 44
ribs
    contusions of, 138
    fractures of, 135–136, 138
Rule of 100, 32–33, 69–70

Safe Kids Campaign, 221
SAM splints, 12
SAMPLE history, 25–26
    in abdominal injuries, 147
    in breathing emergencies, 46
second impact syndrome, 121, 122–124
seizures, 95, 103, 105–106
    causes of, 103
    duration of, 104–105
    fatigue after, 104
    phases of, 103
    protecting patient during, 103–104
    signs of onset of, 104
    types of, 105
Selye, Hans, 195
sensory nerves, 110
sexually transmitted diseases, 157
shivering, 199
shock, 191
    in abdominal injuries, 148
    anatomy and physiology of, 181–182
    assessment of, 23
    causes and mechanisms of, 182
    in cervical spine injuries, 68–69
    examination for, 183–184
    hypovolemic, 135
    management and treatment of, 184–185
    signs and symptoms of, 184
    types of, 182–183
Shockblocker football helmet clip, 80–81
shoulder pads, removal of, 87–89
sickle cell trait, 189–190
signs/symptoms, in SAMPLE history, 26
6-plus-person lift technique, 72–74
skin assessment, 31
soccer equipment safety, 229
sodium loss, 189
soft tissue
    anatomy of, 162–163

injuries to, 177–178
     open, 173–176
spearing, 62
spinal cord, ischemia of, 63
spinal shock, 62, 69
spinal shock cascade, 63
spinal stabilization techniques, 64–65
spine
     cervical, injuries of, 59–89
     injuries of
          assessment for, 24
          establishing airway in, 38–39
          management of, 59–60
               acute, 64–70
               emergency department trauma assess-
                    ment in, 85–89
               facemask removal in, 74–85
               preparing for, 63–64
               protective equipment removal on field
                    in, 70
               transfer and immobilization in, 70–74
          mechanism of, 60–62
          neurophysiology of, 62–63
          prevention of, 63
          zone of injury in, 63
     thoracic, 131
          fractures of, 138–139
          hyperflexion or hyperextension injury of, 138
spleen, 144, 145
     injuries to, 150
     rupture of, 190
splinting (dislocated joint), 165
splints/splinting, 12, 168–169
     of arm, 170
     complications of, 167
     for dislocation, 166
     of forearm and elbow, 169–170, 171
     of fracture, 164–165
     of hand and wrist, 169
     of leg, ankle, and foot, 171–173
     materials for, 167
     principles of, 166
     SAM, 168–170
     of thigh and knee, 170
Sport Concussion Assessment Tool 2 (SCAT2), 115–
     117
sporting rules, for youth athletes, 230
"sports chairs," 13
sports emergency care, definition of, 2
sports emergency care team, 2–3
     members of, 11
Stabilizer loop straps, 81–83
status epilepticus, 104–105
Steri-Strips, 174
sternal fracture/contusion, 137
stomach ulcers, 155–156
strains, 163
stridor, 44
stroke, 55
stupor, 101
subdural hematoma, 109, 113
suction catheters, 42–43
sudden cardiac arrest, 53–54
suicide prevention, 213–214
Suicide Prevention Resource Center Web site, 217
sweating
     hyponatremia and, 189
     rates of and heat exhaustion, 197

syncope, 56, 100–101
     heat, 197
synovial joints, 162, 163

tandem stance test, 119
temperature, in initial assessment, 32
tendons, 163
testicular torsion, 151–152
thalamus, 110
thermal physiology, 195–196
thermometer
     rectal, 198
     tympanic, 32
thigh, splinting of, 170
thoracic injuries, 131, 139–140
     blunt, 132–133
     clinically relevant anatomy for, 131–132
     evaluation and assessment of, 132–139
     penetrating, 132–133
thorax, anatomy of, 131–132
tissue hypoxia, with thoracic injury, 133
Title IX legislation, 221
tonic-clonic seizures, 103, 105
tooth
     avulsed, 177, 178
     broken, 176
tracheal injury, 136–137
traction, of fracture, 164
trailing the action, 20
transfer techniques, in spinal injuries, 70–74
transportation devices, 13
trauma assessment
     in emergency department, 85–89
     rapid, 27
trench foot, 203

unconsciousness, 95, 106
     lack of response in, 96
     medical and substance-related causes of, 102–103
     things to look for in, 103
urinary bladder, injuries to, 151
urinary tract infections, 157

vital signs
     in abdominal injuries, 149
     in cervical spine injuries, 68
     changes with exercise, 28
     normal values of, 28
     obtaining, 27–30
     trending, 32–33

water intoxication, 189
wheelchair, 13
wheezing, 44
wind chill, 200–201
Wolff-Parkinson-White syndrome, 56
wrist, splinting of, 169–170

youth athletes, 236
     emergency action plans for, 233–234
     equipment safety for, 225–229
     field safety for, 224–226
     injuries in
          increased rates of, 221–222
          prevention of, 222–224
     physical and psychological immaturity of, 230–233
     sporting rules for, 230